EMBRACING DIVERSITY

TREATMENT AND CARE IN ADDICTIONS COUNSELING

First Edition

Edited by Tiffany Lee, Ph.D.
Western Michigan University

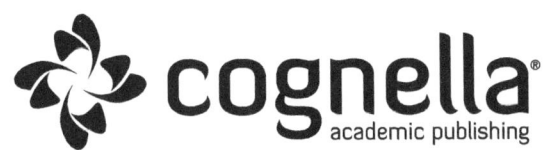

Bassim Hamadeh, CEO and Publisher
Michael Simpson, Vice President of Acquisitions
Jamie Giganti, Managing Editor
Jess Busch, Senior Graphic Designer
John Remington, Acquisitions Editor
Brian Fahey, Licensing Specialist
Mandy Licata, Interior Designer

Copyright © 2015 by Cognella, Inc. All rights reserved. No part of this publication may be reprinted, reproduced, transmitted, or utilized in any form or by any electronic, mechanical, or other means, now known or hereafter invented, including photocopying, microfilming, and recording, or in any information retrieval system without the written permission of Cognella, Inc.

First published in the United States of America in 2015 by Cognella, Inc.

Trademark Notice: Product or corporate names may be trademarks or registered trademarks, and are used only for identification and explanation without intent to infringe.

Cover image: Copyright © 2005 by Laurence's Travels / Flickr / CC BY 2.0.

Printed in the United States of America

ISBN: 978-1-62131-785-2 (pbk) / 978-1-62131-786-9 (br)

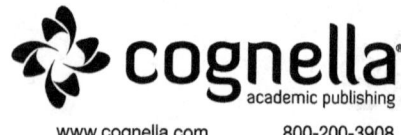

CONTENTS

Introduction — 1

CHAPTER 1
Diversity Concepts and a Discussion of Racism — 13

CHAPTER 2
What It Means to Be White and Privileged — 23

CHAPTER 3
Microaggressions Against Marginalized Groups — 41

CHAPTER 4
Black/African Americans — 53
    Bianca T. L. Fetherson

CHAPTER 5
American Indians — 65
    Andrew Wood, Daniel Gutierrez, Renee Sherrell, and Catherine Griffith

CHAPTER 6
Arab Americans — 79
    Sejal M. Barden and W. Bryce Hagedorn

INTRODUCTION

Addiction is an equal-opportunity disease, inflicting both genders and people of any age, race, religion, education level, sexual orientation, and economic status. All people, however, do not experience substance use, misuse, abuse, and dependency in the same way. The etiology differs among and between groups of people, and everyone does not enter treatment for the same reasons. Treatment efficacy can be affected by cultural variables, and these variables must be taken into account by researchers and clinicians, as well as clients and their family members. In other words, aspects of culture and diversity have vast implications for the delivery and success of substance abuse treatment services provided to special populations.

The term "special populations" has been used in the substance abuse field since the 1970s (Hegamin, Anglin, & Casanova, 2002). By definition, a special population is a subgroup that historically has been underrepresented in substance abuse prevention and treatment research (Polinsky, Hser, & Grella, 1998). The term originated in an effort to address the unique needs of underserved populations and provide appropriate and efficient services to these groups.

Special populations include, but are not limited to, the following subgroups:

Racial and Ethnic Populations:

Black/African Americans   Arab Americans   Asian Americans
Latino Americans   Native Americans

Culturally Diverse Populations:

Women
Older Adults
People within the military
People identifying as spiritual and/or religious
People living in various geographic locations
Adolescents and young adults
People identifying as lesbian, gay, bisexual, transgender
People with disabilities
People who are homeless
People with chronic pain
College students
People who are economically disadvantaged
People living with HIV/AIDS
People in the criminal justice system
People with co-occurring disorders

Most clients have multiple identities and can fit into more than one category of special populations. For instance, a client can present for substance abuse treatment who is:

- A 20-year-old gay partnered Chinese American male who was arrested for driving under the influence and is coming in for an assessment. He recently revealed his sexual orientation to his family, and he reports his family members had a negative reaction to this disclosure. He indicates an increase in alcohol consumption to cope with his feelings.
- A 35-year-old heterosexual married white male who was released from the military a year ago. Two months ago, he was diagnosed with post-traumatic stress disorder and now goes to the Veterans' Affairs center for depression. He reports chronic cannabis use and heavy alcohol consumption.
- A 43-year-old divorced African American female who is required to attend counseling due to involvement with Child Protective Services. Her partner was arrested for domestic violence, and during the incident, police officers found cocaine at the residence.
- A 78-year-old widowed white female who has been prescribed Norco, an opioid pain medication, for the past three years. The client's daughter has noticed her mother feeling "sick" and has been taking more pills than prescribed. Recently, her daughter found her own Vicodin pill bottle empty, and the client admitted taking the medication.
- A 55-year-old divorced Mexican American female who was released from prison last month. She was convicted of manufacturing a methamphetamine lab. She is unemployed, lives at the local shelter, has lost custody of her two children, and has a past diagnosis of bipolar disorder and borderline personality disorder.

Consideration must be given to each identity in an effort to effectively conceptualize clients. Substance abuse counselors should be able to understand how the various multicultural aspects of a person's identity impact not only the use of substances, but also how these aspects correspond with particular barriers, counseling strategies, risk factors, preventive factors, and treatment outcomes.

On the other hand, counselors must be careful with generalizations, as each group is highly heterogeneous. For instance, intragroup differences exist among racial and ethnic groups. Hispanics/Latinos can include Cuban Americans, Mexican Americans, Central and South Americans, and Puerto Rican Americans. A person's country of origin, upbringing, level of acculturation, age, education, religion, and current place of residence are all important to consider (Center for Substance Abuse Treatment, 2006). All of these aspects have the potential to influence worldview, spirituality, community orientation, definition of family, communication styles, boundaries, authority issues, learning styles, views of respect, and attitudes related to helping professionals.

Moreover, a client's identity is fluid and can change over time. For example, a United States–born middle-aged woman was raised by a Mexican-born Catholic father and a Protestant mother born in the United States. As a youth, the woman did not self-identify as a Latina, but over the years developed the identity as a Latina (Loue, 2003). An individual's categorization of self may deviate from what the therapist believes to be the "membership" of various identities. The reactions, behaviors, attitudes, and characteristics of a person may be erroneously attributed to a particular identity, and, in fact, perpetuate stereotypes and misperceptions of a specific population. An Asian saying posits, "All individuals, in many respects, are (a) like no other individuals; (b) like some individuals; and (c) like all other individuals" (Sue & Sue, 2013, p. 41). One's identity has three levels: (1) individual; (2) group; and (3) universal. According to Sue and Sue (2013), individuals have universal commonalities because we are human (e.g., biological and physical similarities); as part of a group identity (e.g., gender, race, sexual orientation), individuals have similarities and differences; and at an individual level, we are all unique (refer to Figure 1 below). In summary, practitioners and researchers must recognize these three aspects of a client's personal identity, as each influences the lived experience of a person.

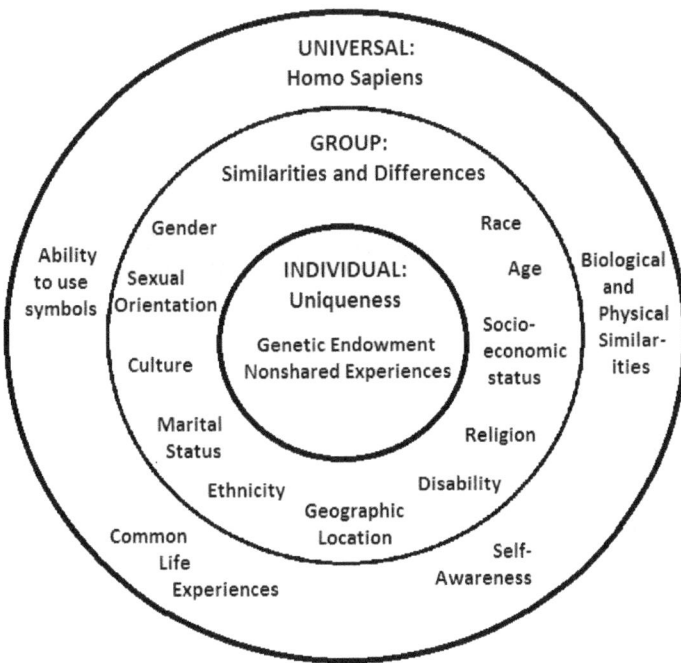

Figure 1: Tripartite Development of Personal Identity.
Adapted from ***Counseling the Culturally Diverse: Theory and Practice*** (Sue & Sue, 2013, p. 42).

RESEARCH ON SPECIAL POPULATIONS

For over 30 years, the National Survey of Substance Abuse Treatment Services (N-SSATS) has collected data on the location and characteristics of addiction treatment facilities and services throughout the United States. In 2011, 90 percent of clients in treatment programs were at outpatient settings; 9 percent of clients were in residential facilities; and 1 percent of clients were in hospital inpatient facilities (Substance Abuse and Mental Health Services Administration [SAMHSA], 2012a). Another noteworthy finding of the N-SSATS in 2011 is that 45 percent of clients in treatment were diagnosed with a co-occurring mental disorder.

N-SSATS researchers also examine the types of presenting substance abuse problem clients identify when in treatment. In 2011, treatment providers reported:

- 44 percent of all clients were in treatment for both alcohol and other drug abuse
- 38 percent of all clients were in treatment for drug abuse only
- 18 percent of all clients were in treatment for abuse of alcohol only

To explore this treatment data further, the author would like to include an overview of admission data that is collected from Treatment Episodes Data Set (TEDS) and analyzed by SAMHSA each year. The TEDS report provides information on the demographic and substance abuse characteristics of admissions to treatment by agencies that report to individual state administrative data systems. (Note: This data includes adults, aged 12 and older). In 2010, there were 1,820,737 substance abuse treatment admissions reported to TEDS (SAMHSA, 2012b). Of those admissions, the two highest racial groups admitted into treatment were: whites (61 percent total; 39 percent males and 21 percent females) and blacks (20 percent total; 14 percent males and 6 percent females) (Refer to Table 1).

Table 1: Substance Abuse Treatment Admissions Rates by Race/Ethnicity in 2010.

RACE/ETHNICITY	PERCENT OF ALL ADMISSIONS
White (non-Hispanic)	60.8
Black (non-Hispanic)	20.1
Hispanic origin	13.1
Mexican	4.4
Puerto Rican	3.7
Cuban	0.2
Other/not specified	4.8
Amer. Indian/Alaska Native	2.4
Asian/Pacific Islander	1.0
Other	2.7

Source: AMHSA / Public Domain.

Substance abuse patterns also differ widely among racial/ethnic subgroups, as indicated by the TEDS data. In Table 2 below, the primary substance of use was divided up by race and ethnicity. Whites were found to be the group that consistently held the highest percentage for each drug category, except for smoked cocaine and PCP. In other words, there were more whites who reported primary problems with alcohol, heroin, marijuana, etc., than did people from other racial or ethnic groups.

Table 2: Primary Substance of Use Indicated at Admission, in 2010.

RACE/ETHNICITY	ALCOHOL ONLY	HEROIN	OTHER OPIATES	SMOKED COCAINE	COCAINE-OTHER ROUTE	MARIJUANA/HASHISH	METH AMPHETAMINE/AMPHET-AMINES	TRAN QUILIZ ERS	SEDA TIVES	HALLU CINO GENS	PCP	INHAL ANTS	OTHER/NONE SPECI FIED
White (non-Hispanic)	67.9	61.5	88.2	35.1	47.4	46.8	67.7	83.4	84.0	67.9	14.2	68.2	60.5
Black (non-Hispanic)	12.7	17.2	3.4	53.5	28.9	30.8	3.4	4.9	5.6	17.4	61.6	9.9	23.3
Hispanic origin	11.7	17.6	4.5	8.1	19.3	16.3	19.0	8.8	6.4	8.4	19.6	13.3	8.6
Mexican	4.8	3.3	1.2	1.5	3.4	5.9	12.8	0.8	1.4	2.1	4.7	6.9	1.1
Puerto Rican	2.1	9.7	0.9	3.1	6.8	3.6	0.4	4.2	1.0	2.2	9.2	1.5	1.8
Cuban	0.2	0.2	0.1	0.2	0.6	0.3	0.1	0.2	0.2	0.2	0.1	0.1	0.2
Other/not specified	4.7	4.3	2.2	3.3	8.5	6.6	5.6	3.7	3.8	3.9	5.6	4.9	5.5
Amer. Indian/Alaska Native	4.1	0.6	1.8	0.9	0.8	1.7	2.3	0.6	1.1	1.7	0.5	5.0	1.5
Asian/Pacific Islander	1.4	0.5	0.5	0.6	0.7	1.1	3.1	0.4	0.7	1.2	0.4	1.2	0.7
Other	2.2	2.7	1.7	1.9	2.9	3.3	4.5	1.9	2.3	3.2	3.7	2.4	5.4
Total Percentage	100	100	100	100	100	100	100	100	100	100	100	100	100

Source: SAMHSA / Public Domain.

Table 3: Race and Ethnic Group Rates of Use by Primary Substance, in 2010

RACE/ETHNICITY	ALCOHOL ONLY	HEROIN	OTHER OPIATES	SMOKED COCAINE	OTHER ROUTE	MARI JUANA/ HASHISH	METH AMPHETAMINE/ AMPHET- AMINES	TRAN QUILIZ ERS	SEDA TIVES	HALLU CINO GENS	PCP	INHAL ANTS	OTHER/ NONE SPECI FIED	TOTAL PERCENTAGE
White (non-Hispanic)	25.3	14.3	12.5	3.3	1.9	14.2	6.9	1.2	0.3	0.1	0.1	0.1	2.1	100
Black (non-Hispanic)	14.3	12.1	1.5	15.3	3.4	28.3	1.0	0.2	0.1	0.1	0.8	*	2.4	100
Hispanic origin	20.3	18.9	3.0	3.6	3.5	23.0	9.0	0.6	0.1	0.1	0.4	0.1	1.4	100
Mexican	24.6	10.7	2.4	1.9	1.9	24.6	18.1	0.1	0.1	*	0.3	0.1	0.5	100
Puerto Rican	12.7	37.1	2.2	4.9	4.4	18.0	0.7	1.0	0.1	0.1	0.6	*	1.0	100
Cuban	22.6	15.1	4.5	6.5	6.5	23.0	3.3	1.0	0.2	0.1	0.2	*	1.6	100
Other/not specified	22.0	12.6	4.0	3.9	4.3	25.3	7.2	0.7	0.2	0.1	0.3	0.1	2.4	100
Amer. Indian/Alaska Native	38.8	3.6	6.5	2.1	0.8	13.5	6.1	0.2	0.1	0.1	0.1	0.2	1.4	100
Asian/Pacific Islander	30.0	6.2	4.2	3.3	1.6	20.3	18.6	0.4	0.2	0.1	0.1	0.1	1.4	100
Other	18.9	14.0	5.4	4.1	2.6	22.7	10.4	0.6	0.2	0.1	0.3	0.1	4.2	100

*Less than .05%

Source: SAMHSA / Public Domain.

The data was also separated out by race and ethnicity to obtain which drugs were used most often (Refer to Table 3). For instance, alcohol was the predominant substance for all racial/ethnic groups (except persons of Puerto Rican origin, where the predominant substance was heroin) (SAMHSA, 2012b). More specifically, alcohol was reported as the primary substance of abuse by almost 40 percent of American Indian/Alaska Native persons at admission. Data also worth noting is related to methamphetamine use. Almost 19 percent of Asian/Pacific Islanders and 18 percent of Mexicans reported methamphetamine as the drug of choice.

The percentages discussed above have meaning, but the readers are encouraged to critically analyze the data presented. These numbers are based on self-report and from a database of information which is put into the system by clinicians at intake. In addition, these are admission reports by clients seeking treatment. What about those who are not admitted? Moreover, usually those seeking addiction services have more severe substance use concerns than those who have not accessed treatment. These are important factors to consider when interpreting this research.

In an effort to meet the needs of all persons entering substance abuse treatment (excluding racial, ethnic, and other cultural considerations), specialized programming has been suggested by researchers and clinicians for decades (Polinsky et al., 1998). Over ten years ago, the 2000 N-SSATS reported approximately 90 percent of facilities offered at least one program designed specifically for certain populations (Olmstead & Sindelar, 2004). In 2011, however, the national survey found a decrease in that percentage; 80 percent of facilities offered at least one special program or group to serve a specific client type (SAMHSA, 2012).

The following is a list of treatment programming found to be available for diverse populations:

- Clients with co-occurring mental and substance abuse disorders (36 percent)
- Adult women (32 percent)
- Persons arrested for DUI or DWI (29 percent)
- Adolescents (28 percent)
- Adult men (25 percent)
- Other criminal justice clients (24 percent)
- Pregnant or postpartum women (13 percent)
- Persons with HIV or AIDS (8 percent)
- Seniors or older adults (6 percent)
- Lesbian, gay, bisexual, or transgender (LGBT) clients (5 percent) (SAMHSA, 2012)

Not only is the specialization of treatment programming suggested, but scholars also recommend offering key services to the various populations in need (Olmstead & Sindelar, 2004). Addiction is considered a primary, progressive problem that causes secondary problems within all life areas such as physical or mental health, unemployment, and housing (Eyrich-Garg, Cacciola, Carise, Lynch, & McLellan, 2008; Friedmann, Lemon, Durkin, & D'Aunno, 2003). In an effort to provide a holistic, recovery-oriented system of care, addiction must be culturally responsive and viewed as a chronic issue (White, 2008). Therefore, treatment services must be grounded in the community and available for those who need comprehensive, wraparound assistance (Friedmann, et al., 2003; Sheedy & Whittner, 2009).

For example, the attractiveness and accessibility of treatment for women are affected by child care and transportation issues (Brady & Ashley, 2005; Green, 2006; Office of Substance Abuse Services, 2004). Thus, programs providing assistance with obtaining these ancillary services increase the likelihood of attracting women who are seeking addiction treatment. Moreover, retention outcomes for women in treatment will improve, as well as their overall functioning, wellness, and quality of life. (Refer to Chapter Nine for the full list of recommended services for women.)

Persons who abuse substances are more at risk for medical issues (e.g., hepatitis, cirrhosis, high blood pressure, cancer, infection with the human immunodeficiency virus [HIV], etc.). According to a literature review by Brown, Kritz, Goldsmith, Bini, Rotrosen, Baker, et al. (2006), 30–40 percent of injection drug users are infected with HIV, and 90 percent have had at least one type of sexually transmitted infection (STI). Due to the increased likelihood of their clients practicing unsanitary injections, as well as unsafe sexual behaviors, treatment programs are encouraged to integrate prevention, intervention, and treatment protocols into their practices. Brown et al. (2006) recommend health services that include:

- provider education
- patient screening and risk assessment
- patient education
- biologic testing
- medical examinations
- counseling
- treatment, and
- treatment monitoring

Other services that treatment personnel are encouraged to provide to specific populations include sign language for persons who are hearing impaired, as well as providing treatment in languages other than English. In 2011, N-SSATS found sign language was offered in 28 percent of all agencies in the study. Moreover, facilities operated by local and state governments were most likely to offer these services (49 and 41 percent, respectively). In 2011, substance abuse treatment was available in languages other than English at 41 percent of all facilities (SAMHSA, 2012). Forty-two percent used only staff counselors who spoke other languages, although 24 percent used both staff counselors and on-call interpreters. To be more specific, Spanish was the most frequently spoken language (94 percent). Services in American Indian/Alaska Native languages were provided by three percent of all facilities where staff counselors provided services in languages other than English. Researchers also determined 26 percent of the agencies provided services in other languages besides Spanish and American Indian/Alaska Native languages.

USING THE TERM "SPECIAL POPULATIONS"

Over the years, there have been discussions related to the appropriate terminology to address specific populations in addictions. Differences even exist with regard to the meaning of the term "diversity" and how research and programming should attend to diversity issues (Loue, 2003). The author would like to take a brief moment to delineate the opposing perspectives. Some scholars suggest several advantages for continued use of the term special populations (Hegamin et al., 2002). The concept of special populations increases the likelihood that therapists will be trained to competently serve all of their clientele. This designation:

- Fosters research agendas to focus on specific groups
- Directs new resources toward treatment services
- Advocates for the consideration of group-based external factors which impact effectiveness of treatment (e.g., cultural beliefs and practices)
- Aids in dispelling myths and stereotypes

The National Institute on Drug Abuse (NIDA) is one of the leading organizations in the field of addiction research. In 1993, NIDA created an office designated to investigate diversity and health disparities and it is called the Special Populations Office (SPO). The SPO has work groups specific to African American, Hispanic, Asian American, Native Hawaiian/Pacific Islander, and American Indian and Alaska Native communities. The SPO aims to:

- Increase the number of underrepresented scholars and researchers actively participating in drug abuse research through outreach, and sponsored career development and research training opportunities;
- Ensure that research addressing minority/health disparity populations are adequately and appropriately represented in NIDA's research programs; and
- Focus on racial/ethnic minority concerns on issues related to drug abuse and addiction (NIDA, n.d.).

While there are advantages to the term's utility—and it is still considered appropriate—there is the potential to marginalize groups outside of the norm (Hegamin et al., 2002; Polinsky et al., 1998). The norm is usually considered white, heterosexual, adult, Christian, economically advantaged, able-bodied males, and it is not expected to become more inclusive. As Lawson and Lawson (2011) indicate in their textbook, *Alcoholism and Substance Abuse in Diverse Populations*, "who is to say who is 'special'?" (p. xxi). If the addiction field continues to label certain groups as "special," the result may be the tendency to segregate these populations. Labels can influence and perpetuate stereotypes, biases, incorrect perceptions, and negative attitudes regarding people who present for substance abuse concerns. Moreover, using the term special populations attaches homogeneity. As discussed earlier, people have multiple identities and these identities may come with unique needs, which may not be attended to if classified under only one of those identities.

After much consideration, the term *specific* is used throughout the text in an effort to more accurately represent persons of diversity. The author is selective on the populations chosen to comprise this text and acknowledges an exclusion of some subgroups (e.g., persons who are homeless, persons living with HIV/AIDS, and persons with spiritual/religious beliefs). As such, the author attempts to address some of these subgroups within other chapters. Moreover, this text was written primarily with counselor trainees in mind. Much of the cited research is from the counselor education literature; however, the information is transferable to the disciplines of social work, criminal justice, sociology, and psychology, as well as the medical and educational fields. As students, teachers, and practitioners, we must continue our journey toward multicultural competency. Thus, in an effort to assist in this process, self-awareness exercises, assessments, and discussion questions exploring diversity issues are scattered throughout the reading. These activities will explore your knowledge, skill, attitudes, awareness, and motivational competencies related

---

PERSONAL IDENTITY QUESTIONNAIRE

1. Who am I? (i.e., what are your identities?)
2. What are your primary racial and cultural backgrounds?
3. How do you experience yourself as a member of these cultural identities?
4. How do you experience other members of these cultural identities?
5. Where were you raised?
6. What were the spiritual beliefs with which you were raised?
7. What are the appropriate gender roles in your culture?
8. What were the most important core values you were raised to follow?
9. What were your beliefs regarding alcohol and substance use when you were growing up? What are they now? How did you develop these beliefs?
10. To whom did people in your culture usually turn to for help?
11. Who had the responsibility of caring for those who became ill (e.g., the individual, family, community, or doctor)?
12. Any reasons why you would have barriers to accessing, retaining, or successfully completing counseling/treatment?
13. Explain why clients from two specific populations may be reluctant to seek out counseling.
14. What two populations do you feel most comfortable interacting with, and why?
15. What two populations do you feel most uncomfortable interacting with, and why?

---

to specific populations.

Before moving on to the first chapter, take about five to ten minutes to complete the Personal Identity Questionnaire and reflect on your answers.

REFERENCES

Brady, T. M., & Ashley, O. S. (Eds.). (2005). *Women in substance abuse treatment: Results from the Alcohol and Drug Services Study (ADSS)* (DHHS Publication No. SMA 04-3968, Analytic Series A-26). Rockville, MD: Substance Abuse and Mental Health Services Administration, Office of Applied Studies.

Brown, L. S., Kritz, S. A., Goldsmith, R. J., Bini, E. J., Rotrosen, J., et al. (2006). Characteristics of substance abuse treatment programs providing services for HIV/AIDS, hepatitis C virus infection, and sexually transmitted infections: The National Drug Abuse Treatment Clinical Trials Network. *Journal of Substance Abuse Treatment, 30*, 315–321.

Center for Substance Abuse Treatment (2006). *Substance Abuse: Clinical Issues in Intensive Outpatient Treatment.* Treatment Improvement Protocol (TIP) Series 47. DHHS Publication No. (SMA) 06-4182. Rockville, MD: Substance Abuse and Mental Health Services Administration.

Eyrich-Garg, K. M., Cacciola, J. S., Carise, D., Lynch, K. G., & McLellan, A. T. (2008). Individual characteristics of the literally homeless, marginally housed, and impoverished in the U.S. substance abuse treatment–seeking sample. *Social Psychiatry and Psychiatric Epidemiology, 43*, 831–842.

Friedmann, P. D., Lemon, S. C., Durkin, E. M., & D'Aunno, T. A. (2003). Trends in comprehensive service availability in outpatient drug abuse treatment. *Journal of Substance Abuse Treatment, 24*, 81–88.

Green, C. A. (2006). Gender and use of substance abuse treatment services. *Alcohol Research and Health, 29*, 55–62.

Hegamin, A. M., Anglin, G., & Casanova, M. (2002). Deconstructing the concept of "special populations." *Journal of Drug Issues, 32*, 825–836.

Lawson, G. W., & Lawson, A. W. (2011). *Alcoholism and substance abuse in diverse populations* (2nd ed.). Austin, TX: PRO-ED, Inc.

Loue, S. (2003). *Diversity issues in substance abuse treatment and research*. New York: Kluwer Academic/Plenum Publishers.

National Institute on Drug Abuse (n.d.). Special Populations Office. Retrieved from http://www.drugabuse.gov/about-nida/organization/offices/office-nida-director-od/special-populations-office-spo

Office of Substance Abuse Services (2004). *Gender differences and their implications for substance use disorder treatment*. Virginia Department of Mental Health, Mental Retardation and Substance Abuse Services.

Olmstead, T., & Sindelar, J. L. (2004). To what extent are key services offered in treatment programs for special populations? *Journal of Substance Abuse Treatment, 27*, 9–15.

Polinsky, M. L., Hser, Y., & Grella, C. E. (1998). Consideration of special populations in the drug treatment system of a large metropolitan area. *Journal of Behavioral Health Services and Research, 25*, 7–21.

Sheedy, C. K., & Whitter, M. (2009). Guiding principles and elements of recovery-oriented systems of care: What do we know from the research? *HHS Publication No.* (SMA) 09-4439. Rockville, MD: Center for Substance Abuse Treatment, Substance Abuse and Mental Health Services Administration.

Substance Abuse and Mental Health Services Administration (2012a). *National Survey of Substance Abuse Treatment Services (N-SSATS): 2011. Data on Substance Abuse Treatment Facilities.* BHSIS Series S-64, HHS Publication No. (SMA) 12-4730. Rockville, MD: Substance Abuse and Mental Health Services Administration, 2012.

Substance Abuse and Mental Health Services Administration (2012b). Center for Behavioral Health Statistics and Quality. *Treatment Episode Data Set (TEDS): 2000–2010. National Admissions to Substance Abuse Treatment Services.* DASIS Series S-61, HHS Publication No. (SMA) 12-4701. Rockville, MD: Substance Abuse and Mental Health Services Administration, 2012.

Sue, D. W., & Sue, D. D. (2013). *Counseling the culturally diverse: Theory and practice* (6th ed.). New York: John Wiley & Sons.

White, W. L. (2008). *Recovery management and recovery-oriented systems of care: Scientific rationale and promising practices*. Rockville, MD: Jointly published by Northeast Addiction Technology Transfer Center, the Great Lakes Addiction Technology Transfer Center, and the Philadelphia Dept. of Behavioral Health.

CHAPTER 1

DIVERSITY CONCEPTS AND A DISCUSSION OF RACISM

All substance abuse counseling is multicultural in nature. Many cultural differences can exist between client and counselor, thereby potentially impacting the efficacy of treatment. These differences include one's identity to various groups such as race, gender, sexual orientation, class, age, etc. Each chapter of this text will address a specific population, but several identities may be discussed within one chapter (e.g., women who also identify as lesbians). The reader can expect the following information will be delivered at some point within the chapters:

- Overview of a specific population (e.g., statistics, prevalence of use, definitions, etc.)
- Substance abuse issues (e.g., etiology, reasons for use, risk factors, stigmas)
- Barriers to treatment
- Resiliency factors
- Screening/assessment tools (e.g., used frequently with or focused on a specific group and any identified diversity concerns associated with these tools)
- Recommendations for treatment and therapeutic considerations
- Self-awareness exercises

Addiction researchers note that the majority of substance abuse therapists are white; however, nearly half of their clients are not (Mulvey, Hubbard, & Hayashi, 2003). Therefore, before discussing the various populations and multicultural counseling competencies, the initial chapters focus on some definitions and key concepts associated with race. Racism, white privilege, and white racial identity will be explored first, and then a brief discussion of sexism, heterosexism, and classism will follow.

Exercise: Take a moment and write a definition for each of these concepts:

Culture
Worldview
Ethnicity
Race

Reflect on this process. Where did you learn these definitions? Which were the hardest to define, and why?

The most obvious cultural differences between the therapist and client are likely to be disparities in gender, race, ethnicity, and age. However, other aspects of diversity are less discernible when you meet a client for the first time. For example, during an intake session, you may sit down with someone who has a disability, is economically disadvantaged, is LGBT, or has different spiritual/religious beliefs and practices from yours. In essence, all of these identities are considered part of a person's culture, but you may not be privy to all of a client's identities unless the client shares this information with you.

Culture is a group of people's way of life. Culture is defined as the thoughts, beliefs, practices, and behaviors of a group in the areas of history, religion, social organization, economic organization, political organization, and collective production (Sue & Sue, 2013). The United Nations Educational, Scientific and Cultural Organization (UNESCO) states culture is the set of distinctive spiritual, material, intellectual, and emotional features of society or a social group, and it encompasses language, food, dress, art, literature, music, lifestyles, value systems, traditions, and beliefs (UNESCO, 2002). In addition, culture is considered to be the sum total of life patterns within a given community over generations, and it also determines who will be oppressed and who will benefit in a particular society (Straussner, 2001).

Culture provides a system in which people:
- set and achieve goals
- make decisions
- solve problems
- define social roles
- emphasize cooperation or competition
- perceive human nature, truth, time orientation, and property
- define identity and individuality (Gambino, n.d.).

Each person is born into a cultural context, and the process of socialization is generally the function of the family and occurs through participation in cultural subgroups (Sue & Sue, 2013). These subgroups influence our **worldview**, which is defined as the perceptions, attitudes, beliefs, and assumptions that individuals and groups hold about the world, including the use of alcohol and other drugs. Sue and Sue (2013) outline two psychological orientations that represent differing worldviews: (1) **locus of control** (internal/external); and (2) **locus of responsibility** (internal/external). Most white middle-class people fall into the internal loci of control and responsibility (e.g., "I am a master of my own fate and I am responsible for my success or lack of success."). A person of color who has external loci of control and responsibility (due to oppression in our society) thinks there is little he or she can do about the injustices and gives up (i.e., learned helplessness), which can also result in mental health concerns (e.g., depression). A person of color can also have an external locus of control and internal locus of responsibility and believe the plight of their own people is due to laziness and stupidity and accept the dominant group's cultural standards (e.g., "It is up to me and society is okay the way it is."). Lastly, a person of color can have an internal locus of control and an external locus of responsibility and believe that he or she can shape events in their life if given a chance (e.g., "I have pride in my identity, and I have control over my life. Society is not okay, and I seek to change it.").

While culture is a global concept, ethnicity is a more focused notion. According to Straussner (2001), the term comes from *ethnos*, which is a Greek word for "people" or "nation" (p. 6). **Ethnicity** refers to a person's identity based on a group's social and cultural heritage passed on to group members from one generation to the next. Often, this term is commonly used interchangeably with the term **race**. How did you define race? Was it similar to ethnicity?

Before discussing what race is, let's look at what race is not. Race is NOT:
- Scientific, biological, or based on genetics
- Neutral or harmless
- The same thing as culture or ethnicity
- Defined by color or other physical attributes
- The same as religious identity (Barndt, 2007).

More than four hundred years ago, in the days of the European colonial expansion, racial identity was imposed and there was a forced process of "lumping" people together (Barndt, 2007, p. 191). This is known as racialization. According to the Dictionary of Human Geography (2009), **racialization** is a process where one group defines another as morally and/or genetically inferior to dominate and oppress others. Therefore, race is a myth, but yet also a reality. It is a societal construct that was designed and used for control and exploitation (Barndt, 2007). In essence, race is a racist concept created to support racism.

When defining race, did you think about how a person looks or include skin color in your definition? Phenotypical features such as skin color, hair texture, or facial structure are interpreted as evidence that two groups are indeed separate "types" of people and are used to strategically demark the boundaries between groups (Dictionary of Human Geography, 2009). To define race based on phenotype is not accurate. A Latino person, for example, can also be of black, white, or Native American racial background and cultures. Thus, racial categorization can negate the various other identities of a person. Through DNA analysis, physical appearance has been found by researchers to determine nothing about a person's ancestry. If you are interested in learning more about this discussion, the author recommends a video called *Race: The Power of an Illusion*, which is available for free on the World Wide Web.

In this text, the concepts of culture, worldview, ethnicity and race are addressed as they relate to each population. The issues associated with substance use, misuse, and abuse must be viewed within the context of a people's past, present, and future. Counselors must take into account the history of our nation. Historical events that have occurred, and incidents that continue to occur, influence: (1) the current environment in which a client lives; (2) the client's mental health status; (3) a client's self-perception, self-esteem, and self-worth; (4) perceptions of others (including you); (5) coping skills; and (6) the consumption of alcohol and other drugs. Exploring addiction as it relates to diversity and specific populations cannot be assessed and interpreted only in terms of prevalence of use and treatment protocols. In order to treat substance use problems effectively, we must not ignore the societal constructs that impact a certain group of people.

RACISM AND PREJUDICE

In an effort to accurately conceptualize the factors impacting alcohol and other drug use by specific populations, counselors should understand the diversity issues that exist within our society. Attempts should be made to empathize with the lived experiences of people who are not identified as white, heterosexual, adult, Christian, economically advantaged, able-bodied males. First, let's take a closer look at racism and prejudice.

Exercise

Take a moment and answer the following questions:

1. How do you define racism?
2. What are five examples of racism?
3. What is prejudice? How is it different from racism?

When defining racism, there are various words or phrases commonly employed, and they can be grouped by category (i.e., individual racism or institutional racism) (Barndt, 2007). Take a look at Table 1.1. Did you include any of the words or phrases outlined below? You were also asked to come up with five examples. These examples can be racist at an individual or systemic level. One example you may have thought of is an overt act of individual racism, such as the use of a racial epithet or slur. Refer to your examples and identify the category for each.

Table 1.1: List of Common Words or Phrases Used to Define Racism

INDIVIDUAL RACISM	INSTITUTIONAL OR SOCIETAL RACISM
Personal prejudice	Systemic power
Bigotry	Institutional discrimination
Hate	Oppression
Bias	Segregation
Personal dislike	Economic inequality
Stereotyping	Political control
Personal belief in superiority	White supremacy

From Joseph Barndt, from *Understanding and Dismantling Racism: The Twenty-First Century Challenge to White America*, p. 56. Copyright © 2007 by Augsburg Fortress.

Source: Joseph Barndt, from *Understanding and Dismantling Racism: The Twenty-First Century Challenge to White America*, p. 56. Copyright © 2007 by Augsburg Fortress.

Three Types of Racism

There are three types of racism: (a) individual; (b) cultural; and (c) institutional (Barndt, 2007; Constantine & Sue, 2006; Helms, 2008; Jones, 1972). **Individual racism** can be viewed as the thoughts, feelings, attitudes, and behaviors of an individual that can be verbal or nonverbal, overt or covert, and intentional or unintentional. While using a racial slur would be considered a verbal, overt, intentional act of racism, saying to a person of color, "When I see you, I don't see color" is a verbal, covert, unintentional act. **Cultural racism** occurs when there is cultural heritage superiority by the dominant group and the imposition of practices and beliefs as the norm. This practice results in the disintegration of the culture of people of color. **Institutional racism** is when the policies, practices, or structures of the educational, governmental, criminal justice, political, medical, economic, corporate, communications and media, and religious systems oppress people of color; thus, whites benefit (Barndt, 2007; Jones, 1997).

Racism-Related Stress

All people experience stress. However, individual, cultural, and institutional racism cause additional stress to people of color. Racism-related stress has negative consequences on emotional, physical, mental, and spiritual health, as well as social connectedness, job performance, academic achievement, and parental functioning (Harrell, 2000). Six types of racism-related stress exist: (1) race-related life events; (2) vicarious racism experiences; (3) daily racism microstressors; (4) chronic-contextual stress; (5) collective experiences of racism; and (6) transgenerational transmission of group traumas (Harrell, 2000).

As a counselor, it is imperative that we explore these stressors with regard to clients who do not identify as white. Review Table 1.2 and hypothesize how these stressors can influence substance use and the treatment of addictions.

Table 1.2: Six Types of Racism-Related Stress

TYPE	DEFINITION	EXAMPLES
Race-related life events	Time limited, have a beginning and an end, may lead to other events, and may occur infrequently	Police harassment Being rejected for a loan Housing discrimination
Vicarious racism experiences	Through observation and report of family members, friends, and strangers	Trayvon Martin Rodney King
Daily racism microstressors	Frequent, subtle, unintentional offenses; most often not confronted; also called microaggressions	Being ignored Being followed while shopping Locking car doors or clutching purse tighter when a person of color walks by
Chronic-contextual stress	Due to social structure, political dynamics, and institutional racism	Prevalence of liquor stores in a neighborhood Out-of-date textbooks in urban public schools
Collective experiences	Cultural-symbolic and sociopolitical manifestations of racism	Economic conditions of one's racial/ethnic group Lack of political representation Media portrayals
Transgenerational transmission	Historical contexts (and traumas) of diverse groups transmitted through discussions, storytelling, and lessons taught to children	Slavery of African people Removal of American Indians from their lands

Adapted from Harrell (2000). A multidimensional conceptualization of racism-related stress: Implications for the well-being of people of color. *American Journal of Orthopsychiatry, 70*, pp. 42–57.

Harrell (2000) suggests incidents occur in daily life that cause stress for all people, regardless of race or ethnicity; however, the frequency, intensity, meaning, and consequences can vary based on one's racial identity. For example, a person is sitting in slow-moving traffic due to a car accident up ahead and thinking about being late for work. Most white people would become anxious and stressed out. However, a person of color may encounter additional stress due to this incident. The person could be concerned about his or her tardiness as a confirmation of a stereotype given to his or her racial or ethnic group (e.g., unprofessional, lazy, or having a poor work ethic).

The six types of racism-related stress can also be compounded for a person of color if he or she is also a member of another oppressed group (Harrell, 2000). If a person of color is a sexual minority, is a woman, is economically disadvantaged, has a disability, or is an older adult, he or she will be placed in "double jeopardy" (Purdie-Vaughns & Eibach, 2008). Researchers have investigated the phenomenon of double jeopardy and argue the lived experiences of this intersection of multiple identities differ qualitatively to the experiences of having only one identity of an oppressed group. Women are oppressed; however, a woman of color in the workplace experiences different stressors than a white woman. The LGBT community also experiences stress from discrimination and oppression, but a black person who is lesbian or gay has different stressors on her or his well-being, as compared to a white person who identifies as lesbian or gay. While interactive effects of multiple cultural identities are experienced (i.e., double jeopardy), when asked to describe the effects specifically, people may have difficulty explaining the interplay, or they may end up focusing more of the explanation on one particular identity (Croteau, Talbot, Lance, & Evans, 2002).

The effect of possessing multiple statuses (both privileged and oppressed identities) has been described as placing a transparency of one color over a transparency of another color. The color of one "is sometimes so strong or pervasive that it completely covers or obscures the other; at other times, overlaying one transparency on top of another merely changes the tint of the original transparency" (Croteau et al., 2002, p. 246). Refer to Figure 1.1 for the following illustration. Imagine if there is a transparency with a blue circle representing a man's racial identification as Latino. This particular man considers his Latino identity to hold much value. At the same time, it is viewed as an oppressed status in America. The other transparency has an orange circle representing his sexual orientation as heterosexual. His sexual orientation does not

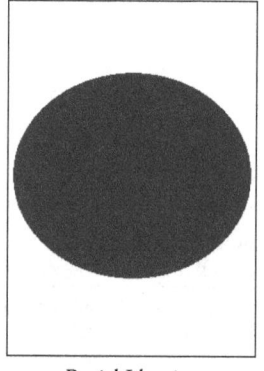
Racial Identity
Latino
Oppressed Status

Sexual Orientation Identity
Heterosexual
Privileged Status

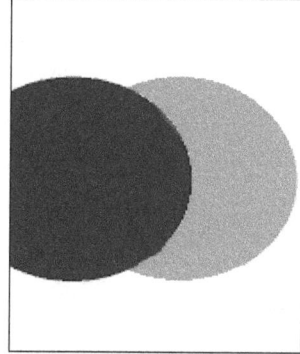
Interplay of Two Identities
Racial Identity Overlaps
Sexual Orientation Identity

Figure 1.1: An example of the interplay between two identities.
Adapted from Croteau et al., 2002.

have much weight on his identification, nor is it recognized often in his daily life. However, identifying as a heterosexual is a privileged status in our country. If the circles were to be placed over one another, the blue circle would cover the orange circle. In essence, the weight, recognition, and value of one (privileged or oppressed) status have the potential to affect the weight, recognition, and value of the other (privileged or oppressed) status.

Reflection Exercises

1. How could racism-related stress play out in therapy?
2. A counselor does not recognize the various types of stress associated with being a member of an oppressed group and does not understand how the stress shapes the lived experiences of a person. What could be the potential consequences?
3. Social scientists assert there is a *cumulative* impact of racism-related stress. In essence, the impact of racism on an individual is larger than the sum of separate events. What does this mean to you?
4. Reflect on the discussion regarding the interplay between identities. How does this play out in your life? The lives of your clients? How could the interplay of identities be correlated with substance use?

Prejudice

How did you define prejudice? How is it different from racism? **Prejudice** can either be favorable or unfavorable in nature and is the expression of bias toward a particular group. The harmful prejudice encompasses the unfounded fears, mistrust, and hatred of a group, and this can include many identities of a single person (e.g., sexual orientation, religion, social status, class, gender, age, etc.). According to Barndt (2007), racial prejudice is not the same thing as racism. **Racial prejudice** is having distorted and unsubstantiated judgments, biases, opinions, and stereotyped beliefs about other racial and ethnic groups. *Everyone can be racially prejudiced, but not everyone can be racist.* Why is this so? People of color do not have the reinforcement by the systems and institutions of our society. In essence, *they do not have power* in our society.

Therefore, racism can be defined as the following equation:

Racism = Racial Prejudice + the Misuse of Power by Systems and Institutions (Barndt, 2007)

As discussed above, institutional racism involves countless systems within our society. In order to be racist, a person must hold prejudice AND abuse or exploit the power generated by our institutions. Consider the ideology that power is a good thing; however, misuse of power is not. There are three ways racism involves the misuse of power (Barndt, 2007). Racism: (1) is a destructive powerful force OVER people of color; (2) provides and preserves power FOR white people; and (3) has the ultimate power to control and destroy EVERYONE.

The absence of power by any group (e.g., women, LGBT, economically disadvantaged, non-Christian, etc.) is a result of oppression. **Oppression** establishes dominance in order to gain benefits and maintain (unearned) privileges or advantages over others. It is seen as a "force that keeps people from self-determination [and] it keeps people from sharing power, sharing goods, and being able to take part in opportunity and wealth" (Hays, Chang, & Dean, 2004, p. 248). The oppression of women, for example, establishes male dominance and provides men power and privilege by dominating, controlling, and exploiting women. The privileges of several dominant groups (i.e., white, heterosexual, able-bodied, and economically advantaged) will be discussed more in depth throughout this text, with white privilege being the first in the next chapter.

Racism Is "Institutionalized"

Historically, institutions and systems have benefited white people, and innumerable laws were created to separate, segregate, discriminate, and control people of color (e.g., Jim Crow laws, Manifest Destiny and the boarding schools for Native American children, the Racial Integrity Act of 1924, and the Naturalization Act of 1790). Institutional racism infers racism transpires *inside* an institution; however, this is not the reality of racism. Barndt (2007) advocates for the use of the term "institutionalized racism" instead. **Institutionalized racism** is *self-perpetuating* and indicates there is an "institutional arrangement that has

Table 1.3: Five Levels of Institutionalized Racism

LEVELS	EXPLANATION	EXAMPLES
PERSONNEL	People who work or volunteer for an institution People authorized to speak, act and implement programs in the institution's name Act as gatekeepers Qualifications, actions and behavior defined by policies	Inequality in numbers, positions and salary Ineffective training on racism and race relations Inadequate supervision, grievance procedures, or conflict resolution Different treatment for whites and people of color
PROGRAMS, PRODUCTS, AND SERVICES	What an institution provides: e.g., food, clothing, technical services, entertainment, etc. Designed to attract, nurture, and retain members, customers or clients	Different quality programs, products, and services for whites than for people of color Policies regarding racism and race relations in personnel, finances, facility use, programs, etc., are absent, not adequate or unenforced
CONSTITUENCY AND COMMUNITY	People served by an institution People who belong to or patronize an institution	Constituency is not representative of the communities of color Communities of color or constituency not adequately or equally served
ORGANIZATIONAL STRUCTURE	Powers of the institution: people in charge, board of directors, managers, etc. Where decisions are made, budgets are decided, people are hired and fired, programs are approved, boundaries are set, etc.	Geographic or organizational boundaries are exclusionary or do not represent people of color People of color do not have power or authority in an institution Institutional structures are accountable to whites and not accountable to people of color
MISSION, PURPOSE, AND IDENTITY	What an institution is for and why it exists Mission, purpose, and identity are defined by constitution, by-laws, belief system, worldview, history and tradition	The original mission, purpose, and organizational structure of every institution in the United States were to serve whites exclusively It is still true today that the values, and worldview of nearly every institution reflects the commitment to serve whites better than people of color

Adapted from *Understanding and Dismantling Racism: The Twenty-First Century Challenge to White America* (Barndt, 2007, p. 168).

been *built into* an institution's purpose, design, and structure" that effectively serves (and is accountable to) one racial group (Barndt, 2007, p. 151). Institutionalized racism can be seen at five different levels: (1) personnel; (2) programs, products, and services; (3) constituency and community; (4) organizational structure; and (5) mission, purpose, and identity. An outline of these levels is displayed above in Table 1.3.

As Barndt (2007) points out, our society is about 50 years after the civil rights movement; some things have improved regarding racism (e.g., segregation laws are gone, equal employment opportunity, affirmative action, economic and educational improvements, the election of President Barack Obama, etc.). Some things have *not* improved (e.g., segregation still exists, whites still have the wealth and power, inequality in the criminal justice system, denial that racism exists, racism is pervasive, but is more subtle and hidden, etc.). Fifty years is only 10 percent of our nation's history, which means 90 percent of our history has involved the creation and perpetuation of white privilege and racism. As discussed above, racism is institutionalized, and the last ten percent of America's history is not enough time to overturn the insidious nature of the racism that was created over hundreds of years.

Reflection Exercise

Take a moment and reflect on how institutionalized racism can be displayed within the five levels of substance abuse treatment centers, as well as the health care systems (e.g., mental and physical health).

REFERENCES

Barndt, J. (2007). *Understanding and dismantling racism: The twenty-first century challenge to white America.* Minneapolis, MN: Fortress Press.

Constantine, M. G., & Sue, D. W. (2006). *Addressing racism: Facilitating cultural competence in mental health and educational settings.* Hoboken, NJ: John Wiley and Sons.

ethnicity. (2009). In *The Dictionary of Human Geography*. Retrieved from http://www.credoreference.com/entry/bkhumgeo/ethnicity on January 7, 2013.

Gambino, B. (n.d.). *Culture and counseling* [PowerPoint slides]. Retrieved from http://mypage.siu.edu/gmieling/493/Chapter%202,%20Culture%20and%20Counseling.ppt

Harrell, S. P. (2000). A multidimensional conceptualization of racism-related stress: Implications for the well-being of people of color. *American Journal of Orthopsychiatry, 70*, 42–57.

Hays, D. G., Chang, C. Y., & Dean, J. K. (2004). White counselors' conceptualization of privilege and oppression: Implications for counselor training. *Counselor Education and Supervision, 43*(4), 242–257.

Helms, J. E. (2008). *Race is a nice thing to have: A guide to being a white person or understanding the white persons in your life.* Alexandria, VA: Microtraining Associates.

Jones, J. M. (1972). *Prejudice and racism.* Reading, MA: Addison-Wesley.

Jones, J. M. (1997). *Prejudice and racism* (2nd ed.). New York: McGraw-Hill.

Mulvey, K. P., Hubbard, S., & Hayashi, S. (2003). A national study of the substance abuse treatment workforce. *Journal of Substance Abuse Treatment, 24*, 51–57.

Purdie-Vaughns, V., & Eibach, R. P. (2008). Intersectional invisibility: The distinctive advantages and disadvantages of multiple subordinate-group identities. *Sex Roles, 59*, 377–391.

Straussner, S. L. (2001). *Ethnocultural factors in substance abuse treatment.* New York: Guilford Press.

Sue, D. W., & Sue, D. D. (2013). *Counseling the culturally diverse: Theory and practice* (6th ed.). New York: John Wiley & Sons.

United Nations Educational, Scientific and Cultural Organization (2002). UNESCO Universal Declaration on Cultural Diversity. Retrieved on March 1, 3013, from http://portal.unesco.org/en/ev.php-URL_ID=13179&URL_DO=DO_TOPIC&URL_SECTION=201.html

CHAPTER 2

WHAT IT MEANS TO BE WHITE AND PRIVILEGED

Citibank in Chicago displayed an advertisement on the side of city buses. The advertisement said: "You were born pre-approved." When I saw that sign, it was clear to me who ... Citibank was addressing. To be born white in our society is to be born pre-approved.

—Joseph Barndt (pastor, author, and antiracism trainer for 30 years)

Whites are born with privileges that support and perpetuate individual, cultural, and institutionalized racism. Some of these privileges can be quite obvious (e.g., having Band-Aids that match skin tone or walking into a room of people and not wondering if there will be another white person present), but many whites lack awareness of these privileges. In fact, whites are taught to not recognize these unearned benefits and advantages (McIntosh, 1995). However, whites must understand what it means to be white in America.

Benefits are given to not only whites, but to other members of dominant groups (e.g., men, heterosexuals, Christians, etc.). These members not only receive benefits, but they also have the absence of barriers. Barriers are put in place with the intention of creating privilege. The collective package of these unearned advantages takes two forms: (1) **negative privilege**, defined simply as the absence of barriers; and (2) **positive privilege**, considered the presence of additional perks that cannot be described in terms of immunities alone (Bailey, 1998). Due to multiple identities, a person can be privileged and also oppressed. While this author recognizes there are other oppressed groups that are denied privileges, this chapter is focused on white privilege. An exploration of sexism, heterosexism, classism, ageism, and ableism will be addressed later in the text.

Dr. Peggy McIntosh, a scholar and social advocate, may be best known for her work titled, "White Privilege: Unpacking the Invisible Knapsack," which was published in 1988. While thinking about male privilege, McIntosh recognized how white privilege is also similarly denied and protected (McIntosh, 1995). She created a list of unearned advantages; Table 2.1 is a short list of some assets in the "invisible knapsack" of "special provisions, maps, passports, codebooks, tools" that whites carry with them on a daily basis (McIntosh, 1995, p. 1).

Table 2.1: White Privileges: Unearned Benefits and Advantages

As a white person:
I can avoid spending time with people whom I was trained to mistrust and who have learned to mistrust my kind or me.
If I should need to move, I can be pretty sure of renting or purchasing housing in an area which I can afford and in which I would want to live.
I am never asked to speak for all the people of my racial group.
I can be pretty sure that my neighbors in such a location will be neutral or pleasant to me.
I can go shopping alone most of the time, pretty well assured that I will not be followed or harassed.
I can turn on the television or open to the front page of the paper and see people of my race widely represented.
I can be pretty sure that if I ask to talk to the "person in charge", I will be facing a person of my race.
If a traffic cop pulls me over or if the IRS audits my tax return, I can be sure I haven't been singled out because of my race.
I can easily buy posters, post-cards, picture books, greeting cards, dolls, toys and children's magazines featuring people of my race.

Adapted from: Peggy McIntosh, "White Privilege: Unpacking the Invisible Knapsack."

In addition to the list above from McIntosh, white people have other assets related to power and privilege that are considered broader in nature. Again, these assets are also not often recognized by people of privilege.

For example, whites have the benefits of obtaining:

- Instant service and attention
- A sense of welcomeness
- The pleasure of being made to feel comfortable
- The freedom of choices
- Financial and economic advantages
- Respect and trust
- Access to and control of institutions
- Quality of education
- Access to products and services
- Safety for their children
- Availability of their choice in housing and employment
- Representation by elected officials
- A lack of being discriminated against because of race
- Protection from police and the courts

- Freedom of movement
- The opportunity to "work hard and earn" advantages/assets
- And maybe most noteworthy, the comfort of being accepted as "normal" (Barndt, 2007, pp. 105 and 213)

The above-mentioned benefits are just the beginning of the long list of privileges from which whites prosper. A speech by a well-known, antiracist activist, Tim Wise (2008), conceptualizes this reality by discussing the literal meaning of the term *underprivileged*. He states that as a society (including behavioral health counselors), we talk about people who are "down and out," and we wish to help those in need. Wise states that the language and terminology we use obscure the relationship between "down" and "up" and suggests there is not a meaning of down without an up.

> We talk about those at the bottom of the hierarchy, not paying attention to the fact that for anyone who is down, someone is above them and they are above them because they are down. We use this language … and when I say we … I'm talking about nice liberal caring service providers. People who just want to help. [They say,] "I just want to help the underprivileged." That's the word we use. (Wise, 2008, p. 7)

Wise urges the discontinuation of the term because there are flaws to its utility. For instance, he states that it is a passively constructed term. Underprivileged "does not imply that anybody did anything to anyone … It's just: There's privilege … There you are under it" (Wise, 2008, p. 7). He goes on to explain how negative events happen in the lives of marginalized people and how these events are the result of oppression.

> That's why we came up with that bumper sticker, "Stuff Happens." That's the G-rated version. That's a bumper sticker that only a straight, white, upper-middle class male could have made. Because anyone who isn't straight, anyone who isn't male, anyone who isn't white, anyone who isn't upper-middle class knows that stuff doesn't just happen. Stuff gets done by people to people. Nothing is a coincidence. Nothing is random. This isn't osmosis. And so we act as if it's this passive thing, but yet that's not the case. (Wise, 2008, p. 8)

The second problem with the word underprivileged, as suggested by Wise, is that it is a relative term. He proposed that if the word underprivileged exists, then, by definition, there must be a term, "overprivileged." Have you heard people discuss overprivilege? And what does it mean? Wise challenged his audience by saying,

> If you don't believe me … punch in [your computer] two little words: the first one, underprivileged. Make no mistake. Your spellcheck is going to recognize that word. It's in their dictionary. They can give you the definition … the synonym … the antonym … the phonetic way in which you should spell it. Now come down one line, type in overprivileged. And watch how fast that little red line pops up. That line that says, "nope, you're an idiot." Making up words that don't exist, try again and get back to us. But if there is an underprivileged, there must be an overprivileged. Why don't we talk about it? Because that would require that we [i.e., white people] acknowledge [being overprivileged].

Other terms like "vulnerable," "at risk," and "underserved" must also be taken into consideration. LeBlanc (1997) encourages us to recognize our paternalistic and patriarchal language and questions if the definitions for these words are used by dominant groups to marginalize people. What are your thoughts?

The recognition or awareness of benefiting from the oppression of others may create uncomfortable, negative feelings (e.g., guilt or anger) and therefore, these types of discussions are avoided in the classroom, counseling sessions, supervision, and daily interactions (Hays & Chang, 2003). A qualitative study conducted by Ancis and Szymanski (2001) examined the awareness of white privilege among white counseling trainees. These researchers interviewed 34 master's level students after they read McIntosh's (1995) article; 31 students were female, three were male. The study took place at a large southeastern university. Ten participants demonstrated a lack of awareness and an outright denial of the existence of privilege (Theme 1). Anger, defensiveness, guilt, selective perception, and a distortion of McIntosh's conditions of privilege were frequently seen. At times, students attributed differential treatment that occurs between whites and other races to nonracial factors. For example, whites have the privilege of not having others question their financial stability because of their phenotype (i.e., white skin color). In reaction to this particular benefit given to whites, one female in the study stated:

> Is it skin color or the appearance of being a member of the socioeconomic class who can afford to shop in this particular location? Have you ever dressed rather shabbily and happened to wander into a high class store? How much assistance did you receive? Did you feel that you were being eyed suspiciously? I have. (Ancis & Szymanski, 2001, p. 555)

This particular student denied that the differential treatment given to whites at stores is due to race, and stated it was due to the perceived socioeconomic status (SES) of a person. She also indicated that a white person can dress in a way that would indicate a lower SES and therefore be overlooked by personnel or viewed as a potential shoplifter. Helms (2008) points out that social class is not race, nor is it SES. **Social class** is a person's subjective evaluation of one's resources, and **SES** is how the person is ranked by indicators chosen by our society (e.g., education, occupation, and income). Someone may consciously choose to change their social class. Later in the text, classism will be explored more in detail. As Ancis and Szymanski (2001) found, some students determined discriminatory acts can be more of a function of class than race, which was a denial of the privileges whites experience on a daily basis.

The second theme found in the reflections of the McIntosh (1995) article was a "demonstrated awareness of white privilege and discrimination" (Ancis & Szymanski, 2001). Many students indicated sadness and disgust and seemed to move beyond their feelings of guilt to a more critical analysis of their privilege. Seven of the 34 students expressed awareness, but accepted no responsibility or stated they were not willing to relinquish these unearned benefits. One student stated that she accepted most of the benefits listed, and she reported it is "part of my world, one that I know and I am comfortable with. I do not wish to change it … maybe I am selfish and unfair but I like being white and what it does for me" (Ancis & Szymanski, 2001, p. 558).

The third theme was "higher-order awareness and commitment to action." Fourteen of the 34 students appeared to express empathy and displayed an awareness of the pervasiveness and systemic nature of racism and privilege. Nine students reported either previous action or a desire to initiate action for social justice. A female student discussed the need for white people to be in uncomfortable or different situations "in order to gain a deeper understanding of what forces lie within us and within society to make up for such a complex web of prejudices and inequities based on such things as race and gender" (Ancis & Szymanski, 2001, p. 660).

Research investigating counselors' reactions to, and recognition of, privilege (e.g., Ancis & Szymanski, 2001) reiterates that awareness (of self and others) are crucial aspects of counselor competency. Recognition of the numerous benefits provided to dominant groups can assist counselors in the ability to create a strong, therapeutic relationship with a client who has an oppressed identity. Awareness is key; however, it is also just as vital for whites not only to recognize privilege, but to abandon these entitlements (Hays, Chang, & Havice, 2008). As stated above, McIntosh (1995) asserts that dominant groups are taught to ignore the positive and negative privileges provided to them. By not acknowledging them, they do not exist, and therefore whites do not have to give them up. Created by oppression, domination, control, and discrimination at a systemic level, these benefits must be made visible. The following metaphor characterizes the invisibility of the large-scale, systemic barriers by members of dominant groups:

> [Oppression is] the experience of being caged in. ... Consider a birdcage. If you look very closely at just one wire, you cannot see the other wires. If your conception of what is before you is determined by this [narrow-minded] focus, you could look at that one wire, up and down the length of it, and be unable to see why a bird would not just fly around the wire ... it is only when you step back, stop looking at the wires one by one, microscopically, and take a macroscopic view of the whole cage, that you can see why the bird does not go anywhere ... (Frye, 1983, p.5)

When the effects of racism and other *-isms* (e.g., sexism, heterosexism, classism, and ableism) are not understood macroscopically as the outcomes of systemic injustices, they are understood microscopically as the exclusive problems of particular people or groups who have made bad decisions, have deficiencies, have poor attitudes, are too sensitive, or are overreacting to an incident (Bailey, 1998). In an effort to have you, the reader, "step back ... and view the whole cage," the privileges of other dominant groups will also be addressed later in this text.

For instance, white, heterosexual, able-bodied, wealthy males are given many advantages, benefits, and tools without awareness. Former Texas governor Ann Richards acknowledged these inequities and the lack of awareness by a particular privileged male when she stated,

> "George Bush was born on third base, but thinks he hit a triple."

Take a moment and think about this quote as it relates to being born into privilege. In America, white children are taught that if you work hard, you will succeed (i.e., make it to home base and score). However, if, as a white person, you are given a knapsack with all the tools for success, then you have a tremendous advantage over others (i.e., being born on third base). Most whites are not aware of their tools provided to them because of their race (i.e., they take credit for hitting a triple). Using the baseball metaphor above, I propose we go even further.

I suggest, because of oppression:

> Many people do not have the opportunity to even make it "on deck."
> If they are given an opportunity to make it on deck,
> they were never provided a bat.
> If they go to bat,
> they are called out after ONE strike, and not three.
> If they strike out,
> it is attributed to being unskilled, lazy players
> who probably were never taught how to bat correctly anyway.
> If they are considered unskilled and lazy,
> then they are not given the opportunity to try out for the team.
> If not given the opportunity to be on the team,
> then why even practice batting?

This metaphor represents: (1) The lack of opportunities provided to marginalized groups; (2) the lack of resources provided to these groups; (3) the uneven playing field and different set of rules based on group membership; (4) the stereotypes created by the lack of opportunities and resources; (5) the systemic barriers set up to impede the success of marginalized groups; and (6) the learned helplessness that is manifested by oppression.

The baseball metaphor helps with conceptualizing privilege and oppression in America. How does this transcend into the counseling room? Counselors are not raised in a bubble. Due to how insidious oppression, racism, and discrimination are in our society, counselors' thoughts, beliefs, and attitudes are undoubtedly impacted. Counselor education researchers have been interested in the conceptualization of privilege and oppression, as well as the personal experiences and reactions that are connected to the development of these two concepts. In one qualitative study, a male counselor discussed his experience and stated,

> It's very easy … for someone of privilege to be oppressive. I am a white, middle-class, heterosexual male. I have to work really hard to understand where I am in this diverse society. How other people view me, or how I subconsciously or automatically view them because they might be different from me. So, it's real easy for me to blend in and just live this life I pretty much have been bred for. (Hays, Chang, & Dean, 2004, p. 252)

How did this individual come to understand his privilege as a white, middle-class, heterosexual male? According to him, he has to "work really hard to understand" his position in society as a man of many privileged statuses. How did he not only become aware, but understand, oppression? How did he shift the biases, prejudicial thoughts, and oppressive (nonverbal and verbal) behaviors from subconscious to conscious? By becoming aware of these thoughts, attitudes, and behaviors, are they no longer automatic?

Hays, Chang, and Dean (2004) generated a framework for explaining the development of awareness. The awareness process is cyclical and has external influences (e.g., government, media, and religion). Family and individual influences also impact the level of awareness one has related to privilege and oppression. The authors suggest that an individual's conceptualization is in response to the perception of these influences.

Cohort effects and historical events can also affect these variables. Internalization of these influences involves an integration of these messages and the perception of the messages and personal experiences. These messages act as a filter for the development of awareness (Hays, Chang, & Dean, 2004). While understanding the development process of recognizing privilege and oppression is important, counselor educators must also focus on (a) helping students gain insight as to the meaning and implications of these realities; and (b) initiate and/or maintain their motivation to take action as an agent for change.

As counselors, we must understand how white privilege plays into the oppression of people of color in our society. In the next section, we will discuss racial identification, how white children are taught not to recognize privilege, and how our society perpetuates stereotypes and negative feelings toward people of color.

Reflection Exercise

1. Refer to the lists of white privileges. What others can you add?
2. What were your emotional reactions to reading about white privilege?
3. What were your thoughts while reading and after reading about privilege?
4. Share this information with another person and have a discussion surrounding privilege.
5. If you are a white person, have you noticed some of these before? Try to imagine being a person of color and having these lived experiences without these privileges. How would this impact your (emotional, physical, mental, and spiritual) well-being?
6. How does white privilege potentially impact substance use? Treatment and counseling strategies? Treatment outcomes? The therapeutic relationship?
7. How does white privilege impact you?

Recommended Video

Tim Wise, *White Privilege*, video, available on YouTube

"LIGHT IS RIGHT": THE MEANING OF SKIN COLOR IN OUR SOCIETY

White privilege is given to people largely based on phenotype; mainly, the color of their skin. Racial identification and socialization occur at a young age, and studies have indicated white children and children of color prefer lighter skin (Clark & Clark, 1940; Gullickson, 2005; Quintana, 1998). The Clark and Clark "doll study" was completed in 1940 and was a ground-breaking investigation regarding racial biases among children. The Clark study looked at children's perceptions of two dolls that were identical, except for their skin tone. Seventy years later, discussions surrounding racial socialization have been brought to millions with the CNN Television show, *Anderson Cooper 360*. Since 2010, CNN news correspondent Anderson Cooper has been involved in presenting a series on children and race. In the CNN *AC360* special in 2010, youth (both white and of color) were shown pictures of children with various skin tones. Children were then asked to "show me the 'bad' child" and "show me the 'good looking' child." The study found children selected the pictures of lighter skin tones for the children perceived as smart, good, nice, good looking and selected the darker skin tones for children perceived as dumb, mean, bad, and ugly (CNN pilot demonstration, 2010). Dr. Margaret Beale Spencer at the University of Chicago was the academic consultant for this study.

The children were also asked to "show me the child who has the skin color you don't want." Anderson Cooper asked one of the black female children (who appeared to be about five years old) to explain why she chose the lighter skin tone as a preference. She responded, "I don't like the way brown looks because … (glanced down at her forearm and paused) … it looks nasty for some reason … (paused) … but I don't know what reason."

As part of the CNN *AC360* series, a new study was commissioned with Dr. Melanie Killen at the University of Maryland entitled *Kids on Race: The Hidden Picture*. This investigation was implemented and aired on television in April, 2012. This particular show included four episodes in which children and adolescents were interviewed to measure their implicit bias, which are biases that children (and adults) hold unbeknownst to themselves. Using modifications of a previously developed instrument by Melanie Killen and Heidi McGlothlin (McGlothlin & Killen, 2006) to measure children's attributions of intentions based on race, the television show depicted children's reaction to ambiguous images involving a black child and a white child. Black and white children (145 at ages 6 and 13 years) were asked, "What's happening in this picture?"; "Are these two children friends?"; and "Would their parents like it if they were friends?"

For example, the children were told to look at the same picture of two students on the playground, as shown below. The only difference is the race of the children. One picture was shown first, and then the other. What do you think a response may have been when a white child was shown the picture on the left and was asked, "What's happening in the picture?" What about a black child's response?

According to CNN, the black first-graders had far more positive interpretations of the images than white first-graders. The majority of the black children were much more likely to say things like, "Chris is helping Alex up off the ground" versus "Chris pushed Alex off the swing." They were also far more likely to think the children pictured are friends and to believe their parents would like them to be friends.

Over the last decade, Dr. Melanie Killen and her colleagues have investigated racial socialization in childhood and adolescence through the use of these ambiguous illustrations. They found that young European-American children attributed more negative bias based on race in the ambiguous pictures then did ethnic minority children, and that this was a function of school composition (McGlothlin & Killen, 2010; McGlothlin, Killen, & Edmonds, 2005). Dr. Killen has stated that racial identity and the

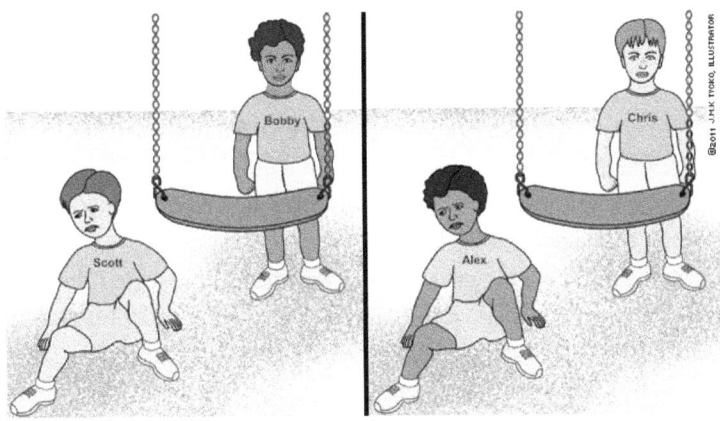

An example of one of the pictures shown to children in the CNN series, *Kids on Race: The Hidden Picture*.
Source: Copyright © 2011 by Joan Tycko. Reprinted with permission.

interpretation of race often begins with the ways parents talk to their kids about race, as she describes in her book on children's racial attitudes (Killen & Rutland, 2011). On the CNN *AC360* show, for example, Dr. Killen stated that "African American parents … are very early on preparing their children for the world of diversity and also for the world of potential discrimination." Dr. Killen asserts that "[Black parents are] certainly talking about issues of race and what it means to be a different race and when it matters and when it doesn't matter." In contrast, the negativity for white children could be more of a result of what *white parents are not saying* to their children. White parents often believe their children are socially colorblind, race is not a necessary issue to address, and talking about race is creating a problem.

Dr. Killen and her colleagues have also looked at biases among adolescents (Killen, Kelly, Richardson, & Jampol, 2010). Below is one of the ambiguous pictures used in their studies. What may have been some responses by white adolescents? Black adolescents? What was your reasoning for these responses?

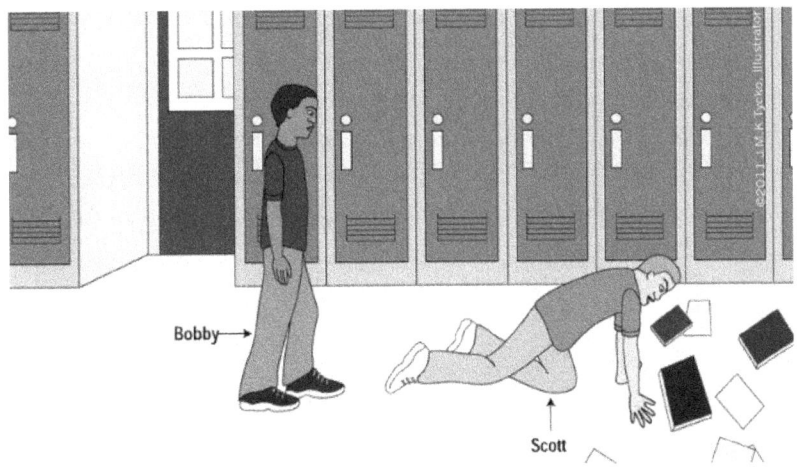

An example of the pictures shown to adolescents in the CNN study on perceptions of race.
Source: Copyright © 2011 by Joan Tycko. Reprinted with permission

Why do children assign negative attributes to others based on skin color? One reason for children's bias and favorable attitudes toward light skin potentially result from our nature to prefer lightness over darkness and also from the cultural messages reinforcing this preference (Quintana, 1998). In America, white represents purity, cleanliness, and goodness, and black is associated with bad, evil, and "nasty" things. For example, angels, brides, and the good guys are dressed in white, while crooks, witches, the grim reaper, and the devil are dressed in black. Another reason is that children identify with their own group, and then, with age, understand that status is associated with race.

Now, think about our everyday language and conversation. How often do we use the term "dark" or "black" to indicate negativity (e.g., dark times, dark ages, black mark, black box warning, black hole, black market) and "light" or "white" to denote positivity (e.g., on a lighter note, seeing the light, Snow White)? The person who holds the most power in our country lives in the White House. Even telling a lie, something considered wrong and immoral, is deemed less harmful…if it is white. What about crime? The non-violent type is considered "white collar" crime. Even one of the most famous quotes by Martin Luther King, Jr. speaks to this dichotomy in the American vernacular.

Darkness cannot drive out darkness: only light can do that. Hate cannot drive out hate: only love can do that.

—Martin Luther King Jr.

In summary, the socialization of race (and racism) begins at an early age (Killen & Rutland, 2011; Quintana, 1998). Our racial identification is not just a label or identifier; it comes with certain cognitive and affective components. Both racist and prejudicial (negative and positive) behaviors result from these components. White helping professionals must free themselves from this cultural conditioning and develop a non-racist identity (Sue & Sue, 2013). In order to do so, race must not be ignored

Reflection Exercise

1. At what age do you remember noticing differences in skin color?
2. What messages about your race were you given by your parents, other family members, teachers, and friends? What messages about other races were you given?
3. In 1995, Supreme Court justice Antonin Scalia made a statement regarding a decision on affirmative action. He stated, "In the eyes of the government, we are just one race here. It is American." Were you ever taught to "not see color" and that everyone was equal, the same, and an American? What are your thoughts about this ideology?

Recommended Videos:

Race: The Power of an Illusion, video, available on YouTube.
CNN series, *Kids on Race: The Hidden Picture*

COLOR BLINDNESS: "BLINDED BY THE WHITE"

Denial of color is really a denial of differences.
The denial of differences is really a denial of power and privilege.
The denial of power and privilege is really a denial of personal benefits that accrue to certain privileged groups by virtue of inequities.
The denial that we profit from racism is really a denial of responsibility for our racism.
Lastly, the denial of our racism is really a denial of the necessity to take action against racism.

—Dr. Derald Wing Sue on the concept of color blindness.

The quote above is from Dr. Derald Wing Sue, a professor and researcher in counselor education, and he is one of the most-cited multicultural scholars of our time. Dr. Sue encourages everyone to see color, including white. White is a color and not invisible. "Color blindness": (1) conveys the message that people of color must assimilate/acculturate to the dominant culture; (2) denies racial and ethnic experiences; (3) denies the person as a racial and cultural being; (4) allows white people to not see whiteness; and (5) avoids the issue of racism and white privilege (Barndt, 2007; Gushue & Constantine, 2007; Sue, 2010). Whites are taught to not see color as a practice of equality, and they do so with good intentions; however, it is a practice that "makes the person [of color] invisible" (Barndt, 2007, p. 89).

What does whiteness mean to you? As a person of color, you may answer this question more easily than whites, and you may have differing thoughts and emotions about whiteness. When whites are asked their heritage, many times they answer with the ethnicity and cultural background of their ancestors (e.g., Irish, German, or English). As a white person, what feelings do you have about being white? Most white people have difficulty describing these feelings (Barndt, 2007). Due to the tendency for discussions of race to be taboo in our society and the discomfort of these discussions, whites are conditioned to not see their color or see the advantages from which they benefit, let alone recognize feelings surrounding their whiteness. Barndt (2007) uses the metaphor of "a fish not knowing it is swimming in water. The environment has become so natural and the privileges have become so internalized in our subconscious that we do not notice them until they are taken away" (p. 89).

Color blindness and race neutrality have roots in the judicial system with the intent to be objective and treat all persons equally, regardless of race. However, ignoring race as a factor in the judicial system, medical community, and behavioral and mental health fields is to ignore the thoughts, behavior, cultural influences, identity, worldview, and the lived experiences of people of color. Barrett and George (2005) assert that color blindness is, in fact, a form of racism.

Color blindness comes in several forms (Helms, 2008; Neville, Lilly, Duran, Lee, & Browne, 2000). As stated previously, **the topic of race is considered taboo** in our society, and this form of color blindness is learned at an early age for white children. A common experience is when a white child points to a dark-skinned child and asks his or her parent, "Why is that kid black?" The parent may become embarrassed and can respond in a way that teaches children: (1) these observations cause anxiety for others; (2) race is to not be discussed; and (3) these types of questions are not to be asked. By not addressing racial issues, whites can "opt out" and not think about or not feel emotions related to privilege, racism, stereotypes, etc. The second form of color blindness is the **invisibility of race**, which is the idea that "everyone is the same" and racial group differences are ignored. The third type was coined **color-evasion** (Neville et al.,

2000) and refers to the rejection of white superiority and the existence of racism by highlighting the ways in which people of color and whites are the same. For example, if someone states, "I don't know why you have to be a hyphenated identity. Why can't you just be American like me?" (Helms, 2008, p. 13). The last form of color blindness is **power-evasion**, and it is the belief that everyone has the same opportunities. Helms (2008) uses the example of someone saying, "My great-grandparents did not have any education or money when they came to this country, but they became the wealthiest people in their community … why can't you?"

If whites engage in verbal and nonverbal behaviors that reflect the four types of color blindness, it may say something about their racial identity development and how they view themselves as racial beings. As discussed previously, socialization occurs at a very young age, and racial identity involves the thoughts, feelings, attitudes, biases, and prejudices we have for people of other races. In the next section, white racial identity will be explored, and the reader is encouraged to consider how racial identity development has implications for multicultural counseling.

Reflection Exercise:

1. What is the impact of color blindness as it relates to the judicial system? Medical community? Behavioral and mental health fields?
2. Regarding the substance abuse field, identify three ways that color blindness can be harmful to a client.

WHITE RACIAL IDENTITY MODEL

The racial socialization of a person is influenced by many factors, including historical events (at individual, family, community, and national levels), economic status, gender, and geographic location (McDermott & Samson, 2005). How would the development of racial identity be different for the following three white people: (1) Someone who grew up in Detroit, Michigan, in a predominantly black community; (2) someone who grew up in an affluent, predominantly white community in Greenwich, Connecticut; and (3) a white person who grew up in an economically disadvantaged, predominantly white community in the foothills of the Appalachian Mountains? How would white privilege be viewed by each person, and how would it be maintained differently in these three areas?

Whiteness is not a static, clearly defined identity. In fact, whiteness is considered a schema, or a pair of eyeglasses through which a person perceives or reacts to other people, situations, and stimuli (Helms, 2008; McDermott & Samson, 2005). These white identity schemas are not necessarily discrete, linear developmental phases with which one progresses. Moreover, a person's emotions, attitudes, and behaviors about race depend on the schema used and do not develop or progress at the same rate (Helms, 2008). If there is a considerable difference between emotions, attitudes, and behaviors about race, the more internal racial tension is experienced. In addition, a white person could have specific attitudes, behaviors, and emotions regarding Latino men, but regard Latina women differently, thus using a different schema when in the presence of a Latino man versus a Latina woman. This same person can also have very different attitudes and emotions when in the presence of an Asian person and exhibit other behaviors due to using a different schema.

In her book, *A Race Is a Nice Thing to Have*, Dr. Janet Helms (2008) outlines the process of white racial identity development. She indicates that a person can use more than one schema at a time, but most whites have a preference for one particular set of eyeglasses. The model put forth by Dr. Helms is the most widely used and accepted; therefore, it will be the only white identity framework presented. However, there are other identity models that are also well known and cited frequently (e.g., a five-stage development proposed by Hardiman, 1982, or the White Racial Consciousness Types proposed by Rowe, Bennett, and Atkinson, 1994). Helms (2008) asserts there are six schemas (not linear stages) of white identity development. The first three schemas maintain the status quo and relate to internalizing racism. These schemas involve the evolution of self-protective strategies that preserve the benefits of white privilege. The last three schemas require challenging white racial socialization norms and are correlated with progression toward a nonracist identity.

The first schema is **contact**. This set of eyeglasses is characterized by color blindness, denial, innocence, and ignorance. The person has satisfaction with the status quo and is oblivious to racial issues, racism, and his or her participation in racist thoughts and actions. A person who uses this schema in a particular situation may indicate the following: "There are no race problems in the United States"; "I do not discuss the characteristics of white people in public settings"; or "I personally do not notice what race a person is." The second schema is **disintegration**. A person uses this pair of eyeglasses when denial, ignorance, and color blindness no longer work, and he or she recognizes that inequalities exist. The person believes she is not racist, acknowledges there are benefits to being white, and considers these benefits to be at risk. She becomes conflicted because of the moral dilemma between (a) the desire for continued group membership as a white person; and (b) humanism. Thus, guilt, shame, anxiety, and helplessness are often experienced. As a result, people can avoid thinking about racial issues, and reality can be skewed, and the victims of racism are blamed (e.g., "People get what they deserve and/or earn; if they do not have anything, then they did not earn anything"; or "There is nothing I can do myself to solve society's racial problems."). The third schema is **reintegration**. Although he is now consciously white, the person regresses, in a sense. In this schema, the person is highly protective of white privilege; there is hostility, anger, or intolerance for other groups; whites are believed to be superior; stereotypes are endorsed; and he blames people of color (e.g., "The white race will be polluted by interracial marriage"; "Most blacks and Latinos are criminals, and that is why there is a disproportionate number of them in prison"; "People of color complain too much about perceived injustices.").

Advancement toward a nonracist identity involves the last three schemas (Helms, 2008). **Pseudo-independent** is a schema that still involves the belief that the white culture is better than others, but not intentionally so. The person may indicate she "feels as comfortable around (people of color) as she does around whites." A person in the pseudo-independent schema takes responsibility for helping others to think, feel, and behave in order to be accepted by (white) society. He recognizes that white people are responsible for racism, but does not acknowledge any personal responsibility for it and may not know how to articulate the ways he has benefited from racism. There is an intellectualized interest in racial issues, but it lacks an emotional attachment.

The next schema is **immersion-emersion**. A person is actively attempting to redefine her whiteness through self-exploration. She may feel anger toward other white people and attempts to find other whites who think about race in the same way. An increased experiential and affective understanding is

Table 2.2: White Identity and the Degree of Racial Comfort

	DEGREE OF RACIAL COMFORT		
	ANTI-DIVERSITY	**DIVERSITY DÉTENTE**	**PRO-DIVERSITY**
Relationship to Whiteness	Consciously acknowledges whiteness Takes an ethnocentric perspective	Actively questions white superiority, but still holds a white perspective Holds some degree of uncertainty and discomfort about racial identity Has let go of racist identity, but has not developed nonracist identity Sees white responsibility for racism May be viewed with suspicion by whites who see him/her as violating racial norms	Is comfortable with own whiteness Is able to apply definitions of race and whiteness to self-image and behaviors
Relationship to Non-Whiteness	Believes racial stereotypes.	Recognizes society treats people of color differently Has the feeling of being caught between white world and "non-white" one Tends toward more paternalistic encounters with people of color. May be viewed with suspicion by people of color, seeing him/her as having and advancing white mores	Comfortable with people of color Values a pluralistic society Seeks opportunities to learn from other groups Loses need to see group memberships as positive or negative, idealized, or denigrated
Behaviors and Cognitions	May express views actively: overtly hostile May express views passively: avoiding contact with other groups May not give voice to these feelings until he/she feels personally threatened Guilt or anxiety sublimated; transformed into feelings of fear and anger	Centered on intellectualization—emotions about race tend to be submerged Looks to people of color to explain racism/offer solutions Prone to behave unconsciously according to racist assumptions Experiences anger and/or guilt as motivating factors in dealings with race Seeks out new information regarding racial issues to lower anxiety, not out of commitment to antiracism or personal development Dissonance exists between previously held ethnocentric beliefs and new information View of self as moral is contradicted by realization that he/she is benefiting racism May try to change his/her beliefs, but may only have racist society as model	Realistic view of race, the effects of racism, and the actions which can be taken to be effective Has a sense of internalization about his/her approach to race Is motivated by a moral consciousness Does not approach identity issues out of anger or guilt Has the ability to identify and abandon racism Can exhibit behaviors that are active (e.g., organizes events to protest racism) Can exhibit behaviors that are passive (e.g., contributes to organizations that fight racism) Continuously open to new ideas about race and culture Emotions that were suppressed resurface/may have cognitive and emotional restructuring

Adapted from: Peter DiCaprio, "A Framework for Understanding White Identity Development."

also now present. One may even be embarrassed as she becomes aware of the previous ineptness and may become quite critical of herself and others. **Autonomy** is the last schema and is referred to as "racial self-actualization" (Helms, 2008, p. 85). The person accepts his whiteness and allows the racial part to influence other aspects of his life (e.g., "My whiteness is an important part of who I am."). Opportunities to actively confront racism are sought out. He values diversity, has less feelings of guilt, and is no longer fearful, intimidated, or uncomfortable with the reality of racial issues (Sue & Sue, 2013).

For years, researchers have studied racial identity and attitudes toward diversity (Croll, 2007; Goren & Plaut, 2012). Social scientists suggest a person has a relationship to their whiteness, as well as a relationship to non-whiteness. For instance, white anti-racism activists and white Neo-Nazis do not think of their whiteness in the same way (Goren & Plaut, 2012). In essence, there is a degree of racial comfort associated with one's identity development. After analyzing various racial identity developmental models, DiCaprio (2012) created a list of traits which are correlated to one's degree of racial comfort. Three traits were proposed: (1) anti-diversity; (2) diversity détente; and (3) pro-diversity. In the Table 2.2 above, behaviors and cognitions are also included as they relate to the degree of racial comfort. As you can see, the contents correspond with the schemas of the white identity development model by Helms.

How does white racial identity influence the working alliance in therapy? The importance of recognizing these developmental factors play a crucial part in multicultural competency of white counselors (Burkard, Juarez-Huffaker, & Ajmere, 2003; Gushue & Constantine, 2007). There is no clear-cut way of determining how your racial identity development and your comfort levels with racially and ethnically dissimilar clients impact your skills as a therapist. Gushue and Constantine (2007) studied 177 white counseling trainees and suggest that less advanced white racial identity statuses (e.g., color-blind attitudes) are correlated with more overt forms of racism.

Unfortunately, one common limitation of research is the inability to generalize findings. However, the implications for (a) having a low level of racial identity and (b) discomfort with people of color are crucial to multicultural competence. These two concepts can have a negative impact on the therapeutic relationship, and, in fact, cause harm to the client. In the next chapter, we discuss microaggressions, which can be the result of less advanced white identity development, as well as biases and prejudices toward other marginalized groups.

Reflection Exercises

If you are a white therapist, self-awareness is essential to becoming not only a multicultural competent counselor, but also to progress toward racial self-actualization. In an effort to overcome sociocultural conditioning and make whiteness visible to you, the author suggests the following:
1. Recognize that all whites are racist, whether knowingly or unknowingly. As a white person, work on accepting your whiteness, but define it in a non-defensive and nonracist manner. How you perceive yourself as a racial being seems to correlate strongly with how you perceive and respond to racial stimuli.
2. Spend time with healthy and strong people from another culture or racial group. Awareness and competency stem from lived experiences and understanding the reality of our racist society and the lived experiences of people of color.
3. When is the last time you attended a cultural event, meeting, or activity led by another racial or ethnic group? Make sure to stretch yourself and be out of your comfort zone. Be aware of your whiteness.

4. When around people of color, pay attention to your feelings of disparity. How do you feel different? Pay attention to feelings of uneasiness and fear, and ask yourself, "Where are these feelings coming from?" Take note of your thoughts, assumptions, biases, and stereotypes as well. Do not dismiss, avoid, or make excuses for them. Confront them, attach meaning to them, and attempt to unlearn the misinformation causing these thoughts or feelings.
5. Make a personal commitment to take action. Counselors are to be advocates for the client, not only in the individual counseling sessions, but also in their community and in the public arena. Social justice will be discussed later in the text, but you are encouraged to notice how you can be a change agent. Be accountable for making a difference at a personal and systemic level (adapted from Sue & Sue, 2013).

Recommended Video

Race is a Nice Thing to Have, an interview of Janet Helms. Microtraining video.

REFERENCES

Ancis, J. R., & Szymanski, D. M. (2001). Awareness of white privilege among white counseling trainees. *Counseling Psychologist, 29*, 548–569.

Bailey, A. (1998). Privilege: Expanding on Marilyn Frye's "oppression." *Journal of Social Philosophy, 2*(3), 104–119.

Barndt, J. (2007). *Understanding and dismantling racism: The twenty-first century challenge to white America.* Minneapolis, MN: Fortress Press.

Barrett, K. H., & George, W. H. (2005). Judicial color blindness, race neutrality, and modern racism: How psychologists can help the courts understand race matters. In K. H. Barrett & W. H. George (Eds.), *Race, culture, psychology and law* (pp. 31–46). Thousand Oaks, CA: Sage.

Burkard, A., Juarez-Huffaker, M., & Ajmere, K. (2003). White racial identity attitudes as a predictor of cross-cultural working alliances. *Journal of Multicultural Counseling and Development, 31*, 226–244.

Clark, K. B., & Clark, M. K. (1940). Skin color as a factor in racial identification of Negro preschool children. *Journal of Social Psychology, 11*, 159–169.

CNN Pilot Demonstration (2010). Retrieved on January 17, 2013, from http://i2.cdn.turner.com/cnn/2010/images/05/13/expanded_results_methods_cnn.pdf

Croll, P. R. (2007). Modeling determinants of white racial identity: Results from a new national survey. *Social Forces, 86*, 613–642.

DiCaprio, P. (2012). A framework for understanding white racial identity development. Retrieved on March 3, 2013, from http://triadllc.com/pdf/DiCaprio.pdf

Frye, M. (1983). *The Politics of Reality*. Trumansburg, NY: Crossing Press.

Goren, M. J., & Plaut, V. C. (2012). Identity form matters: White racial identity and attitudes toward diversity. *Self and Identity, 11*(2), 237–254.

Gullickson, A. (2005). The significance of color declines: A re-analysis of skin tone differentials in post–civil rights America. *Social Forces, 81*, 157–180.

Gushue, G. V., & Constantine, M. G. (2007). Color-blind racial attitudes and white racial identity attitudes in psychology trainees. *Professional Psychology: Research and Practice, 38*(3), 321–328.

Hardiman, R. (1982). White identity development: A process-oriented model for describing the racial consciousness of white Americans. *Dissertation Abstracts International, 43, 01.* (UMI No. 8351619)

Hays, D. G., & Chang, C. Y. (2003). White privilege, oppression, and racial identity development: Implications for supervision. *Counselor Education and Supervision, 43*(2), 134–145.

Hays, D. G., Chang, C. Y., & Dean, J. K. (2004). White counselors' conceptualization of privilege and oppression: Implications for counselor training. *Counselor Education and Supervision, 43*(4), 242–257.

Hays, D. G., Chang, C. Y., & Havice, P. (2008). White racial identity statuses as predictors of white privilege awareness. *Humanistic Counseling, Education, and Development, 47,* 234–246.

Helms, J. E. (2008). *Race is a nice thing to have: A guide to being a white person or understanding the white persons in your life.* Alexandria, VA: Microtraining Associates.

McDermott, M., & Samson, F. L. (2005). White racial and ethnic identity in the United States. *Annual Review of Sociology, 31,* 245–261.

McIntosh, P. (1995). White privilege and male privilege: A personal account of coming to see correspondences through work in women's studies. In M. L. Andersen & P. H. Collins (Eds.), *Race, class, and gender: An anthology* (2nd ed., pp. 76–87). Belmont, CA: Wadsworth.

Neville, H. A., Lilly, R. L., Duran, G., Lee, R. M., & Browne, L. (2000). Construction and initial validation of the color-blind racial attitudes scale (CoBRAS). *Journal of Counseling Psychology, 47,* 59–70.

Quintana, S. M. (1998). Children's developmental understanding of ethnicity and race. *Applied and Preventative Psychology, 7,* 27–45.

Rowe, W., Bennett, S. K., & Atkinson, D. R. (1994). White racial identity models: A critique and alternative proposal. *Counseling Psychologist, 22,* 129–146.

Sue, D. W. (2010). *Microaggressions in everyday life: Race, gender and sexual orientation.* Hoboken, NJ: John Wiley & Sons.

Sue, D. W., & Sue, D. D. (2013). *Counseling the culturally diverse: Theory and practice* (6th ed.). New York: John Wiley & Sons.

Wise, T. (2008). *The pathology of privilege: Racism, white denial, and inequality.* Media Education Foundation. [Transcript] Retrieved from http://www.mediaed.org/assets/products/137/transcript_137.pdf

CHAPTER 3

MICROAGGRESSIONS AGAINST MARGINALIZED GROUPS

In the previous two chapters, the author focused on issues related to people of color. In this chapter, the reader is encouraged to also incorporate other populations into the conceptualization and reflection of the material. Many people are often marginalized, and thus exist on the "margins," or outer limits, of social desirability, awareness, and appreciation (Sue, 2010). People are pushed to the outer limits because of identities, associations, experiences, and environments (LeBlanc, 1997). Therefore, they are confined to the edge of our systems and encounter exclusion and social injustice. As stated previously, the inequities between groups are so deeply ingrained in our society they are practically invisible. Most people of privilege are unaware of the myriad of benefits they receive and do not recognize the barriers or marginalization of others. Due to this lack of consciousness, subtle forms of racism, sexism, heterosexism, classism, and ableism occur unbeknownst to the oppressor. These acts are called microaggressions, also referred to as microstressors (Harrell, 2000; Sue, 2010).

Microaggressions are brief and everyday verbal, behavioral, and environmental indignities, whether intentional or unintentional, that communicate hostile, derogatory, or negative slights and insults to the target person or group (Sue, 2010). Perpetrators are usually unaware that they have engaged in an exchange that demeans the recipient of the communication. Microaggressions may be more influential than overt forms of racism, sexism, and heterosexism. More specifically, these slights and insults have more impact on anger, frustration, self-esteem, well-being, and standard of living (Sue, Capodilupo, et al., 2007). As a result, microaggressions figuratively cause "a slow death by a thousand cuts" (Sue, 2010, p. 66).

Exercise

Read the following examples of microaggressions. Determine what the hidden message(s) are for each. What does it convey to the victim of the microaggression?

1. A gay adolescent is frequently uncomfortable when fellow classmates describe silly or stupid behavior by saying, "that's gay."
    Hidden message?
2. A friendly neighbor states to a Jewish mother, "Merry Christmas."
    Hidden message?
3. A blind man reports that, when people speak to him, they often raise their voices.
    Hidden message?

4. A woman tells someone, "I don't trust him, he's an Arab." The person replies, "No. He's a decent family man, a citizen …"
   Hidden message?

5. A man describes a politician and states, "You have your first mainstream African American who is articulate and bright and clean and a nice-looking guy. I mean, that's a storybook man."
   Hidden message?

Possible hidden messages:

1. Homosexuality is deviant, wrong, silly, or stupid.
2. Everyone is Christian.
3. A person with a disability is defined as lesser in all aspects of functioning.
4. Arab American males are not trustworthy, good people, family men, or citizens. (Note: The first statement was made by a woman in the audience at a presidential political rally. The response was from Senator John McCain, the Republican presidential candidate.)
5. Most blacks are unintelligent, inarticulate, dirty, and unattractive, and this black politician is the exception. (Note: The statement was made by Vice President Joe Biden in reference to President Barack Obama.)

Adapted from *Microaggressions in Everyday Life: Race, Gender and Sexual Orientation* (Sue, 2010).

Microaggressions can be expressed in behaviors, both verbal and nonverbal, but they can be present in the environment as well (Sue, 2010). An example of an environmental microaggression: a female employee walks into a conference room and takes note of the various pictures of the past presidents of the company, all of whom are men. The message is clear for her: you are not welcome here, and no matter how hard you work, there exists a glass ceiling. Environmental microaggressions are also displayed through symbols or mascots. Sports teams have used (mis)representations of Native Americans for decades (e.g., Florida State Seminoles, Atlanta Braves, and Cleveland Indians), and controversy continues regarding the perpetuation of stereotypes (King & Springwood, 2001). Therapists should be aware of the manifestations of microaggressions, as they can occur in treatment. Continual exploration of one's thoughts, beliefs, biases, and prejudices is essential to avoid being the perpetrator of such acts.

Reflection Exercise

What nonverbal microaggressions can occur in the counseling environment (for a woman, person of color, or sexual minority)? Think about how documents, pictures, posters, etc., can convey microaggressions. How does the lack of group representation constitute a microaggression, and what message is that sending clients?

Types of Microaggressions

There are three types of microaggressions: (1) microassaults; (2) microinsults; and (3) microinvalidations (Sue, 2010; Sue et al., 2007). Refer to Figure 1 below for an outline of racial microaggressions; however, the taxonomy is the same for gender and sexual orientation. **Microassaults** are conscious and deliberate acts meant to cause harm, intimidate, threaten, and make the person feel unwanted and unsafe (e.g., using the term "fag" or laughing at or telling a joke about women). **Microinsults** are subtle snubs, and the perpetrator is often not aware of the insult (e.g., a female doctor is mistaken for a nurse or saying to an Asian person "Why are you so quiet? Speak up more."). **Microinvalidations** deny the reality of a person by negating the thoughts, feelings, or experiences of someone (e.g., asking a person of color, "Where are you from?" or making the statement, "Everyone can succeed if you just work hard enough.").

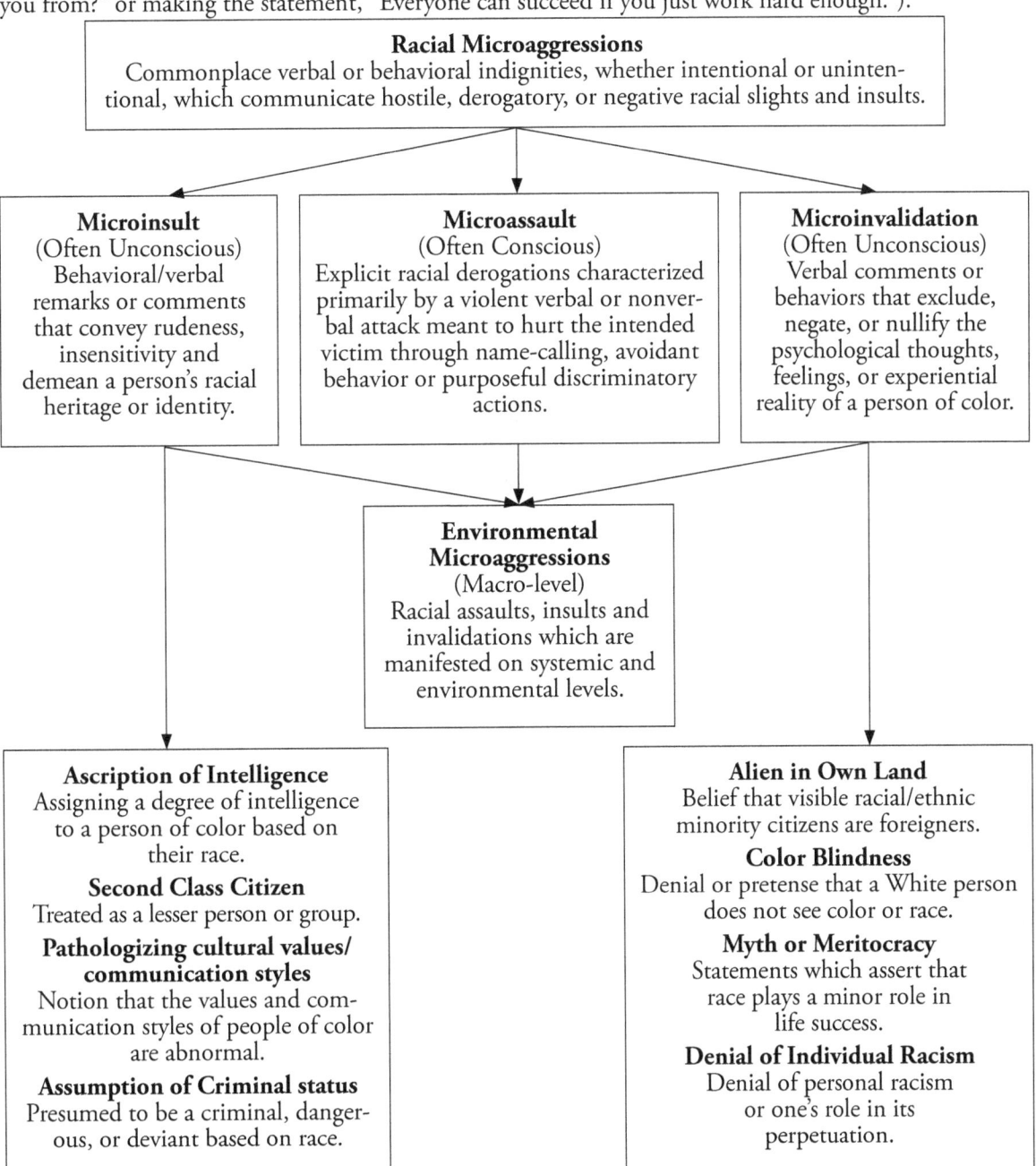

Figure 3.1: Categories of and Relationships Among Racial Microaggressions

Source: Derald Wing Sue, et al., from American Psychologist, vol. 62, no. 4, p. 278. Copyright © 2007 by American Psychological Association. Reprinted with permission.

Table 3.1: Examples of Racial Microaggressions

THEME	MICROAGGRESSION	MESSAGE
Alien in own land When Asian Americans and Latino Americans are assumed to be foreign-born	"Where are you from?" "Where were you born?" "You speak good English." A person asking an Asian American to teach them words in their native language	You are not American. You are a foreigner.
Ascription of intelligence Assigning intelligence to a person of color on the basis of their race	"You are a credit to your race." "You are so articulate." Asking an Asian person to help with a math or science problem	People of color are generally not as intelligent as Whites. It is unusual for someone of your race to be intelligent. All Asians are intelligent and good in math/sciences.
Color blindness Statements that indicate that a White person does not want to acknowledge race	"When I look at you, I don't see color." "America is a melting pot." "There is only one race, the human race."	Denying a person of color's racial/ethnic experiences. Assimilate/acculturate to the dominant culture. Denying the individual as a racial/cultural being.
Criminality/assumption of criminal status A person of color is presumed to be dangerous, criminal, or deviant on the basis of their race	A White man or woman clutching their purse or checking their wallet as a Black or Latino approaches or passes A store owner following a customer of color around the store A White person waits to ride the next elevator when a person of color is on it	You are a criminal. You are going to steal/ You are poor/ You do not belong. You are dangerous.
Denial of individual racism A statement made when Whites deny their racial biases	"I'm not racist. I have several Black Friends." "As a woman, I know what you go through as a racial minority."	I am immune to racism because I have friends of color. Your racial oppression is no different than my gender oppression. I can't be a racist. I'm like you.
Myth of meritocracy Statements which assert that race does not play a role in life successes	"I believe the most qualified person should get the job." "Everyone can succeed in this society, if they work hard enough."	People of color are given extra unfair benefits because of their race. People of color are lazy and/or incompetent and need to work harder.
Pathologizing cultural values/communication styles The notion that the values and communication styles of the dominant/White culture are ideal	Asking a Black person: "Why do you have to be so loud/animated? Just calm down." To an Asian or Latino person: "Why are you so quiet? We want to know what you think. Be more verbal." "Speak up more." Dismissing an individual who brings up race/culture in work/school setting	Assimilate to dominant culture. Leave your cultural baggage outside.

Source: From Sue et al. (2007). Racial microaggressions in everyday life: Implications for clinical practice. *American Psychologist*, 62(4), p. 276.

The messages conveyed to the victim of microaggressions can fall under various categories or "themes." Figure 3.1 and Table 3.1 provide examples of these themes with regard to racial microaggressions. However, the same messages can be delivered to women, sexual minorities, persons with economic disadvantages, and persons with disabilities. For instance, a heterosexual male states, "I am not homophobic, I have several gay friends" falls under the same "Denial" theme as saying, "I am not racist. I have several black friends." Moreover, the theme of "Second-Class Citizen" can be seen by people of various oppressed groups. A person of color may be mistaken for a service worker, or a woman states she works for the local university, and it is assumed she is an office coordinator and not a professor. Consider the "myth of meritocracy," which asserts all groups have the same opportunity to succeed. It tends to blame the oppressed groups for having deficiencies which result in poverty, unemployment, and lower educational achievement. A common idiom used in our vernacular is, "The cream of the crop rises to the top." Is this truth for someone who is not male? Not white? Not heterosexual?

Therapists who may take on the color-blind perspective (e.g., Helms's Contact status) discriminate against women, have prejudice toward people in the LGBT community, hold biases toward economically disadvantaged persons, or display intolerance for persons with disabilities, can view microaggressions as harmless "misunderstandings." Often, clients are viewed as being too sensitive. If this were to occur, inappropriate treatment goals can be created. For instance, a therapist could discuss the development of coping skills for these "instances" when they present in the future (Gushue & Constantine, 2007).

In an effort to avoid microaggressions and generate suitable treatment goals for our clients, we must first become aware of our emotions, biases, prejudices, attitudes, and behaviors for the privileged and for the oppressed. In the previous chapters, race and ethnicity were the foci of discussion. Before moving on to examine specific populations and the implications for substance abuse and treatment methodology, the privileges for other dominant groups will be briefly explored. The author will concentrate on three areas of discrimination: (1) sexism; (2) heterosexism; and (3) classism. There are chapters devoted to women, the LGBT population, and the economically disadvantaged; however, for the purposes of self-exploration and awareness, this author wishes to take a moment and address these concepts before proceeding.

SEXISM

Females in our society have been historically disadvantaged by being underpaid and undervalued, and they live in a place that "distorts a woman's personality, limits her potential, and threatens her physical and psychological well-being" (Berg, 2006, p. 970). Like other marginalized groups, women can experience oppression on an individual and systemic level. **Sexism** has been defined as "any attitude, action, or institutional structure which subordinates, restricts, or discriminates against a person or group because of their sex, gender role, or sexual preference" (O'Neil, 1980, p. 62). As discussed previously about racist events, women also frequently experience overt and covert acts of sexism on a daily basis. In fact, Berg (2006) surveyed 382 women and found 100 percent of the sample experienced some form of sexism in the past year. More specifically, in a lifetime, the women reported hearing sexist jokes (98 percent), being sexually harassed (94 percent), and experiencing sexism by employers (87 percent).

Forms of sexism can vary from hostile to subtle, including aggression, intimidation, objectification, stereotyping, harassment, and exclusion. For example, sexism is present in our everyday language and can differ in nature. An instance of **hostile sexism** is when a man calls a woman an "aggressive bitch" (Bosson,

Pinel, & Vanello, 2010). Bosson et al. (2010) also report that there are acts of **benevolent sexism**, such as when a man calls a woman a "sweet girl." How is this statement considered sexist?

Not only is sexism entrenched in our spoken jargon and vernacular, but it is also in writing; quite blatantly, at times. How often have we walked by or driven past a sign warning us that there are "Men at Work" and never thought twice about this microaggression? Over 20 years ago, a counselor educator took note of these written offenses and published an article called *He/She/They/It?: Implied Sexism in Speech and Print* (Wilcoxon, 1989). This author explored the sexist language in our society and the implications for counselors and their clients. For instance, instead of using words like "mankind, manmade, and manpower," we should say "humankind, manufactured/synthetic, and human power/muscle power." In addition, gender symmetry should be employed when appropriate (e.g., layperson, spokesperson, chairperson, and salesperson). Counselors must also be aware of implied sexism when talking to clients. How would the following statement be sexist to a female client? "Oh, wow, so as a working mother, you have a lot to handle …" Moreover, think of how we use the terms "feminine" and "womanly" versus "masculine" and "manly." What connotations do these words have, and how do we tend to use them in our conversations, media, etc.? Wilcoxon addressed these concerns over 20 years ago, so our assumption is sexist language has decreased. As a society, we have been more cognizant of the insidious nature of sexism. In your opinion, what is the current state of sexism in the United States?

The "masculine mystique" has contributed to the perpetuation of sexism in America and negatively affects both genders (O'Neil, 1980). This value system is based on rigid stereotypes related to masculinity and femininity. The following are some examples of the underlying assumptions of masculinity in our society:

- Men are biologically superior to women; therefore, men have a greater human potential than women.
- Masculinity (versus femininity) is the more valued form of gender identity.
- Expressing vulnerability and emotions are signs of femininity and should be avoided by men, especially in the presence of other men. Also known as restrictive emotionality.
- Interpersonal communication showing emotion indicates weakness and a lack of control.
- Men's work and career success are measures of masculinity (and self-worth), as women's caretaking of the home and children are measures of femininity.
- Women are not fulfilled without children, and they innately know more about children than men (O'Neil, 1980, p. 76).

This socialization process causes the internalization of sexism by both men and women. For instance, the ideology that women are to dominated, protected, and subordinated is supported by the assumptions outlined above, and both sexes have internalized this ideology. The daily injustices and inequities between the sexes can be considered "insidious traumas" (Berg, 2006, p. 971) and have negative effects on a woman's quality of life. Women can experience psychological distress, disordered eating, lowered self-esteem, anger, and feelings of powerlessness, and display symptoms of post-traumatic stress, depression, and anxiety (Moradi & Funderburk, 2006; Zucker & Landry, 2007). Sexism is correlated with the desire to escape these negative effects via chemical substances (Bright, Osborne, & Greif, 2011). The prevalence of substance use and gender differences is well documented and researched. Extreme acts of sexism such as sexual abuse and domestic violence are strongly tied to substance misuse. Later in the text, the issues facing women in substance abuse treatment, such as sexual trauma, domestic violence, mental health concerns, and relationship status will be discussed in more detail.

Reflection Exercise

Males have benefits and advantages due to their gender. Reflect on the following statements and decide if they are accurate assertions.

1. Men automatically have more opportunities than women in employment and education.
2. Men are at an advantage because they hold most of the positions of power in society.
3. Men must be willing to give up their privileged status in order for men and women to be truly equal.
4. Laws that protect women from discrimination in employment and education are no longer needed.
5. Affirmative action policies require employers to hire unqualified women over qualified men.
6. Women have to learn they are entitled to no special consideration and must make it strictly on merit (adapted from Case, 2007).

HETEROSEXISM

Heterosexuality is not only defined by sexual activity (Sue & Sue, 2013). For the purposes of this text, heterosexuals (or "straight" people) are classified as those having affectional and sexual attraction to only the opposite sex. Heterosexuals have the comforts of not being excluded from the norm. The privileged status of heterosexuality in our society allows countless advantages to straight individuals. For instance, heterosexuals have the "right" to marry and adopt children, gain tax and insurance benefits, and obtain assets and protection in regard to military service, inheritance, hospital visitations, etc. (Gonsiorek, 1991; Rocco & Gallagher, 2006; Simoni & Walters, 2001). Moreover, using the terms "husband," "wife," "boyfriend," and "girlfriend"—without a second thought—is an aspect of privilege, as most people do not consider the term "partner" to be all-inclusive. To illustrate the numerous "straight privileges" that exist in the United States, a list is delineated below.

As a straight person …

- If I pick up a magazine, watch TV, or play music, I can be certain my sexual orientation will be represented.
- I do not have to fear that if my family or friends find out about my sexual orientation there will be economic, emotional, physical, or psychological consequences.
- I am not accused of being abused, warped, or psychologically confused because of my sexual orientation.
- I can go home from most meetings, classes, and conversations without feeling excluded, fearful, attacked, isolated, outnumbered, unheard, held at a distance, stereotyped, or feared because of my sexual orientation.
- I am never asked to speak for everyone who is heterosexual.
- People don't ask why I chose to be heterosexual.
- I don't have to defend my heterosexuality.
- I can easily find a religious community that will not exclude me for being heterosexual.

- I can count on finding a therapist or doctor willing and able to talk about my sexuality.
- My masculinity/femininity is not challenged because of my sexual orientation.
- I am not identified by my sexual orientation.
- I can walk in public with my significant other and not have people do a double-take or stare.
- I'm not grouped because of my sexual orientation.
- People can use terms that describe my sexual orientation and mean positive things (e.g., "straight as an arrow," "standing up straight" or "straightened out") instead of demeaning terms (i.e., "eww, that's gay," or being "queer").
- I am considered "normal." (Adapted from Earlham College, n.d.)

Unfortunately, many heterosexual people do not recognize how sexual orientation status comes into play in their own lives, the lives of others who are lesbian, gay, bisexual, or transgender (LGBT), and the systems and institutions of our society. This lack of awareness may not be only ignorance to heterosexual privilege, but heterosexuals can also be in denial of their own **homophobia**. Homophobia is considered the fear, hatred, and prejudice at an individual level. As a result, persons in the LGBT community are subject to microaggressions quite frequently by well-intentioned heterosexuals. Thus, counselors are urged to explore heterosexism and the implications for therapy.

Heterosexism involves (1) homophobia; and (2) the cultural and institutional levels of oppression (i.e., denial of rights and privileges on a social level). This type of oppression results from considering heterosexuality as the norm and superior to other sexual orientations (Simoni & Walters, 2001). Heterosexist attitudes have been shown to correspond with sexual identity development. In addition to developing a racial identity, people also develop an identity related to their sexual orientation. Researchers have shown heterosexuals transition through statuses similar to the White Racial Identity Model (Helms, 2008), and the lower the status, the more likely heterosexuals are to hold negative stereotypes/attitudes (Simoni & Walters, 2001). Moreover, these heterosexist stereotypes/attitudes are held by men more frequently than women (Davies, 2004). Why would you think this may be the case?

Due to heterosexism, LGBT people face discrimination and are marginalized in our society. The prejudice, harassment, rejection, hatred, and threats of violence against sexual minorities influence psychological health and well-being (Szymanski, 2005). For instance, if LGBT individuals internalize the stigmas and negative attitudes/assumptions about homosexuality (i.e., **internalized heterosexism**), then feelings ranging from self-doubt to self-hatred can result (Szymanski, West, & Meyer, 2008). In an effort to increase the quality of life for this population, continued research is recommended. More specifically, investigators can focus on the availability and impact of community, family, and social supports; LGBT and heterosexual identity development; and the coping strategies employed by LGBT people. Later in the text, these aspects will be addressed and information provided regarding the substance use, misuse, and dependency among individuals who identify as LGBT.

Reflection Exercises

1. What is your level of exposure, interaction, and comfort with the LGBT population?
2. Do you think the prevalence of substance use would differ between people who identify as LGBT and heterosexuals? Why or why not? Do you think there are any differences in the use of certain substances between the two groups?

3. What therapeutic considerations do you think counselors need to be aware of when treating the LGBT population? As a group, there are similarities; however, what would be the different considerations when treating lesbian women, gay men, bisexual women, bisexual men, etc.?

CLASSISM

Researchers are not necessarily in agreement on the definition of social class, and they indicate it is a difficult concept to understand. However, class is becoming more prominent in the counseling literature related to diversity and social justice issues (Pincus & Sokoloff, 2008). For the purposes of this text, the author uses the phrase *working class* in lieu of *lower class*. Before addressing the marginalization and oppression of people based on class, the author suggests completing the exercise below.

Exercise

Take a moment and answer the following questions:
1. How would you define the "middle-class" population?
2. What are five indicators used to define class in our society (e.g., income)?
3. What three words or phrases are used for those of working-class status?
4. As a child, which class status was your family? How about your class status currently? What criteria were used?

Defining working, middle, and upper class can be difficult; however, we all probably agree that status, power, and access to resources vary depending on class categorization. How did you define middle class? Some people may self-identify as middle class when they make $25,000, and some may self-identify as middle class when they make $100,000. Income can be one way to identify social class status, but other criteria may also include education level, occupation, where one lives, etc. To illustrate this point, do you have the same thoughts and attitudes toward every person who makes $50,000 (e.g., a factory worker,

Table 3.2: Indicators of Class

Income (Personal or Parents')	Resource Capital
Inherited or Earned Wealth	Cohort and Peer Groups
Employed or Unemployed	Home or Car Ownership
Occupation (Personal or Parents')	Lifestyle
Prestige of Occupation (Personal or Parents')	Having Insurance or Medicaid Political Power
Education (Location and Level)	Marital Status
Residence Location (Neighborhood, City, or State)	Clothing Language, Accent, Vernacular
Vacation (Ability to take it, and where)	Eating Habits (What kind, and where)

Adapted from Helms (2008) and Lott (2012)

middle school teacher, or police officer)? What about if the person is married to a doctor? What if the person has a high school education versus a master's degree?

Socioeconomic status is often used interchangeably with class; there are many words, phrases, or indicators associated with this concept. In fact, researchers found over 400 terms that people use to convey social class (Liu, Ali, et al., 2004). What five indicators did you think of for question 2 above? Are any of your indicators listed in Table 3.2? This author will use the definitions proposed by Helms (2008), which designate class as a *person's subjective evaluation of one's resources* (i.e., self-identification) and socioeconomic status (SES) as class assignment or *how the person is ranked by indicators chosen by our society* (e.g., income, occupation, and education).

The worldview and life experiences may vary by class. Based on the economic culture in which one lives, there tends to be a worldview on aspects of social connections, cultural tastes, etiquette, lifestyles, and relationships with property (Liu & Arguello, 2006). The environment shapes our views on **human capital** (e.g., education, occupation, physical attributes, and interpersonal skills), **social capital** (e.g., peers and professional networks), and **cultural capital** (e.g., leisure time, traveling) (Liu, Soleck, Hopps, Dunston, & Pickett, 2004). Liu et al. (2004) suggest some forms of human, social, and cultural capitals are more valued, encouraged, and used. For those in the middle class, leisure time allows for exercise, vacation, hobbies, and attending to the interests of their children and is an expected part of the middle-class lifestyle (Lott, 2012). Leisure time, however, is considered a privilege by many. Worldview and life experiences, based on these forms of capital, influence one's vernacular. For example, the term *winter* has been used as a verb by wealthy college students who spend vacations in other countries (Lott, 2012).

Through socialization, a person's perceptions, thoughts, beliefs, attitudes, and stereotypes of others are learned. These positive and negative thoughts, beliefs, etc. are related to people *within* one's class and those considered *outside* of one's class. The social devaluation, prejudice, and discrimination associated with class are aspects of **classism**. In question 3, you were asked to identify three words or phrases used to describe those of working class status. You may have indicated "blue collar" or "less educated." Some other more derogatory, classist terms you may have heard include "white trash," "trailer trash," "hillbilly," "welfare recipients," or "Wal-Mart shoppers." Attributes are commonly associated with those in the working class such as being lazy, irresponsible, unattractive, overweight, of poor hygiene, inarticulate, unlawful, untrustworthy, or impolite (Liu, et al., 2004; Lott, 2012; Moss, 2003; Smith, 2008). As far as substance use, one may hold the (inaccurate) belief that it is more prevalent among people who have certain education levels, attire, location of residences, or occupations. Remember the myth of meritocracy? This holds true not only for race, but for class. In America, all men and women are created equal and have the same opportunity for social class mobility. If one works hard, the expectation is that prosperity will follow. Unfortunately, we know that our school, criminal justice, and health care systems are not set up for everyone to succeed with equivalent efforts (Reiman & Leighton, 2010). On the other hand, not all worldviews stress upward mobility, individualism, material acquisition, and industriousness (Liu et al., 2004). Therefore, negative attitudes toward those who do not hold that same worldview can result. This type of classism is called **downward classism** and occurs when prejudice and discriminatory behavior is directed at those who are perceived as "below" the person (Liu et al., 2004). Downward classism is the type of oppression that most people think of regarding class. However, there are three other identified types of classism. **Upward classism** is when people who are perceived as higher class are referred to as "snobs" or "elitists," and they are not considered warm, friendly people. **Lateral classism** is referred to as a "keeping up with the Joneses" mentality and when people of the same class attempt to maintain the lifestyle of that specific economic status. A person feels pressured to continue to dress a certain way, accumulate material possessions, and participate in certain leisure activities in order to not be discriminated against or marginalized by others in their social cohort. Lastly, **internalized classism** is the internal conflict a person experiences that comes from the inability to meet the demands of one's economic culture and may result in feelings of depression, anxiety, frustration, and feelings of failure (Liu et al., 2004).

In summary, classism is not an isolated phenomenon; the intersections between race, sex, sexual orientation, age, ability, etc., must all be taken into account. Microaggressions occur without intention by the perpetrator, but can harm the recipient's psychological well-being. Starting with the next chapter, a specific population will be presented. The author encourages the reader to consider these complex intersections and how these have implications for counseling. In each chapter, the reader will be presented with an overview of statistics and definitions; substance abuse issues, such as etiology, risk factors, stigmas, and barriers to treatment; the utility of screening/assessment tools with the certain population; resiliency factors; and recommendations for treatment and therapeutic considerations. After all the populations are discussed, the author will conclude with a chapter that addresses social justice and multicultural competency concerns.

REFERENCES

Berg, S. H. (2006). Everyday sexism and post-traumatic stress disorder in women: A correlational survey. *Violence Against Women, 12*, 970–988.

Bosson, J. K., Pinel, E. C., & Vandello, J. A. (2010). The emotional impact of ambivalent sexism: Forecasts versus real experiences. *Sex Roles, 62*, 520–531.

Bright, C. L., Osborne, V. A., & Greif, G. L. (2011). One dozen considerations when working with women in substance abuse groups. *Journal of Psychoactive Drugs, 43*, 64–68.

Case, K. A. (2007). Raising male privilege awareness and reducing sexism: An evaluation of diversity courses. *Psychology of Women Quarterly, 31*, 426–435.

Davies, M. (2004). Correlates of negative attitudes toward gay men: Sexism, male role norms, and male sexuality. *Journal of Sex Research, 41*, 259–266.

Earlham College (n.d.). Daily effects of straight privilege. Retrieved from http://www.cs.earlham.edu/~hyrax/personal/files/student_res/straightprivilege.htm

Gonsiorek, J. C. (1991). The empirical basis for the demise of the illness model of homosexuality. In J. C. Gonsiorek & J. D. Weinrich (Eds.), *Homosexuality: Research implications for public policy* (pp. 115–136). Newbury Park, CA: Sage.

Harrell, S. P. (2000). A multidimensional conceptualization of racism-related stress: Implications for the well-being of people of color. *American Journal of Orthopsychiatry, 70*, 42–57.

Helms, J. E. (2008). *Race is a nice thing to have: A guide to being a white person or understanding the white persons in your life*. Alexandria, VA: Microtraining Associates.

King, C. R., & Springwood, C. F. (2001). *Team Spirits: The Native American Mascots Controversy*. Lincoln: University of Nebraska Press.

LeBlanc, R. G. (1997). Definitions of oppression. *Nursing Inquiry, 4*, 257–261.

Liu, W. M., & Arguello, J. L. (2006). Using social class and classism in counseling. *Counseling and Human Development, 29*(3), 1–10.

Liu, W. M., Ali, S. R., Soleck, G., Hopps, J., Dunston, K., & Pickett, T. (2004). Using social class in counseling psychology research. *Journal of Counseling Psychology, 51*, 3–18.

Liu, W. M., Soleck, G., Hopps, J., Dunston, K., & Pickett, T. (2004). A new framework to understand social class in counseling: The social class worldview model and modern classism theory. *Journal of Multicultural Counseling and Development, 32*(2), 95–122.

MacDonald, M., & Wright, N. E. (2002). Cigarette smoking and the disenfranchisement of adolescent girls: A discourse of resistance? *Health Care for Women International, 23*, 281–305.

McIntosh, P. (1995). White privilege and male privilege: A personal account of coming to see correspondences through work in women's studies. In M. L. Andersen & P. H. Collins (Eds.), *Race, class, and gender: An anthology* (2nd ed., pp. 76–87). Belmont, CA: Wadsworth.

Moradi, B., & Funderburk, J. R. (2006). Roles of perceived sexist events and perceived social support in the mental health of women seeking counseling. *Journal of Counseling Psychology, 53*, 464–473.

Moss, K. (2003). *The color of class: Poor whites and the paradox of privilege.* Philadelphia: University of Pennsylvania Press.

O'Neil, J. M. (1980). Male sex role conflicts, sexism, and masculinity: Psychological implications for men, women, and the counseling psychologist. *Counseling Psychologist, 9*(2), 61–80.

Reiman, J., & Leighton, P. (2010). *The rich get richer and the poor get prison: Ideology, class, and criminal justice* (9th ed.). Boston: Allyn & Bacon.

Rocco, T. S., & Gallagher, S. J. (2006). Straight privilege and moral/izing: Issues in career development. *New Directions for Adult and Continuing Education, 112*, 29–39.

Simoni, J. M., & Walters, K. L. (2001). Heterosexual identity and heterosexism: Recognizing privilege to reduce prejudice. *Journal of Homosexuality, 41*, 157–172.

Smith, L. (2008). Positioning classism within counseling psychology's social justice agenda. *Counseling Psychologist, 36*, 895–924.

Sue, D. W. (2010). *Microaggressions in everyday life: Race, gender and sexual orientation.* Hoboken, NJ: John Wiley & Sons.

Sue, D. W., & Sue, D. D. (2013). *Counseling the culturally diverse: Theory and practice* (6th ed.). New York: John Wiley & Sons.

Sue, D. W., Capodilupo, C. M., Torino, G. C., Bucceri, J. M., Holder, A. M., Nadal, K. L., & Esquilin, M. (2007). Racial microaggressions in everyday life: Implications for clinical practice. *American Psychologist, 62*(4), p. 278.

Szymanski, D. M. (2005). Heterosexism and sexism as correlates of psychological distress in lesbians. *Journal of Counseling and Development, 83*, 355–360.

Szymanski, D. M., Kashubeck-West, S., & Meyer, J. (2008). Internalized heterosexism: A historical and theoretical overview. *Counseling Psychologist, 36*, 510–524.

Wilcoxon, S. A. (1989). He/she/they/it?: Implied sexism in speech and print. *Journal of Counseling and Development, 68*, 114–116.

Zucker, A. N., & Landry, L. J. (2007). Embodied discrimination: The relation of sexism and distress to women's drinking and smoking behaviors. *Sex Roles, 56*, 193–203.

CHAPTER 4

BLACK/AFRICAN AMERICANS

By Bianca T. L. Fetherson

According to the 2012 United States (U.S.) Census Bureau, 13.1 percent of the American population identified as black or African American. Blacks or African Americans are people having origins in any of the black racial groups of Africa (U.S. Census Bureau, 2012). This includes cultural groups (e.g., Africans, African Americans, Afro-Caribbean, and Hispanic blacks) that vary in language, customs, and acculturation. In spite of their variation, these individuals are often perceived as monolithic and incessantly recognized as nothing more than a racial group (Howard, 2003). Case in point—the terms *colored*, *Negro*, *black*, *Afro-American*, and *African American* have all been used to racially categorize individuals with African ancestry. These racial terms are used consistently and interchangeably in our society, thus generalizing those of African descent without considering their cultural identity. This generalization can be damaging to their psychological well-being (Britt, 2004). The term "black/African American" is much more befitting to recognize the sociocultural aspects of this population, as well as the within and the between group heterogeneity that exists. Therefore, this author will use the term black/African American throughout the chapter as a way to not racialize those with African ancestries and in an attempt to include all cultural groups within this population.

Repeated exposure to racism and discrimination has been linked to anxiety, depression, and substance use disorders in black/African Americans (Pierre & Mahalik, 2005). Hence, this chapter is very much focused on highlighting and addressing the psycho-socioeconomic aspects of substance use–related problems in the black/African American population. To begin, an overview of this population is presented in the next section, including incarceration rates and substance use trends and patterns.

STATISTICS

Among the black/African American population, there are more males born than females. However, black/African American females outnumber males by the time they reach 15 to 29 years old, partly due to homicide, suicide, and substance abuse (Baker & Bell, 1999; U.S. Census Bureau, 2011). In fact, black/African American males are more prone to be victims of a violent crime than any other racial group (Toldson, 2012).

Still, black/African American males are incarcerated at a rate that is seven times the rate of their white male counterparts (Allen, 2013; Mukku, Benson, Alam, Richie, & Bailey, 2012; Toldson, 2012). Black/African American women are also eight times more likely than white women to be in prison (Vassall-Fall, 2003). One study investigated the health aspects of black/African American female inmates and found that three percent reported testing positive for HIV; nearly all of them previously used illicit drugs and had a history of physical and/or sexual abuse (Roberts & Carlton-LaNey, 2000, Substance Abuse and Mental Health Services Administration [SAMHSA], 2005). Incarceration rates have also been examined over the years and the increase of black/African Americans behind bars is staggering. In fact, the incarceration rates among black/African Americans exploded by 500 percent between 1986 and 2004. Black/African Americans are disproportionately represented in drug arrests and prison sentences nationwide (Allen, 2013; Costen, 2009). For example, of the 225,242 individuals serving time in state prisons for drug-related offenses in 2011, black/African American males made up 45 percent, whereas white males comprised just 30 percent (Knafo, 2013). Even more, black/African Americans without any previous history of a substance use disorder have a higher risk of using and developing a substance use disorder once they leave the prison system (Mukku et al., 2012).

Researchers have investigated substance use rates among adolescents ages 12 to 17 and found black/African American adolescents have lower rates of use as compared with their peers. For instance, black/African American youth had lower rates of cigarette use (5.8 versus 10.2 percent), alcohol use (10.5 versus 16.0 percent), marijuana use (6.5 versus 6.9 percent), and nonmedical use of prescription drugs (2.9 versus 3.3 percent) (National Survey on Drug Use and Health, 2012). Despite black/African American adolescents abstaining from alcohol and other drugs at higher rates than the national average, approximately 8.9 percent of black/African American individuals aged 12 or older (22.2 million) were classified with having a substance use disorder in the past year (National Survey on Drug Use and Health, 2012). Moreover, SAMHSA reported about 21 percent of the 1.8 million admissions to publicly funded substance abuse treatment programs were by black/African Americans (National Institute on Drug Abuse, 2011).

ETIOLOGY AND PREDICTORS OF SUBSTANCE USE-RELATED PROBLEMS IN BLACK/AFRICAN AMERICANS

Racism is fashioned in the social trends, dynamics, and echelons of dominance in a society that produce intended and foreseen effects on individuals without power (Domhoff, 2009). Substance use has been found to be linked with the effects of racism. For example, black/African Americans have reported alcohol, tobacco, and continuous marijuana and crack-cocaine use as a way to cope with the manifestations of race-related stress (Gibbons et al., 2010; Martin, Tuch, & Roman, 2003). Yet, there are countless black/African Americans who do not succumb to alcohol and/or other drug use to deal with the consequent emotional and psychological traumas of racism. With that being said, substance use trends and patterns differ greatly across black/African Americans, mainly because of access, means, and function.

Access

The pattern of substance use and the subsequent issues among black/African Americans are highly associated with the availability and accessibility of alcohol and other drugs in their immediate environment. LaVeist and Wallace (2000) at Johns Hopkins School of Public Health determined that black/African American low-income neighborhoods were eight times more likely to have liquor stores than white or racially integrated neighborhoods. Similarly, the availability of illicit drugs is far greater in low-income urban black/African American communities compared to (a) low- and higher-income predominantly white areas; and (b) higher-income areas of other black/African Americans (Romley, Cohen, Ringel, & Strum, 2007).

The creation and maintenance of inner-city neighborhoods through racial segregation ensure the availability of drugs by transforming neighborhoods into physically deteriorated areas. These areas tend to have higher rates of poverty, unemployment, and single-female-headed households (Ludwig et al., 2012; Massey, 1990). The stress from living in inner-city neighborhoods remains positively linked to the underpinnings of substance use-related problems in the black/African American community (Britt, 2004). As one black/African American, thirty-something female stated, "How am I supposed to maintain sobriety when the dope man is next door and the liquor store is around the corner. I can't just move, my minimum wage job doesn't pay enough to live anywhere else."

Means

The majority of white America believes that if black/African Americans just work hard and stop living in the past and playing the race card, then they, too, can live the American dream (Bonilla-Silva, 2003). If this were so, then the economic plight faced by many black/African Americans would have improved after the demise of legal segregation. Even with the considerable gains from the civil rights movements and subsequent first U.S. black/African American president, there has been very little improvement in the economic situation of black/African Americans (Harris, 2010). The Pew Economic Mobility Project revealed a great number of middle-class black/African American children have grown up to be worse off economically than their parents (Austin, 2009). In fact, 10.7 million black/African Americans lived below the poverty line in 2010 (U.S. Bureau of the Census, Income, Poverty, and Health Insurance Coverage in the United States, 2010). The unemployment rates of black/African American adults 25 years of age and older is usually twice that of their white counterparts (Harris, 2010). Moreover, the median income for employed black/African Americans continues to be 55 percent that of whites. Investigations were done which examined the opportunities for employment among black/African Americans and found inequities in these opportunities. For instance, researchers have shown blacks/African Americans can possess the same education, qualifications, experience, and interviewing styles as a white applicant—and the white applicant is much more likely to be offered the job (Austin, 2009).

Due to the scarce job opportunities, meager education, poverty, illiteracy, increased access to drugs, and the stressors of the urban lifestyle experienced by the black/African American community, the risk of substance use is higher (Britt, 2004). There is very little research on the substance use–related problems for black/African Americans who have attained educational and economic wealth. However, multiple population-based and epidemiological studies have identified specific stressors and individual-level variables that are predictive of substance use and abuse among black/African Americans (Mays, Cochran, & Barnes, 2007; Minior, Galea, Stuber, Ahern, & Ompad, 2003; Sinha, 2008). When the lack of income is no longer a mediating factor in black/African Americans' alcohol and drug use, pervasive racism and perceived discrimination continues to be. Regardless of their educational and economic background, black/African Americans endure countless everyday stressors and chronic strains that are unique to their racial group membership (Settles, 2006). Over and over again, the stress from race-based discrimination outweighed levels of income as a risk factor in the development of addiction and in addiction relapse vulnerability for black/African Americans (Gibbons et al., 2010; Sinha, 2008).

Function

The use of alcohol and other drugs can function as a form of escapism and as a coping mechanism for many black/African Americans. For instance, one black/African American 23-year-old male described using marijuana to deal with the stress of not finding a job and as a way to "calm my anxiety" about not being able to provide for his wife and daughter. As told by another 55-year-old black/African American man,

> I drank every day for years to deal with the pressure of being the only Black manager. I felt like I was on display, that my every move was watched and somehow if I failed that would prove the white man right; that Blacks can't be leaders.

Substance use can be circular in nature. More specifically, alcohol and other drug use can impact how one functions at home, work, school, etc. This impairment in functioning can contribute to the continued use of substances and the development of substance use disorders. However, many people can continue to use without severe impairment in their quality of life or they may not acknowledge how dysfunctional their lives have become. A 48-year-old black/African American male explains his denial of having a problem with cocaine use by stating,

> I didn't look like the typical crackhead, skinny, strung out, and feening. I had a job, a great job, I went to work every day. I took care of my responsibilities. It wasn't until I had a heart attack and needed a pacemaker and a fibrillator that I realized my use was a drug problem.

Black/African Americans may also use alcohol and other drugs to cope with the agony of self-stigma. *Self-stigma* is an underreported condition in which individuals internalize and agree with the social myths, prejudices, and stereotypes about themselves and whatever social group they belong to (Health, 2010; Lucoma, Kohlenberg, Hayes, Bunting, & Rye, 2008). Self-stigma involves three steps: (1) awareness of the stereotype; (2) agreement with it; and (3) applying it to oneself (Corrigan, Larson, & Rüsch, 2009). Self-stigma in the black/African American population lingers from slavery and is a resultant of the "lie of Black inferiority" (Arid, 2008). The "lie of Black inferiority" boldly asserts that black/African American people are not as beautiful, valuable, intelligent, or capable as any other people, in particular white people (Aird, 2008). Self-stigma among black/African Americans is displayed in the media (e.g., the highly aggressive, sexual black/African American male savage or the angry, hard-to-tame black/African American female), in the Eurocentric standards of beauty (e.g., anything that is white is good and beautiful, while anything, including hair, that is black/African American or black-like is bad and detestable), in education (e.g., the overwhelming numbers of black/African American boys in remedial or special education classes), and in politics (e.g., the persistent discrimination and suppression of black/African American voters) (Aird, 2008; Gilchrist & Jackson, 2012; Horsey, 2013; Reese, 2013). As a result, black/African Americans experience a diminished self-worth and self-efficacy, a lower quality of life, and are dissuaded from pursuing the kinds of opportunities that are fundamental to achieving life goals (Luoma et al., 2008). When enacted, self-stigma remains as an effectual tool in black/African Americans developing an inferiority complex that fosters self-hatred and maladaptive behaviors like substance abuse (Aird, 2008; Bonilla-Silva, 2003; Burrell, 2010).

RESILIENCY, BLACK/AFRICAN AMERICANS, AND RECOVERY

Black/African Americans suffering from racial battle fatigue are more likely to use alcohol and other drugs to deal with chronic exposure to discrimination and oppression. Racial battle fatigue results from the psychological, physiological, emotional, and cultural responses to repeated incidents of racism and being in constant contact with racially hostile environments (Smith, Allen, & Danley, 2007). Nevertheless, black/African Americans have consistently proven to be tenacious and resilient. In order to buffer racial battle fatigue, many have developed a cultural reality and worldview grounded in: (a) a strong religious belief system; (b) a collective social orientation; (c) strong family/kinship bonds; (d) communalism; (e) psychological flexibility; (f) affective expressiveness; and (g) a present-time orientation (Utsey, Hook, Fischer, & Belvet, 2008).

There is a variety of spiritual and religious beliefs (e.g., Christianity, Islam, Buddhism) that black/African Americans employ to prevail over racism and race-related stress to experience a healthy quality of life (Brown, 2008). Additionally, strong family/kinship bonds aid their adaptability, alleviate maladaptive coping, and increase their chances for well-being (Utsey, Bolden, Lanier, & Williams, 2007). Through strong kinship bonds, black/African Americans who are able to develop a positive self-concept learn self-efficacy and refute self-stigma. Furthermore, black/African Americans who flexibly and resourcefully adapt to internal and external stressors are likely to be shielded from the effects of race-related stress. Black/African Americans who possess self-awareness, openness, and have the capacity to maintain an optimistic attitude diminish their risk and vulnerability to developing substance-related problems (Brown, 2008; Utsey et al., 2008; Watkins, 2012). Plus, black/African Americans with a present-time orientation tend to accept what is out of their control (e.g., the disease of addiction) and commit to actions that improve and enrich their lives (e.g., accessing substance abuse treatment). Resiliency in black/African Americans gives them the wherewithal to conquer all types of challenges such as racism, discrimination, traumas, and substance abuse–related issues and spring forward stronger, wiser, and empowered.

BARRIERS TO BLACK/AFRICAN AMERICANS SEEKING AND RECEIVING TREATMENT

Although resiliency factors are core to the survival of black/African Americans, they can also serve as a hindrance in their willingness to seek and/or participate in substance abuse treatment services. For example, plenty of black/African Americans believe: (a) prayer alone can heal their addiction; (b) family concerns should be resolved within the family; (c) suffering is the plight of black/African American life; and therefore (d) seeking treatment and asking for help is a sign of weakness (Lim, 2008; Thompson, Bazile, & Akbar, 2004). With the lack of knowledge regarding addiction, it is rather difficult for some black/African Americans to discern when their use is a problem that requires professional help. Therefore, many black/African Americans with substance use disorders are unsuspecting and think they do not have a diagnosable illness. Besides, a great deal of black/African Americans may be even less aware that applicable psychological treatments exist for their specific addiction problem (Williams, 2011).

For those black/African Americans who realize the benefit of treatment, there is still a concern whether substance abuse counselors possess enough knowledge to accept and understand them. Often, they fear they will be misdiagnosed, labeled, and brainwashed (Brown, 2008; Thompson et al., 2004; Williams, 2011, 2013). This mistrust is historically and culturally rooted in slavery and has been strongly associated with the help-seeking attitudes and treatment retention among black/African Americans with substance use disorders. As a result of the historical experiences and contemporary social injustices, quite a few black/African Americans have tremendous difficulty accessing and completing treatment (Madison-Colmore & Moore, 2002). Most black/African Americans avoid substance abuse services altogether, fearing racist and discriminatory treatment. Several experts in the substance abuse field have attributed the underutilization of outpatient and residential treatment services and the premature termination from therapy by black/African Americans to cultural insensitivity and multicultural incompetency of the counselor and the substance abuse program (Barber et al., 2001; Campbell, Weisner, & Sterling, 2006; Castro & Garfinkle, 2003; Dais & Ancis, 2012).

AFROCENTRIC ACCEPTANCE AND COMMITMENT THERAPY (AACT): A CULTURALLY RESPONSIVE SUBSTANCE ABUSE TREATMENT FOR BLACK/AFRICAN AMERICANS

Historically, substance abuse treatment programs hardly recognized cultural variables as possible determinants of substance use and/or as essential components of these programs (Castro & Alarcón, 2002). Nonetheless, cultural factors are expected to impact countless aspects of the substance abuse treatment process (Dais & Ancis, 2012). Thus, substance abuse counselors must attend to cultural factors by using therapeutic approaches that take cultural variables into consideration. Acceptance and Commitment Therapy (ACT) is one model that can be adapted in an effort to conceptualize the lived experiences of black/African Americans. ACT is comprised of the following principles: (a) acceptance; (b) contact with the present moment; (c) observing the self; (d) values; and (e) committed action (Hayes & Smith, 2005). This author proposes a theoretical substance abuse treatment model which embeds the ACT principles into an Afrocentric worldview. This model is called Afrocentric Acceptance and Commitment Therapy (AACT) and can be used with black/African Americans with substance use disorders.

Key Concepts of the AACT Model

In this section, four philosophical underpinnings of AACT will be addressed. First, AACT acknowledges and accepts that racism and discrimination are real lived experiences rooted in history (e.g., slavery) and manifested constantly through social contexts (e.g., education, employment, and housing). Second, AACT posits repeated exposure to racism, oppression, and discrimination impedes valued living. Also, the adverse effects that result from repeated exposure are catalysts to maladaptive behaviors like alcohol and drug use. Third, the self-efficacy of black/African Americans is said to be learned. For example, social situations can influence Black/African Americans' beliefs about their capabilities to perform and be successful. Self-efficacy is also enacted and regulated by contextual features of the situation. One example of a contextual feature that would impact self-efficacy is the cultural insensitivity displayed in a substance abuse treatment program. As a result of this insensitivity, the black/African American client's capacity for recovery is negatively influenced. Last, AACT suggests black/African Americans' self-determination: (a) aids in their ability to

AACT Understanding of Racism

Racism and discrimination are ongoing dynamic actions rooted in historically and situationally defined social contexts. Repeated exposure impedes valued living, and consequent adverse effects are catalysts to maladaptive behaviors such as alcohol and other drug use.

AACT Conceptualization of Black/African Americans' Self-Efficacy

The self-efficacy of black/African Americans is *learned*, *enacted*, and *regulated* by contextual features of a situation, which can foster self-acceptance or self-stigma.

AACT Theory on Recovery for Black/African Americans

The self-determination of black/African Americans aids in their ability to clarify personal values and to take action on them, brings more vitality and meaning to their lives, increases their psychological flexibility, and empowers their capacity for recovery.

Figure 4.1: AACT Model's Conceptualization of Substance Use-Related Issues in the Black/African American Community (Hayes & Smith, 2005; Lumoa et al., 2008)

clarify personal values and to take action on them; (b) brings more vitality and meaning to their lives; (c) increases their psychological flexibility; and finally (d) empowers their capacity for recovery.

AACT proposes that the aforementioned processes are interconnected and very much active at each phase of the recovery process (i.e., use, sobriety, relapse prevention) for black/African Americans. Refer to Figure 4.1 for an illustration of how AACT understands the connection between racism and substance use.

AACT Interventions

AACT denotes the following attitudes, thoughts, and interventions as being culturally responsive to the treatment needs of black/African Americans with substance use disorders:

- An approach that is genuine and open, expresses empathy, and seeks clarification allows black/African American clients to tell their story, hold on to their dignity while asking for help, and be the experts on their problems and necessary solutions.
- Acknowledge multiple aspects of black/African American clients' cultural identity (e.g., gender, sexuality).
- When working with black/African American clients, avoid generalizations and stereotypes (e.g., all black/African Americans with substance use disorders are poor and come from single-female-headed households). Always take time to get to know the client.
- Integrate cultural values, such as spirituality/religiosity, in the substance abuse assessment and therapeutic process. By doing so, it (a) acknowledges what is important to the client; (b) fosters trust; and (c) creates a safe place to discuss spiritual beliefs without being labeled or misdiagnosed.

- Appropriate self-disclosure may increase trust and build the therapeutic alliance.
- Collectivism has been strongly identified as a cultural orientation for black/African Americans. When assessing and conceptualizing substance use issues with black/African Americans, consider the individual in relation to social roles, obligations, and situational restrictions. Empathetically understand and facilitate the recovery process within the context of the culture.
- Assist black/African American clients with acquiring the tools to effectively cope with cultural barriers to recovery (e.g., helping them link to community resources to assist with accessibility, legal issues, costs of treatment).
- Appreciate the clients' verbal communication. This is likely to increase black/African American clients' level of engagement and participation in the therapeutic process.
- Attend to sources of stress that are likely contributors to the clients' substance use–related issues.

Working from an AACT framework facilitates unconditional positive regard and an awareness of the complexity and impact of substance use–related issues in the black/African American population. Substance abuse professionals who empathically address the cultural needs of black/African Americans with substance use disorders will be better prepared to support these individuals in their recovery process.

Reflection and Self-Awareness Exercises

1. Identify two or three areas of growth that would assist you in being more culturally responsive when working with black/African American clients.
2. How do you incorporate black/African American clients' cultural identities in your assessment and case conceptualization of their substance use disorder?
3. How do you consider cultural mistrust when seeking self-disclosure from the client?
4. How do you (or would you) attend to cultural similarities and differences between you and your black/African American client?
5. Are there any attitudes, emotions, and behaviors you hold that could impede your ability to have unconditional positive regard for black/African American clients with substance use problems?

REFERENCES

Aird, E. G. (2008). Toward a renaissance for the African American family: Confronting the lie of black inferiority. *Emory Law Journal, 58*, 7–21.

Allen, F. (2013). Drug abuse, African Americans and jail. Retrieved from http://www.tsdmemphis.com/index.php/opinion/9742-drug-abuse-african-americans-and-jail

Austin, A. (2009). Three lessons about black poverty. *Economic Policy Institute*. Washington, DC.

Baker, F. M., & Bell, C. C. (1999). Issues in the psychiatric treatment of African Americans. *Psychiatric Services, 50*(30), 362–368.

Barber, J. P., Lester, L., Gallop, R., Critis-Christoph, P., Frank, A., Weiss, R. D., et al. (2001). Therapeutic alliance as a predictor of outcome and retention in the national institute on drug abuse collaborative cocaine treatment study. *Journal of Counseling and Clinical Psychology, 69*(1), 119–124.

Bonilla-Silva, E. (2003). "New racism", color-blind racism, and the future of whiteness in America. In A. Doane & E. Bonilla-Silva (Eds.), *White out: The continuing significance of racism*. New York: Taylor and Francis Books, Inc.

Britt, A. B. (2004). African Americans, substance abuse and spirituality. Retrieved from http://www.minoritynurse.com/article/african-americans-substance-abuse-and-spirituality

Brown, D. L. (2008). African American resiliency: Examining racial socialization and social support as protective factors. *Journal of Black Psychology, 34*(1), 32–48.

Burrell, T. (2010). *Brainwashed: Challenging the myth of Black inferiority*. New York: Smiley Books.

Campbell, C. I., Weisner, C., & Sterling, S. (2006). Adolescents entering chemical dependency treatment in private managed care: Ethnic differences in treatment initiation and retention. *Journal of Adolescent Health, 38*(4), 343–350.

Castro, F. G., & Alarcon, E. H. (2002). Integrating cultural variables into drug abuse prevention and treatment with racial/ethnic minorities. *Journal of Drug Issues, 32*, 783–811.

Castro, F. G., & Garfinkle, J. (2003). Critical issues in the development of culturally relevant substance abuse treatments for specific minority groups. *Alcoholism: Clinical and Experimental Research, 27*, 1381–1388.

Corrigan, P. W., Larson, J. E., & Rüsch, N. L. (2009). Self-stigma and the "why try" effect: Impact on life goals and evidence-based practices. *World Psychiatry, 8*, 75–81.

Domhoff, G. W. (2009). *Who rules America? Challenges to corporate and class dominance* (6th ed.). New York: McGraw-Hill.

Gibbons, F. X., Etcheverry, P. E., Stock, M. L., Gerrard, M., Weng, C-Y., Kiviniemi, M., & O'Hara, R. E. (2010). Exploring the link between racial discrimination and substance use: What mediates? What buffers? *Journal of Personality and Social Psychology, 99*(5), 785–801.

Gilchrist, E., & Jackson, R. (2012). Articulating the heuristic value of African American communication studies. *Review of Communication, 12*(3), 237–250.

Harris, A. L. (2010). The economic and educational state of Black Americans in the 21st century: Should we be optimistic or concerned? *Review of Black Political Economy, 37*(3), 241–252. doi:10.1007/s12114-010-9065-z

Hayes, S. C., & Smith, S. (2005). *Get out of my mind and into your life: The new acceptance and commitment therapy*. Oakland, CA: New Harbinger.

Health.com. *How self-stigma hurts people with depression* (September 14, 2010). Retrieved from http://www.health.com/health/condition-article/0,,20425884,00.html

Horsey, D. (2013). Supreme Court ignores new voting rights discrimination. *Los Angeles Times*. Retrieved from http://articles.latimes.com/2013/jun/28/nation/la-na-tt-new-voting-rights-discrimination-20130628

Howard, D. L. (2003). Culturally competent treatment of African American clients among a national sample of outpatient substance abuse treatment units. *Journal of Substance Abuse Treatment, 24*, 89–102.

Knafo, S. (2013). When it comes to illicit drug use, white America does the crime, black America gets the time. Retrieved from http://m.huffpost.com/us/entry/394136/

LaVeist, T. A., & Wallace, J. M. (2000). Health risk and inequitable distribution of liquor stores in African American neighborhoods. *Social Science & Medicine, 51*(4), 613–617.

Lim, R. F. (2008, September 23). *Cultural issues in substance abuse treatment*. 38th semiannual Substance Abuse Research Consortium (SAR) meeting, Sacramento, CA.

Ludwig, J., Duncan, G. J., Gennetian, L. A., Katz, L. F., Kessler, R. C., Kling, J. R., & Sanbonmatsu, L. (2012). Neighborhood effects on the long-term well-being of low-income adults. *Science, 337*(6101), 1505–1510.

Luoma, J. B., Kohlenberg, B. S., Hayes, S. C., Bunting, K., & Rye, A. K. (2008). Reducing self-stigma in substance abuse through acceptance and commitment therapy: Model, manual development, and pilot outcomes. *Addiction, Research, and Theory, 16*(2), 149–165.

Madison-Colmore, O., & Moore, J. L. (2002). Using the H.I.S. model in counseling African-American men. *Journal of Men's Studies, 10*(2), 197–208.

Martin, J. K., Tuch, S. A., & Roman, P. M. (2003). Problem drinking patterns among African Americans: The impacts of reports of discrimination, perceptions of prejudice, and "risky" coping strategies. *Journal of Health & Social Behavior, 44*(3), 408–425.

Massey, D. S. (1990). American apartheid: Segregation and the making of the underclass. *American Journal of Sociology, 96*(2), 329–357.

Mays, V. M., Cochran, S. D., & Barnes, N. W. (2007). Race, race-based discrimination, and health outcomes among African Americans. *Annual Review of Psychology, 58*, 201–225.

Minior, T., Galea, S., Stuber, J., Ahern J., & Ompad, D. (2003). Racial differences in discrimination experiences and responses among minority substance users. *Ethnicity and Disease, 13*(4), 521–527.

Mukku, V. K., Benson, T. G., Alam, F., Richie, W. D., & Bailey, R. K. (2012). Overview of substance use disorders and incarceration of African American males. *Frontiers in Psychiatry, 3*, 98. doi:10.3389/fpsyt.2012.00098

National Institute on Drug Abuse. (2011). *Treatment statistics*. U.S. Department of Health and Human Services. Retrieved from www.drugabuse.gov

National Survey on Drug Use and Health. (2012). *Substance use among Black adults*. Substance Abuse and Mental Health Services Administration (SAMHSA). Retrieved from http://store.samhsa.gov/product/Substance-Use-among-Black-Adults/NSDUH10-0218

Pierre, M. R., & Mahalik, J. R. (2005). Examining African self-consciousness and Black racial identity as predictors of Black men's psychological well-being. *Cultural Diversity and Ethnic Minority Psychology, 11*, 28–40.

Reese, R. (2013). Trayvon Martin and the myth of black inferiority. *Huffington Post*.

Romley, J. A., Cohen, D., Ringel, J., & Strum, R. (2007). Alcohol and environmental justice: The density of liquor stores and bars in urban neighborhoods in the United States. *Journal of Studies on Alcohol and Drugs, 68*, 48–55.

Settles, I. H. (2006). Use of an intersectional framework to understand Black women's racial and gender identities. *Sex Roles, 54*(9–10), 589–601.

Sinha, R. (2008). Chronic stress, drug use and vulnerability to addiction. *Annals of the New York Academy of Sciences, 1141*, 105–130.

Smith, W., Allen, W., & Danley, L. (2007). "Assume the position … you fit the description": Psychosocial experiences and racial battle fatigue among African American male college students. *American Behavioral Scientist, 51*, 551–578.

Thompson, V. L., Bazile, A., & Akbar, M. (2004). African Americans' perceptions of psychotherapy and psychotherapists. *Professional Psychological Research and Practice, 35*, 19–26.

U.S. Census Bureau. (2012). The Census Bureau's population estimates program. Retrieved from http://www.census.gov/population/race/data/black.html

U.S. Census Bureau. (2011). Race. Retrieved from http://www.census.gov/population/race/

U.S. Census Bureau, Income, Poverty, and Health Insurance Coverage in the United States. (2010). Retrieved from http://www.census.gov/prod/2011pubs/p60-239.pdf

Utsey, S. O., Bolden, M. A., Lanier, Y., & Williams, O. (2007). Examining the role of culture-specific coping as a predictor of resilient outcomes in African Americans from high-risk urban communities. *Journal of Black Psychology, 33*, 75–93.

Utsey, S. O., Hook, J. N., Fischer, N., & Belvet, B. (2008). Cultural orientation, ego resilience, and optimism as predictors of subjective well-being in African Americans. *Journal of Positive Psychology, 3*(3), 202–210.

Watkins, N. L. (2012). Disarming microaggressions: How black college students self-regulate racial stressors within predominately with institutions (Doctoral Dissertation). Retrieved from http://hdl.handle.net/10022/AC:P:14170

Williams, M. T. (November 2, 2011). Why African Americans avoid psychotherapy. Retrieved from http://www.psychologytoday.com/blog/colorblind/201111/why-african-americans-avoid-psychotherapy/

Williams, M. T. (August 31, 2013). How well-meaning therapists commit racism. Retrieved from http://www.psychologytoday.com/blog/culturally-speaking/201308/how-well-meaning-therapists-commit-racism

CHAPTER 5

AMERICAN INDIANS

By Andrew Wood, Daniel Gutierrez, Renee Sherrell, and Catherine Griffith

INTRODUCTION

This chapter will describe issues that counselors should consider when providing therapy to American Indian clients with substance abuse concerns. For the purposes of this chapter, the authors will use the term "American Indian" to refer to individuals belonging to the indigenous tribes of the continental United States and Alaska (e.g., Native Americans, Alaska Natives, and specific tribal designations). We use the term "American Indian" rather than the more common term "Native American" due to the prevalence of the term "American Indian" in counseling literature. Further, the term "American Indian" will refer to all who self-identify as being of American Indian descent. First, the authors provide an overview of the population. Next, a discussion of the particular substance abuse issues American Indian clients may encounter is presented, followed by an overview of this population's resiliency and protective factors. Screening and assessment issues applicable to American Indian clients are then addressed. Lastly, the authors approach treatment considerations and barriers to treatment that are unique to American Indian clients. At the end of the chapter, individual and group exercises are included in an effort to foster self-awareness and critical thinking with respect to this specific population.

OVERVIEW OF POPULATION

The 2010 United States Census defined American Indians as "a person having origins in any of the original peoples of North and South America (including Central America) and who maintains tribal affiliation or community attachment" (U.S. Census Bureau, 2012, p. 2). The origins of American Indians in the United States can be traced back to before the colonization by Europeans (Gone & Trimble, 2012). There are approximately 5.2 million individuals who identify as American Indian (either solely or with another race), and their population is increasing more than the national population of the United States (Gone & Trimble, 2012). Those who identify as American Indian may qualify in various ways. Individuals can personally identify as American Indian, while specific tribes require additional qualifications to belong to that tribe. The Bureau of Indian Affairs, for example, requires individuals to trace back to a lineal American Indian ancestor (e.g., parent or distant ancestor) who is or was a member of the tribe they wish to join ("A Guide to Tracing American Indian and Alaska Native Ancestry," n.d.). There are over 500 tribal entities among the American Indian population, each having distinct characteristics (e.g., language, practices, and philosophy; Bureau of Indian Affairs, 2012; Gone & Trimble, 2012). Despite these differences, American Indian tribes also share numerous traits, characteristics, and experiences (Young & Joe, 2009). Included among these shared experiences is historical mistreatment by European Americans in the United States (Brave Heart, 2003; Gone, 2009). An awareness of key cultural differences and similarities empower substance abuse counselors to serve the American Indian population effectively.

One cultural factor that must be considered when treating American Indian clients is historical trauma (Brave Heart, Chase, Elkins, & Altschul, 2011). Brave Heart (2003) defines historical trauma as "cumulative emotional and psychological wounding, over the lifespan and across generations, emanating from massive group trauma experiences" (p. 7). Historical trauma has roots in instances of oppression, hardship, humiliation, and marginalization that the American Indian population has experienced (Evans-Campbell, 2008). Events that have contributed to historical trauma include forced boarding school attendance, outlawing of religious or spiritual practices, dumping of radioactive materials on American Indian land, flooding of those lands, and the introduction of disease into American Indian communities (Evans-Campbell, 2008). Also of major significance is forced relocation. The most widely known example of this type of historical trauma is the Trail of Tears, a forced relocation of Cherokee individuals from the southeast region of the United States to the Oklahoma area. This instance followed the relocation of other tribes (e.g., Seminole, Creek, Chickasaw, and Choctaw). These forced relocations resulted in the deaths of thousands of American Indians. In conceptualizing historical trauma, it is important to remember that individuals can experience this issue differently, depending on their own history (Brave Heart et al., 2011). It should also be noted that historical trauma can apply to particular tribes for specific reasons. In other words, an event may be historically traumatic to one tribe, but not to another tribe (Evans-Campbell, 2008). Not surprisingly, those who continue to face aspects of historical trauma (e.g., past movement from tribal homelands to remote areas and present-day movement from tribal reservations to suburbia), tend to feel more historical trauma and subsequently engage in increased instances of substance use than those who have not reexperienced historical trauma (Wiechelt, Gryczynski, Johnson, & Caldwell, 2012). It is important to be aware of issues that cause recollections of historical trauma, as they could affect the counseling relationship (e.g., suggestion of alternate schooling or intolerance of religious practices).

The number of American Indian individuals seeking substance abuse–related care is nearly double the general United States (Substance Abuse and Mental Health Services Administration [SAMHSA], 2010). Researchers with SAMHSA estimate 18 percent of American Indians are in need of substance abuse treatment. In particular, American Indian adolescents (ages 12–17) have the highest rate of substance use among adolescents of any other race or ethnicity in the United States (Wu, Woody, Yang, Pan, & Blazer, 2011). In addition, American Indian individuals tend to engage in risky substance use behaviors (e.g., binge drinking) more often than the national population (SAMHSA, 2010). In fact, over the past 30 years, the American Indian population has had the highest rate of mortality related to substance use of any racial or ethnic group in the United States (Indian Health Service, 2004).

The basis for some of these issues (e.g., need for substance abuse treatment and high mortality rates) could be linked to a multitude of disparities (Gone & Trimble, 2012). Such disparities include having

(a) lower income; (b) less education; and (c) limited access to adequate mental-health care, especially for those living on rural tribal reservations. In addition, issues surrounding the process of adapting to mainstream American culture (e.g., acculturation) while also living in an American Indian culture may also be present (LaFromboise, Albright, & Harris, 2010).

This section provides an overview of the American Indian population, including statistics that justify the need to address substance abuse issues specific to this population. As the reader continues with this chapter, the authors suggest remembering American Indians constitute a large group that contains multiple smaller groups. Each group has individual differences to which counselors must attend. Thus, counselors should be aware of differences between clients at the group and individual levels (Beals et al., 2005).

SUBSTANCE ABUSE ISSUES

The reasons why American Indian individuals turn to using alcohol and other substances at an alarming rate is a complicated issue, and could stem from a number of sources. One etiological theory is historical influence, such as the introduction of alcohol to American Indians by the U.S. colonists and the rate at which colonists consumed alcohol (Lamarine, 1988). According to Lamarine, the novelty of alcohol existed for American Indians, but the colonists did not impart the restraint with which to use alcohol or the general risks of abusing alcohol. Others have posited substance use by American Indians could relate to communal aspects of the various American Indian cultures (Legha & Novins, 2012). Community is incredibly important to this population; thus, characteristics that improve community (e.g., sharing, generosity, consideration, and modesty) are highly valued and encouraged. Peer pressure, therefore, may play a role in American Indians' increased substance use. If individuals are offered alcohol, they are encouraged to share and be considerate of the offering that is made to them, so as to not disrespect the other person and potentially harm the community (Legha & Novins, 2012).

Stigma may also play a role in the increased substance use by American Indians. American Indian communities can stigmatize substance abuse treatment due to the importance placed on pride in American Indian cultures. Johnson, Gryczynski, and Wiechelt (2007) found some American Indian individuals do not seek professional help with substance use issues due to feelings of shame, which can lead to risky behaviors (e.g., needle sharing or binge drinking). American Indian individuals may seek help by consulting with cultural leaders, rather than seeking professional help outside of their tribe (Dickerson & Johnson, 2011).

Risk factors specific to the American Indian population can also exacerbate substance use issues, particularly alcohol use. Binge drinking among the American Indian population occurs more often than in any other racial or ethnic group in the United States (see Figure 5.1 below, SAMHSA, 2010). Among American Indians, a large proportion of young people are using and abusing alcohol. Due to the prevalence of young American Indians using alcohol, mortality rates are higher in this population. In fact, the Indian Health Service (2004) reported there were approximately 0.3 alcohol-related deaths (per 100,000) among American Indian individuals aged 5–14, whereas the national sample was much smaller at 0.05 deaths per 100,000 individuals aged 5–14.

Several other factors can increase substance use rates among American Indian individuals (Kunitz, 2008). Such factors include: (a) changes in social organizations (e.g., the American Indian population becoming younger and establishing trends of substance abuse); (b) increasing access (e.g., improved roads to travel from rural tribal reservations to more urban areas and access to media via television and

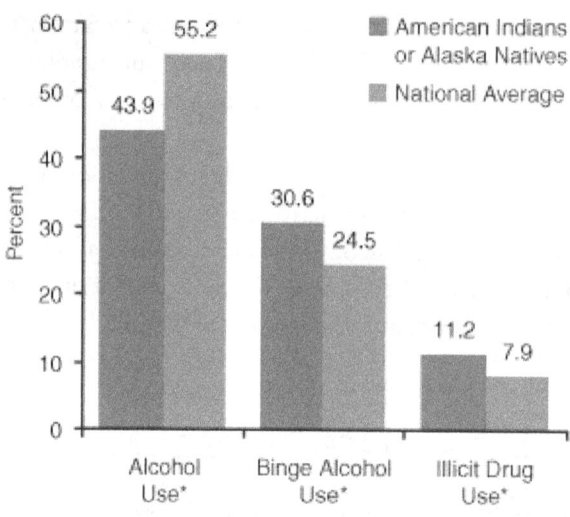

Figure 5.1: Past Month Substance Use among American Indians or Alaska Natives Aged 18 or Older Compared with the National Average: 2004 to 2008
Source: SAMHSA / Public Domain.

the Internet); and (c) diagnosis of conduct disorder in those under 15 years of age (Kunitz, 2008). The common use of substances within American Indian cultures for spiritual practices can also be a risk factor. For instance, the use of peyote in spiritual practices can be seen as harmful by those in mental health fields (Halpern, 2005). The assumption that substance use for spiritual practices is harmful could negatively affect American Indian clients' by perpetuating stereotypes and dismissing their cultural beliefs (Johnson, Bartgis, Worley, Hellman, & Burkhart, 2010; Myhra, 2011).

In summary, numerous substance abuse issues can harm American Indians. Historical issues, the stigma of substance abuse treatment, the young age at which American Indians tend to start using substances, and other reasons can all lead to increased substance abuse in the American Indian population. As substance abuse issues have been detailed in this section, it is important to consider resiliency and protective factors that may be present among American Indian clients.

RESILIENCY AND PROTECTIVE FACTORS

Given the overwhelming diversity of American Indian cultures, it is difficult to describe resiliency and preventive factors that are common among all individuals. The material presented is instead a broad description of traits that are regularly observed among the majority of tribes. Therefore, it is important for substance abuse counselors to explore the protective factors that are unique for their clients.

The roles of families are often paramount in American Indian cultures, with extended family members playing core roles in one another's lives. Family therapist Terry Tafoya (1989) describes how: (a) cousins are often referred to as brother and sister; (b) siblings of both parents and grandparents share in the responsibility of child caregiving; and (c) families seldom make distinctions between blood relatives and those inducted by marriage. Sometimes, families also include tribal healers and other nonrelated people (e.g., close friends; Brucker & Perry, 1998). Additionally, grandparents often fulfill the role of primary guides and disciplinarians. These large family systems work together to solve problems, and American Indians with substance abuse concerns will generally have access to large networks of support.

American Indians often identify strongly with their tribe, seeing themselves as "we" rather than "I," a key trait of collectivistic cultures (Sutton & Broken Nose, 2005). Sue and Sue (2012) explain that providing support to others and sharing resources with one another is an important value in many tribes, as is cooperation and putting the needs of others before themselves. American Indians also typically have great reverence for the wisdom and knowledge of elders in their community, and respect their guidance and advice (Sue & Sue, 1999). Part of treatment with American Indians may involve determining whether elders will be able to support the client during the recovery process (Coyhis, 2000).

Spirituality also plays an important role in the healing process of many American Indians (Navarro, Wilson, Berger, & Taylor, 1997). The American Indian Religious Freedom Act of 1978 ensures that communities may engage in religious and spiritual practices without fear of government interference, resulting in the increasing popularity of incorporating traditional culture in life, health, illness, and healing (Johnson & Cameron, 2001). Buchwald, Beals, and Manson (2000) revealed in their study of 871 American Indian primary care patients that two-thirds of the participants regularly employed traditional healing practices and thought such interventions greatly improved their health. Furthermore, in a study of American Indians seeking services at an urban clinic, 38 percent reported concurrent work with a native healer in order to amplify treatment. Of those not currently collaborating with a native healer, approximately 90 percent stated they would strongly consider doing so in the near future (Marbella, Harris, Deihr, Ignace, & Ignace, 1998). Consequently, part of offering culturally competent services may involve collaborating with spiritual leaders and healers, just as one would with other traditional health care providers.

In summary, because practices and worldviews of a tribe may differ significantly from one another, a substance abuse counselor will need to explore the unique nuances of the individual's culture. Ask about family ties, spirituality and practices, and access to resources. All the while, a counselor should affirm existing strengths (Sutton & Broken Nose, 2005). Keeping in mind resiliency and protective factors that are present for the majority of American Indians may help guide the direction of treatment as strengths are explored.

SCREENING AND ASSESSMENTS

Research on mental health and substance abuse among American Indians is restricted by the small size of the population and by its diverse heterogeneity (American Psychiatric Association, 2010). Often, within the American Indian population, physical ailments and psychological issues are not differentiated from one another. Therefore, American Indians may display emotional distress in a manner that is inconsistent with standard diagnostic symptoms, making the use of the *Diagnostic and Statistical Manual of Mental Disorders* difficult and potentially inappropriate (Urban Indian Health Commission, 2007).

Challenges add to the difficulty in assessing American Indians for substance use, such as (a) economic obstacles (e.g., cost or lack of insurance); (b) mental illness stigma; (c) limited culturally appropriate services; (d) mistrust of health care providers; (e) scarcity of data and research on American Indians; (f) a shortage of appropriate interventions; and (g) high turnover rates for mental health professionals (Legha & Novins, 2012). Researchers have sought to develop new models of assessment and treatment for the American Indian population (Gone, 2011; Johnson et al., 2010; Morgan & Freeman, 2009). However, these attempts have been criticized due to limitations in generalizability, randomization, and heterogeneity, which indicate further research is required.

Despite these challenges in substance abuse assessment, Beals et al. (2006) suggest American Indians actively seek help, which includes traditional healing practices, as well as 12-step programs. In their study, they found that 38 percent of American Indians diagnosed with substance use disorders sought services for alcohol and drug problems. Furthermore, the majority of American Indians feel most comfortable receiving services from a combination of 12-step programs, biomedical providers, and traditional healers (Beals et al., 2006).

Help seeking from traditional healers is common among the American Indian culture (Gone, 2011; Walls, Johnson, Whitbeck, & Hoyt, 2006). Traditional healers in American Indian cultures usually focus on holistic approaches to healing, one that includes a sense of connectedness with place and land and does not include a typical Western view of problem identification (Beals et al., 2005). Additionally, most healers do not incorporate traditional mental health assessments in their treatments. As a result, Beals et al. (2005) suggest service providers assessing American Indians for substance abuse may find success when incorporating some of the strengths and protective factors of American Indian cultures. These include: (a) a strong identification with culture; (b) importance of family; (c) traditional health practices (such as ceremonies); (d) adaptability; and (e) emphasis on the wisdom of elders. The following section on treatment considerations covers these factors in greater depth.

In conclusion, research on American Indian cultures and American Indian clients suggests a need for appropriate substance abuse assessment (Walls et al., 2006). Services that incorporate culturally sensitive approaches with traditional informal methods appear to better serve the mental health and substance abuse assessment needs of American Indians (Beals et al., 2006; Gone, 2011). A deeper understanding of the specific cultures—in addition to the importance of socioeconomic variables such as education, salary, and status—could also help to appropriately serve American Indian clients (Walls et al., 2006). Lastly, substance abuse assessment may be more appropriate when referencing American Indian values (e.g., respect for all living creatures) and traditional practices (e.g., rituals and ceremonies) that promote connection with higher principles (Navarro et al., 1997). Assessing for substance abuse among American Indians can be challenging. Therefore, making carefully regarded treatment considerations is vital in the effort to provide the most appropriate services.

TREATMENT CONSIDERATIONS

In considering the statistics regarding substance use and the alarming rate of health-related consequences, the importance of substance use treatment becomes increasingly clear (Indian Health Service, 2004). However, in order to provide effective treatment and understand the underlying concerns of those with addictions, substance abuse counselors must pay close attention to certain contextual factors, such as cultural and spiritual beliefs (Garret & Carroll, 2000). Researchers demonstrate that American Indians, like many other cultural groups, experience high levels of distrust and fear of traditional evidence-based treatment practices (Larios, Wright, Jernstrom, Lebron, & Sorensen, 2011). Moreover, treatment practices deemed as evidence based tend to ignore salient client characteristics (e.g., the input of tribal elders, cultural knowledge, and participant satisfaction) that may significantly moderate and mediate treatment outcomes (Nebelkopf et al., 2011). Thus, well-informed and effective substance abuse counselors must select and adapt culturally appropriate treatments.

One common mistake made by substance abuse counselors is the instant referral to 12-step programs at the onset of substance abuse treatment. Recommending a 12-step program such as Alcoholics Anonymous (AA) may be an appropriate suggestion. However, before recommending 12-step programs, it is important to process the underlying spiritual philosophy of AA with clients first (Carvajal & Young, 2009; Garret & Carroll, 2000), and then help clients select a 12-step group that comfortably fits their worldview.

One culturally appropriate version of a 12-step program is White Bison (Moore & Coyhis, 2010). Like AA, White Bison operates under a specific philosophy and a set of traditions. However, the White Bison philosophy describes an American Indian understanding of a higher power (e.g., Mother Earth, the natural order, or the Supreme Being), the importance of community in recovery, and encourages leadership. In addition, the White Bison philosophy includes four laws of change: (a) change is from within; (b) in order for development to occur, it must be preceded by a vision; (c) a great learning must take place; and (d) you must create a Healing Forest (for more information, see www.whitebison.org). Through this culturally informed framework, White Bison, Inc. offers several noteworthy resources to aid in the recovery and "wellbriety" of American Indians, including an adaptation of the original text of AA to include stories of American Indian individuals overcoming addiction (Coyhis, & White, 2002). Likewise, AA meetings conducted for American Indians are often adapted to be more consistent with American Indian cultures. For instance, meetings typically start and end late, include family members, have longer periods of socialization, and replace the concept of powerlessness with an emphasis on acquiring power over personal and tribal life (Coyhis & White, 2002). These modifications to the traditional AA program offer American Indian clients a program more consistent with their values, which may increase their likelihood of engaging in treatment.

To this end, Garret and Carroll (2000) make several other clinical recommendations, which include:

- Avoid firm handshakes because they are seen as a show of power
- Show hospitality by offering the client a snack or a beverage
- Use silence at the beginning of each session to place the client at ease
- Make an effort to understand the client's level of acculturation by informally assessing values, geographic residence, tribal affiliation, and nonverbal cues
- Match the client's level of eye contact. Some clients may interpret too much eye contact as aggressive or arrogant
- Establish a trusting relationship by keeping commitments and promises
- Respect the client's choice and offer helpful alternatives through empathic collaboration.

Legha and Novins (2012) further investigated clinical considerations for working with American Indian communities, concluding that treatment programs integrating culturally based care do so in two ways: (a) by integrating specific cultural practices; and (b) adapting Western methods into culturally

Table 5.1

SUGGESTED PRACTICES THAT REFLECT AMERICAN INDIAN FOUNDATIONAL BELIEFS (LEGHA & NOVINS, 2012)
• Have an open-door policy
• Emphasize respectful relationships
• Involve family and community members
• Be flexible with the client
• Be cognizant of challenges faced by some clients (e.g., access to transportation, language barriers, and financial constraints)

acceptable approaches. They suggested several practices that reflect American Indian foundational beliefs, which can be found in Table 5.1 above. In essence, to be effective in treating American Indians with substance abuse issues, counselors should make efforts to understand their clients' cultural world, and then integrate and honor their values and beliefs in treatment.

Some approaches that researchers have modified to be culturally congruent for American Indian clients include: (a) Motivational Interviewing (Gilder et al., 2011; Venner, Feldstein, & Mescalero, 2006); (b) the previously mentioned 12-step program, White Bison (Moore & Coyhis, 2010); and (c) neurofeedback (Kelley, 1997). In addition, some scholars have suggested integrating American Indian practices such as the *sweat lodge* (e.g., a steam bath purification ritual), the *Sun Dance* (e.g., a native dance in honor of the sun), *Talking Circles* (e.g., an intertribal method of communicating where a talisman is passed to signify who is allowed to speak), and *smudging* (Chong, Fortier, & Morris, 2009; Garret et al., 2011). Smudging is a traditional cleansing ceremony where one burns sacred herbs and leaves. Smudging practitioners believe that the smoke attaches itself to negative thoughts and emotions, and cleanses those who participate in the ritual. Each native tribe practices smudging differently; however, congregants typically partake in a prayer, and the smoke is positioned so it ascends in a specific direction. Given the powerful symbolism and the spiritual intensity of these rituals, one can easily see how the integration of these spiritual and cultural practices into clinical work can have therapeutic benefits (Garret et al., 2011).

To summarize, when working with American Indian clients, substance abuse counselors must equip themselves with an understanding of their clients' worldviews. By doing so, counselors build a therapeutic relationship and help engage clients in treatment. Interventions employed during treatment should be culturally appropriate and reflect the foundational beliefs of clients. For instance, researchers have modified several approaches, such as Motivational Interviewing (Gilder et al., 2011; Venner, Feldstein, & Mescalero, 2006)) and neurofeedback (Kelley, 1997) to be more culturally responsive. Furthermore, traditional practices (e.g., smudging and sweat lodges) can also be included in treatment. Next, the authors consider the barriers to treatment that counselors may face at the outset of substance abuse counseling.

BARRIERS TO TREATMENT

Understanding the help-seeking behaviors of American Indians and the concurrent barriers that influence these actions is an important part of conceptualizing substance abuse concerns. Sociocultural factors play a vital role in the clients' decision to obtain treatment, as does a history of distrust for dominant culture practices. Contact with Europeans, for example, has resulted in profound historical traumas, as the efforts to eliminate and assimilate indigenous peoples caused the loss of native lands, tore families apart, and denigrated tribal languages, customs, and spiritual practices (La Due, 1994). Even in the 1950s and 1960s, the federal government was relocating American Indians from their homes and families to urban centers, resulting in a spike in substance abuse, suicide, violence, teen pregnancies, school dropouts, and unemployment (La Due, 1994; Tafoya & Del Vecchio, 2005).

Naturally, the factors and events discussed have resulted in a general skepticism for non–American Indian care providers, passed down through generations of oppressed peoples. Too often, missionaries, teachers, and counselors have attempted to help American Indians by imposing their own value systems, which has led to misgivings about the therapeutic process (Sutton & Broken Nose, 2005). Consequently, American Indians may feel hesitant and conflicted about seeking out mental health services when needed. Walls et al. (2006) found in a study of 865 American Indians from the northern Midwest that only 33 percent of respondents reported it would be "very or extremely effective" to speak with a counselor. Instead, participants indicated it would be very or extremely effective to speak with a family member (71 percent) or tribal elder (59 percent). Participants also highly rated the following practices: (a) offering tobacco and praying; (b) seeing a traditional healer; and (c) participating in ceremonies, sweat lodges, and healing circles. Furthermore, professional services located off reservation were seen as least effective of all (Walls et al., 2006). Duran and Duran (1995) suggest counselors acknowledge historical inequities and validate the resulting harm experienced because of oppression. Consequently, clients may feel empowered by understanding that their substance abuse issues may at least partially stem from external forces.

Economic obstacles represent another barrier in the ability to seek treatment. The unemployment rate for American Indians is 14.6 percent, approximately double that of white, non-Hispanic Americans (Bureau of Labor Statistics, 2012). Poverty rates and the proportion of individuals without health insurance are higher for American Indians, and education attainment is generally lower (Sarche & Spicer, 2008). Access to mental health care is also greatly decreased in rural, isolated areas, where many American Indians live (Johnson & Cameron, 2001). Other barriers exist within the medical system itself, such as: (a) a lack of funding and subsequent understaffing; (b) inconsistent availability of services; (c) cultural insensitivities on the part of the providers; (d) staff burnout; (e) fear of litigation; and (f) needing to comply with organizational requirements (e.g., manualized treatment modalities) that are not necessarily suited to the American Indian population (Rodenhauser, 1994).

Finally, American Indians who follow the traditional spiritual practices of their community may have difficulty participating in AA, as this organization's tenets derive from a primarily European, Christian point of view (Coyhis, 2000; Duran & Duran, 1995). An alternative such as White Bison or the wellbriety movement "integrates the medicine wheel with the twelve-step teachings of AA to adapt substance abuse recovery to Native American culture" (Krestan, 2000, p. 36).

CONCLUSIONS

In concluding this chapter, the authors hope to convey the specific needs of American Indian clients in substance abuse counseling. American Indian clients are at an increased risk of substance use that could lead to addiction issues. Due to risk factors unique to American Indian clients (along with the stigma associated with seeking professional help), it is a counselor's duty to reach out to the American Indian population. Reaching out can begin by becoming familiar with American Indian tribes in your practice area. Counselors could also seek the help of tribal leaders in American Indian communities to start a partnership to aid American Indian clients. Finally, counselors can follow some of the treatment considerations discussed in this chapter in an effort to help American Indian clients feel comfortable in counseling situations.

Group Exercises

1. In groups of three or four, generate a list of questions you could ask a client that would help you to assess for the following factors: (a) level of acculturation; (b) feelings about participating in traditional counseling; and (c) existing strengths and current protective factors. If time permits, take turns role-playing counselor and client with the questions you wrote down. Remaining group members will observe and provide feedback.
2. Find a recent journal article on incorporating traditional healing ceremonies/practices in working with American Indians. In a group, discuss the articles. Share your ideas about how to apply suggestions from the articles specifically to substance abuse treatment with this population.

Self-Awareness Exercise

1. What stereotypes are most prevalent in the media about American Indians? What stereotypes do you hold about American Indians? What microaggressions (e.g., subtle insults) may result because of these stereotypes?

Reflection Questions

1. What are some characteristics about American Indians that make them different from other racial/ethnic groups? What specific substance abuse issues must you be aware of concerning this population?
2. What American Indian groups (i.e., tribes) are in your area? How would you tailor treatment to the specific groups in your area?
3. Do you think there are any substance abuse issues (e.g., using the medical model or the sociocultural model to describe substance use to clients) that will be met with differing levels of resistance when counseling American Indian clients?

REFERENCES

American Psychiatric Association. (2010). Mental health disparities: American Indians and Alaska Natives. Retrieved from APA Office of Minority and National Affairs website: http:www.psych.org

Beals, J., Manson, S. M., Whitesell, N. R., Spicer, P., Novins, D. K., & Mitchell, C. M. (2005). Prevalence of DSM-IV disorders and attendant help-seeking in two American Indian reservation populations. *Archives of General Psychiatry, 62*(1), 99–108.

Beals, J., Novins, D. K., Spicer, P., Whitesell, N. R., Mitchell, C. M., & Manson, S. M. (2006). Help seeking for substance use problems in two American Indian reservation populations, *Psychiatric Services, 57*(4), 512–520.

Brave Heart, M. Y. H. (2003). The historical trauma response among Natives and its relationship with substance abuse: A Lakota illustration. *Journal of Psychoactive Drugs, 35*(1), 7–13.

Brave Heart, M. Y. H. (2011). Historical trauma among indigenous peoples of the Americas: Concepts, research, and clinical considerations. *Journal of Psychoactive Drugs, 43*(4), 282–290.

Brucker, P. S., & Perry, B. J. (1998). American Indians: Presenting concerns and considerations for family therapists. *American Journal of Family Therapy, 26*(4), 307–320.

Buckwald, D. S., Beals, J., & Manson, S. M. (2000). Use of traditional healing among Native Americans in a primary care setting. *Medical Care, 38*, 1191–1199.

Bureau of Indian Affairs (n.d.). A guide to tracing American Indian and Alaska Native ancestry. Retrieved June 19, 2013, from http://www.bia.gov/cs/groups/public/documents/text/idc-002619.pdf

Bureau of Indian Affairs (2012). Indian entities recognized and eligible to receive services from the Bureau of Indian Affairs. Retrieved February 20, 2013, from http://www.bia.gov/cs/groups/public/documents/text/idc-020700.pdf

Bureau of Labor Statistics, U.S. Department of Labor. (2012, September 5). Racial and ethnic characteristics of the U.S. labor force, 2011. In *Editor's Desk*. Retrieved February 28, 2013, from http://www.bls.gov/opub/ted/2012/ted_20120905.htm

Carvajal, S., & Young, R. S. (2009). Culturally based substance abuse treatment for American Indians/Alaska Natives and Latinos. *Journal of Ethnicity in Substance Abuse, 8*, 207–222.

Chong, J., Fortier, Y., & Morris, T. L. (2009). Cultural practices and spiritual development for women in a Native American alcohol and drug treatment program. *Journal of Ethnicity in Substance Abuse, 8*, 261–282.

Coyhis, D. (2000). Culturally specific addiction recovery for Native Americans. In J. Krestan, (Ed.), *Bridges to recovery: Addiction, family therapy, and multicultural treatment* (pp. 77–114). New York: Free Press.

Coyhis, D., & White, W. L. (2002). Addiction and recovery in Native America: Lost history, enduring lessons. *Counselor, 3*(5), 16–20.

Dickerson, D. L., & Johnson, C. L. (2011). Design of a behavioral health program for urban American Indian/Alaska Native youths: A community informed approach. *Journal of Psychoactive Drugs, 43*(4), 337–342.

Duran, E., & Duran, B. (1995). *Native American postcolonial psychology*. Albany: State University of New York Press.

Evans-Campbell, T. (2008). Historical trauma in American Indian/Native Alaska communities: A multilevel framework for exploring impacts on individuals, families, and communities. *Journal of Interpersonal Violence, 23*(3), 316–338.

Garret, M. T., Torres-Rivera, E., Brubaker, M., Portman, T. A., Brotherton, D., West-Olantunji, C., Grayshield, L. (2011). Crying for a vision: The Native American sweat lodge ceremony as therapeutic intervention. *Journal of Counseling and Development, 89*, 318–325.

Garret, M. T., & Carroll, J. J. (2000). Mending the broken circle: Treatment of substance dependence among Native Americans. *Journal of Counseling and Development, 78*, 379–387.

Gilder, D. A., Luna, J. A., Calac, D., Moore, R. S., Monti, P. M., & Ehlers, C. L. (2011). Acceptability of the use of motivational interviewing to reduce underage drinking in a Native American community. *Substance Use and Misuse, 46*, 836–842.

Gone, J. P. (2011). The red road to wellness: Cultural reclamation in a Native First Nations community treatment center. *American Journal of Community Psychology, 47*, 187–202.

Gone, J. P. (2009). A community-based treatment for Native American historical trauma: Prospects for evidence-based practice. *Journal of Consulting and Clinical Psychology, 77*(4), 751–762.

Gone, J. P., & Trimble, J. E. (2012). American Indian and Alaska Native mental health: Diverse perspectives on enduring disparities. *Annual Review of Clinical Psychology, 8*, 131–160.

Halpern, J. H., Sherwood, A. R., Hudson, J. I., Yurgelun-Todd, D., & Pope, H. G. (2005). Psychological and cognitive effects of long-term peyote use among Native Americans. *Biological Psychiatry, 58*, 624–631.

Indian Health Service. (2004) Trends in Indian Health 2002–2003 Edition. http://www.ihs.gov/ihs_stats/index.cfm?module=hqPubTrends03

Johnson, C. V., Bartgis, J., Worley, J. A., Hellman, C. M., & Burkhart, R. (2010). Urban Indian voices: A community-based participatory research health and needs assessment. *American Indian and Alaska Native Mental Health Research: Journal of the National Center, 17*(1), 49–70.

Johnson, J. L., & Cameron, M. (2001). Barriers to providing effective mental health services to American Indians. *Mental Health Services Research, 3*(4), 215–223.

Johnson, J. L., Gryczynski, J., &Wiechelt, S. A. (2007). HIV/AIDS, substance abuse, and hepatitis prevention needs of Native Americans living in Baltimore: In their own words. *AIDS Education and Prevention, 19*(6), 531–544.

Kelley, M. J. (1997). "Native Americans, neurofeedback, and substance abuse theory": Three-year outcome of alpha/theta neurofeedback training in the treatment of problem drinking among Diné (Navajo) People. *Journal of Neurotherapy: Investigations in Neuromodulation, Neurofeedback and Applied Neuroscience, 3*, 24–60.

Krestan, J. A., (2000). Addiction, power, and powerlessness. In J. A. Krestan, (Ed.), *Bridges to recovery: Addiction, family therapy, and multicultural treatment* (pp. 15–44). New York: Free Press.

Kunitz, S. J. (2008). Risk factors for polydrug use in a Native American population. *Substance Use and Misuse, 43*, 331–339.

La Due, R. (1994). Coyote returns: Twenty sweats does not an Indian expert make, bringing ethics alive. *Feminist Ethics in Psychotherapy Practice, 15*(1), 93–111.

LaFromboise, T. D., Albright, K., & Harris, A. (2010). Patterns of hopelessness among American Indian adolescents: Relationships by levels of acculturation and residence. *Cultural Diversity and Ethnic Minority Psychology, 16*(1), 68–76.

Lamarine, R. J. (1988). Alcohol abuse among Native Americans. *Journal of Community Health, 13*(3), 143–155.

Larios, S. E., Wright, S., Jernstrom, A., Lebron, D., & Sorensen, J. L. (2011). Evidence-based practices, attitudes, and beliefs in substance abuse treatment programs serving American Indians and Alaska Natives: A qualitative study. *Journal of Psychoactive Drugs, 43*(4), 355–359.

Legha, R. K., & Novins, D. (2012). The role of culture in substance abuse treatment programs for American Indian and Alaska Native communities. *Psychiatric Services, 63*(7), 686–692.

Marbella, A. M., Harris, M. C., Diehr, S., Ignace, G., & Ignace, G. (1998). Use of Native American healers among Native American patients in an urban Native American health center. *Archives of Family Medicine, 7*, 182–185.

Moore, D., & Coyhis, D. (2010). The multicultural wellbriety peer recovery support program: Two decades of community-based recovery. *Alcoholism Treatment Quarterly, 28*(3), 273–292.

Morgan, R., & Freeman, L. (2009). The healing of our people: Substance abuse and historical trauma. *Substance Use and Misuse, 44*, 84–98.

Myhra, L. L. (2011). "It runs in the family": Intergenerational transmission of historical trauma among urban American Indians and Alaska Natives in culturally specific sobriety maintenance programs. *American Indian and Alaska Native Mental Health Research, 18*(2), 17–40.

Navarro, J., Wilson, S., Berger, L. R., & Taylor, T. (1997). Substance abuse and spirituality: A program for Native American students. *American Journal of Health Behavior, 21*(1), 3–11.

Nebelkopf, E., King, J., Wright, S., Schweigman, K., Lucero, E., Habte-Michael, T., & Cervantes, T. (2011). Growing roots: Native American evidence-based practices. *Journal of Psychoactive Drugs, 43*(4), 263–268.

Rodenhauser, P. (1994). Cultural barriers to mental health care delivery in Alaska. *Journal of Mental Health Administration, 21*(1), 60–70.

Sarche, M., & Spicer P., (2008). Poverty and health disparities for American Indian and Alaska Native children: Current knowledge and future prospects. *Annals of the New York Academy Of Sciences, 1136*, 126–136.

Substance Abuse and Mental Health Services Administration, Office of Applied Studies. (2010). NSDUH Report: Substance Use among American Indian or Alaska Native Adults. Rockville, MD.

Sue, D. W., & Sue, D. (2012). *Counseling the culturally diverse: Theory and practice* (6th ed.). Hoboken, NJ: John Wiley & Sons Inc.

Sutton C. T., & Broken Nose, M. A. (2005). American Indian families: An overview. In M. McGolderick, J. Giordano, & J. K. Pearce, (Eds.), *Ethnicity and family therapy* (3rd ed., pp. 43–54) New York: Guilford Press.

Tafoya, N., & Del Vecchio, A. (2005). Back to the future: An examination of the Native American holocaust. In M. McGolderick, J. Giordano, & J. K. Pearce, (Eds.), *Ethnicity and family therapy* (3rd ed., pp. 55–63) New York: Guilford Press.

Tafoya, T. (1989).Coyote's eyes: Native cognition styles. *Journal of American Indian Education* [Special issue], 29–40.

Urban Indian Health Commission. (2007) Invisible Tribes: Urban Indians and Their Health in a Changing World. www.rwjf.org/pr/product.jsp?id= 23193

U.S. Census Bureau. (2012). American Indian and Alaska Native Population: 2010. Retrieved from http://www.census.gov/prod/cen2010/briefs/c2010br-10.pdf

Venner, K. L., Feldstein, S. W., & Tafoya, N. (2006). Native American motivational interviewing: Weaving Native American and western practices—A manual for counselors in Native American communities. Retrieved from http://www.quantumunitsed.com/materials/5722_native%20america%20and%20motivational%20interviewing.pdf

Walls, M. L., Johnson, K. D., Whitbeck, L. B., & Hoyt, D. R. (2006). Mental health and substance abuse services preferences among American Indian people of the northern Midwest. *Community Mental Health Journal, 42*(6), 521–535.

Wiechelt, S. A., Gryczynski, J., Johnson, J. L., & Caldwell, D. (2012). Historical trauma among urban American Indians: Impact on substance abuse and family cohesion. *Journal of Loss and Trauma, 17*, 319–336.

Wu, L., Woody, G. E., Yang, C., Pan, J., & Blazer, D. G. (2011). Racial/ethnic variations in substance-abuse related disorders among adolescents in the United States. *Archives of General Psychiatry, 68*(11), 1176–1185.

Young, R. S., & Joe, J. R. (2009). Some thoughts about the epidemiology of alcohol and drug use among American Indian/Alaska Native populations. *Journal of Ethnicity in Substance Abuse, 8*(3), 223–241.

CHAPTER 6

ARAB AMERICANS

By Sejal M. Barden and W. Bryce Hagedorn

OVERVIEW OF POPULATION

Arab Americans have roots in the Middle East, North Africa, and the Arabic Peninsula. Not officially classified as a minority group, Arab Americans are a cultural group with unique values, norms, and beliefs (Moradi & Hasan, 2004). The Arab Anti-Discrimination Committee (ADC) defines *Arab* as "a cultural and linguistic term that includes people who share the Arabic language and Arabic culture" (ADC, n.d.). Unfortunately, this limited definition fails to acknowledge many Arab Americans who do not speak or understand the Arabic language. The authors, therefore, suggest the adoption of an alternate definition that describes Arab Americans as Americans whose ancestors originated from any one of 22 Arabic countries. These 22 countries include: Algeria, Bahrain, the Comoros Islands, Djibouti, Egypt, Iran, Jordan, Kuwait, Lebanon, Libya, Morocco, Mauritania, Oman, Palestine, Qatar, Saudi Arabia, Somalia, Sudan, Syria, Tunisia, the United Arab Emirates, and Yemen (Moradi & Hasan, 2004).

According to the U.S. Census Bureau (2010), over 1.7 million Americans living in the United States are of Arab descent. However, according to the Arab American Institute (AAI), actual population percentages are around 5.1 million persons (AAI, n.d). Historically, the U.S. Census Bureau has undercounted this population based on lack of knowledge, such as excluding certain subgroups from recognized Arabic-speaking countries (e.g., Somali and Sudanese). In addition to the diversity in country of origin, Arab Americans are greatly diverse in social class, level of education, native dialect, religion, acculturation, and time of immigration. Although Arab Americans are heterogeneous in many respects, some common values include the central role of family, respect for elders, prioritizing family ties over personal successes, and the importance of religious faith (Moradi & Hasan, 2004). Both areas of diversity and common values will be explored further in this chapter as they relate to addiction service needs for Arab Americans. In the next section, an overview of Arab American worldviews that may influence the engagement in services is provided.

ARAB AMERICAN WORLDVIEWS

Several cultural values (e.g., acculturation, family, and religion) contribute to Arab Americans' worldviews. The following section is a brief overview of these cultural values and is provided to assist counselors in working with Arab American clients.

Acculturation

Several factors influence the experiences of acculturation by Arab Americans, to include country of origin, length of time in the United States, reasons for immigration, separation of family, capability to visit or return to their home country, ability to speak English, and/or the presence of a distinct accent (Erickson & Timimi, 2001). Similarly, a family's educational level and socioeconomic status in their home country (i.e., "status") can be very different following immigration. For example, someone who was a medical doctor in her home country and then immigrates to American suddenly finds the only available job to be a custodian in a hospital: one can assume the pressures this would create and how it would contribute to families' acculturation and related stress.

Counselors are encouraged to assess levels of acculturation within individuals and between family members. For example, generational gaps exist that can negatively impact relationships. Arab American children born in the United States often do not feel the same cultural connections to their heritage as their parents do, which may create conflict and upheaval within the family system. On the other hand, a younger generation may desire stronger cultural connections to their roots and find it difficult to develop these connections. Another example of acculturation-related stress includes the challenges associated with feeling disconnected from one's community, which can result in difficulties adhering to traditional customs and religious ceremonies. In sum, counselors may want to assess adjustment difficulties and the presence or lack of community support when conceptualizing the role that acculturation plays on mental health and substance abuse issues (Erickson & Timimi, 2001).

Family

In addition to acculturation and ethnic identity, several other cultural factors influence Arab Americans' worldviews. Families are central to Arab societies and tend to be patriarchal. Fathers of the nuclear family are considered to be strong and powerful authority figures that make all decisions for the family. Arab societies are hierarchical and authoritarian in nature, with adults being perceived as the ultimate source of knowledge, wisdom, and power: elders are highly regarded and seen as knowledgeable and wise (Al-Krenawi & Graham, 2000). This viewpoint is found in many fables, expressed through common sayings such as, "Wisdom is found among adults," or "A day older in age is equal to a year older in understanding" (as cited in Al-Krenawi & Graham, 2000, p. 11). Furthermore, Arab Americans consider family honor and status as prioritized goals. As such, the idea of considering one's personal needs in any given situation may cause feelings of confusion and guilt, perceiving such individuation as having betrayed the family system (Erickson & Timimi, 2001).

Even with gender roles appearing oppressive and rigid at times, the centrality of family can be a real strength for Arab families. The pursuit of family honor has been found to encourage hard work, educational attainment, and economic advancement (Erickson & Timimi, 2001). To avoid bringing shame or dishonor to the family, individuals tend to avoid engaging in substance abuse and other criminal behavior, which can serve as a protective factor.

Religion

Similar to family, religion often plays a central role in the lives and worldviews of Arab Americans. Many Arab Americans are Muslim, or followers of Islam. Interestingly, Islam shares many beliefs and traits similar to, and based on, the same religious foundations as Christianity and Judaism. As such, Islam shares the belief in the sacred history of the Bible, adherence to the Ten Commandments, and a belief in one God (or *Allah*). Muslim religious practices are different from Christian practices in that they include: (a) an emphasis on the teachings and authority of Muhammad rather than on the teachings of Jesus; (b) specific dietary restrictions; (c) prayer five times per day; (d) worship services at a mosque led by an imam on the Sabbath (which is Friday); (e) fasting during the daylight hours of the holy month of Ramadan; and (f) one pilgrimage (if possible) to Mecca to pray and worship. Therefore, it is imperative for counselors to understand the importance of religion and values, beliefs, and worldviews when working with clients from Arab American backgrounds (Erickson & Timimi, 2001). Furthermore, while family and religion are central to Arab American worldviews, several barriers continue to perpetuate underutilization of addiction treatment services by Arab Americans. The authors provide a brief overview of such barriers in the next section.

BARRIERS TO TREATMENT

Several cultural barriers, including stigma, gender, ethnicity, and communication, contribute to the underutilization of addiction treatment services for Arab Americans. More specifically, barriers influencing Arab Americans may include feeling intimidated by the mental health care system, experiencing stigma (both internally and externally) for seeking emotional support, encountering language difficulties, and having previously worked with culturally insensitive counselors and other mental health professionals (Abi-Hashem, 2008). It is up to the culturally competent counselor to help her or his clients to work through these significant barriers.

Clients from Arab societies tend to have negative views of mental health and addiction treatment services, causing underutilization, early termination, and mistrust of helping professionals. Some of these negative views are formed by gender differences. For example, seeking addiction treatment for females of Arabian descent can be particularly stigmatizing in that it may damage their potential to get married (as they may be viewed as having "mental problems"), increase their risk of divorce and separation, and may be used as leverage for men of the Muslim faith to obtain a second wife (Al-Krenawi & Graham, 2000). On the other hand, given that Arab societies are patriarchal in nature, Arab men may have difficulty accepting and respecting directions from a female counselor. When working with couples and families, counselors are encouraged to address the males first and acknowledge their power as head of the family, while paying particular attention to not disrupting hierarchical patterns or gender roles within their client families.

Another barrier to treatment includes Arab communication styles and preference for privacy within families. Communication is often formal, impersonal, and restrained, with little emphasis on personal problems and feelings due to perceptions of being disloyal, weak, or both (Al-Issa, 1990). Self-exploration, client insight, and client affect are particularly difficult if perceived to damage family reputation or family honor. Furthermore, communication barriers are challenging based on miscommunications between clients and counselors. A lack of understanding of verbal and nonverbal behaviors can lead to incorrect assessments and unsuitable techniques. Consequently, to most effectively work with this population, it is imperative for counselors to understand the worldviews of Arab clients, as well as their own personal beliefs and values. Keeping the aforementioned sections in mind, the authors now transition into discussing substance abuse and treatment recommendations for Arab Americans in the remainder of this chapter.

SUBSTANCE ABUSE ISSUES

Research related to alcohol and other drug (AOD) use behaviors among Arab Americans is quite limited, partly resulting from inaccessibility to such populations (due in part to religious and/or foreign governmental interventions) and resulting from the personal absence of admittance of AODs (for the same reasons) (Arfken, Kubiak, & Farrag, 2009). Even less is known about the engagement of Arab Americans with addictive behaviors (gambling, sexuality, eating, and other behaviors), but Abi-Hashem (2008) noted some concerns about the scarcity of treatment opportunities for these behaviors due to the lack of admittance. Closer to home, AOD use has traditionally been restricted among the Arab population in America because of religious restrictions, limited access, and stigmatization.

Perhaps more than any other cultural group noted in this text, Arab American clients face a form of stigma that counselors must be ready to help them navigate, particularly given the aforementioned fact that Arab Americans already have a perceived stigma in seeking addiction treatment services. Within the Arabian culture, substance abuse is considered to be highly shameful on both a personal and familial level (Arfken, Kubiak, & Farrag, 2009). For those who ascribe to the Muslim religion and moral code, such behaviors are actually forbidden and bring grave consequences to the transgressor (Michalak, Trocki, & Bond, 2007). Michalak et al. (2007) note that the Qur'an prohibits the use of alcohol (and by association, any recreational drug), going so far as denoting it to be an abomination before Allah. Further, the authors noted that the Prophet Muhammad spoke to the curse of God falling upon anyone who associated with alcohol in any way, be it through the production, distribution, reception, transportation, or service of the drug. As a result of their unwillingness to admit to using substances due to their alcohol-restrictive culture/religion of origin, it is important for counselors to determine if this denial is more a cultural phenomenon, the result of the substance use itself (as denial is a classic symptom of substance abuse), or a combination thereof (Arfken et al., 2009).

Upon moving to the United States, Arab Americans experience additional risk factors, most notably marginalization, acculturation, and de-culturalization (a process whereby clients feel alienated both from the culture of their country of origin and the culture of the United States) (Amer & Hovey, 2007). Similar to other cultural groups for which AOD use is a problem, additional risk factors include (a) unstable family lives; (b) influences of peer-use patterns; and (c) favorable attitudes toward substances by the dominant media (Azaiza, Bar-Hamburger, & Moran, 2008). Interestingly, the "American" portion of "Arab American" may be the biggest risk factor for clients. More specifically, as noted earlier, whereas substance abuse has not been a concern for Arabs in their countries of origin, when they begin life in the United States, they gain the exposure, availability, and opportunity that they previously lacked.

Given that Arab Americans are relatively new to the phenomenon of substance abuse (and its associated problems), they may be more prone to legal consequences than other cultural groups. That is, whereas native-born Americans (without the Arabian moral/religious restrictions) often hear about the dangers of drinking alcohol and driving in their teenage years as a part of such programs as D.A.R.E. (Drug Abuse Resistance Education) or M.A.D.D. (Mothers Against Drunk Driving), Arab Americans may have missed these educational opportunities, since the topic of alcohol use is avoided. Therefore, when Arab Americans choose to consume alcohol, they may do so with little regard for their ability to operate an automobile. The study by Arfken et al. (2009) verified this predicament when they noted that more than 43 percent of Arab Americans who entered publicly funded treatment for substance abuse did so as a result of involvement with the legal system (compared to 10 percent of African Americans, 26 percent for Caucasians, 37 percent for Hispanics, and 23 percent for all other admissions). Therefore, for those working with the Arab American population, an emphasis on education and prevention would predictably lower these numbers.

The lack of attention to the AOD abuse of Arab Americans has led to a dearth of culturally specific assessment instruments, a predicament noted by Karam, Yabroudi, and Melhem (2002). Therefore, one must be mindful of the use of standardized screening and assessment instruments because almost all of the instruments used in the United States have been created for, and thus normed on, Euro-American clients. Whereas translating assessments into the native language of one's clients is a significant step toward being culturally sensitive, many of the American concepts found in such instruments do not transfer to the various Arabic languages. Given that there are two general groups to consider when working with Arab Americans (those who have recently moved to the United States and those who were born in and/or have been living in America for a while), assessing can take two different formats. Abi-Hashem (2008) suggests counselors use projective type assessment instruments for those who have recently immigrated to the United States (as well as for those who do not have a high level of education). On the other hand, for English-speaking and well-educated clients, the more common substance abuse inventories may work favorably.

Studies like those done by Abou-Saleh, Ghubash, and Daradkeh (2001) demonstrate the utility of expanding the use of assessment questions related to AOD use. These authors found that when participants were asked directly about their AOD use, they reported extremely low rates of use. But when asked about household problems that can be attributed to AOD use, participants' responses quadrupled. The need to expand assessment questions coupled with the lack of culturally sensitive assessment instruments that can circumvent the denial expressed by Arab American clients is clear; therefore, the current authors advocate for the creation of a modified instrument that can help clients speak about their AOD use.

Perhaps one of the most clinically used and researched assessment instruments in addiction counseling is the CAGE clinical interview, developed by Ewing and Rouse in 1970 (Ewing, 1984). Each of the four letters remind the assessor of clinically relevant questions to ask their AOD-using clients to determine the severity of their substance use disorder (the more questions answered affirmatively, the more severe the disorder). Below, the current authors offer a culturally altered version of the CAGE for work with Arab American clients, with the express caveat that this version has not been tested on an Arab American population. Rather, the authors tried to capture the intent of the four original questions while remaining cognizant of the cultural influences experienced by Arabian clients.

- Original question to ascertain the client's desire to control, cut back, or stop AOD use:
  - *Have you ever felt as though you should **C**ut down on your substance use?*
  - *Adapted question:*
    - *Has your use of AOD **C**ut off your connections to those things you hold dear?*
- Original question to ascertain the interpersonal impacts of AOD use:
  - *Have you ever felt **A**nnoyed by someone who was criticizing your substance use?*
  - *Adapted question:*
    - *Are you **A**shamed of how your use of AOD has impacted people close to you?*
- Original question to ascertain the personal impacts of AOD use:
  - *Do you ever feel **G**uilty about your substance use?*
  - *This question needs no adaptation.*
- Original question to ascertain the presence of withdrawal:
  - *Do you ever use the substance in the morning to steady your nerves or to get rid of a hangover (**E**ye opener)?*
  - *Adapted question:*
    - *Have your **E**yes been opened to the amount of substances that you're using to obtain the same effect?*

As Arab American clients find themselves struggling more and more with AOD and other addictive behaviors, the need for culturally competent care becomes more apparent. In the next section, the authors provide our recommendations for treating Arabian clients.

RECOMMENDATIONS FOR TREATMENT

In light of the aforementioned unique cultural considerations, characteristics, and challenges, working with Arab American clients who struggle with addictive disorders requires culturally sensitive settings and culturally competent clinicians. Before moving into the needed competencies for counselors, the authors offer several suggestions that can help establish a clinical environment where Arab American clients will feel comfortable enough to engage in the therapeutic process.

Clinical Environment

There are many aspects to creating an inviting environment for Arab American clients to find recovery. First, to address the stigma experienced by Arab American clients, Arfken et al. (2009) note the clinical efficacy of posting signs which read, *Addiction Is a Disease, Not a Disgrace* in both Arabic and English throughout the facility. Similarly, treatment centers that avoid confrontation as a primary modality and instead espouse respect for all clients will experience more favorable results with these clients. Third, Arfken et al. (2009) recommend that a shared language is crucial in connecting with Arabian clients. Given the multitude of countries sharing an "Arabian" designation, this may present quite the challenge, but even when staff members make an effort at connecting by using clients' primary language, treatment outcomes can be improved.

A final environmental suggestion was made by Dwairy (2006), who notes the need to respect Arab American clients' (particularly those of the Muslim religion) need to pray five times per day. Thus, it would be important for addiction facilities to (a) provide a setting where such praying can occur that is distraction free; and (b) avoid scheduling sessions at times that would interfere with such observances. Similarly, Muslim clients are called to fast (go without food) during the month of Ramadan, which occurs during the ninth month in the Islamic calendar (this typically occurs during the months of June, July, or August for a period of 30 days—consult the Internet for the correct days of each year, as it changes). This information is important for counselors working with Arab American clients who have addictive relationships with food or who have tended to substitute addictions. Before one confronts an observed maladaptive eating pattern, be sure to check the calendar and inquire as to the religious observances of your clients.

Culturally Competent Clinicians

It is imperative that culturally competent counselors create a change-friendly environment for working with Arab American clients who struggle with addictive disorders. Abi-Hashem (2008) offers several suggestions to work with Arab American clients in general, which the current authors adapted to working in the area of addiction counseling. These suggestions are ordered into the following categories: preclinical awareness, making the initial connection/establishing trust, appropriate approaches and techniques, moving into the therapeutic realm, and general caveats.

Preclinical Awareness

Prior to beginning any therapeutic work with Arab American clients, Abi-Hashem (2008) advises that counselors remain cognizant of the fact that the term "Arab American" encompasses individuals with a wide variety of religions, educational backgrounds, social classes, personal histories, and worldviews. When it comes to addiction counseling, while counselors do their best to remain culturally sensitive, the *culture of addiction* (i.e., addicted clients tend to act fairly similarly as a result of their disease) can be so pervasive that it is often easy to overlook the unique characteristics of each client. Counselors will need to be vigilant to remain cognizant of impacts of both the culture of their clients and the culture of addiction in their work with clients.

The Initial Connection/Establishing Trust

Abi-Hashem (2008) offers several suggestions, which, when used appropriately, can help counselors to initially bond/establish trust with their clients. These include addressing differences, establishing commonalities, and balancing professionalism and approachability. First, it is important to recognize and address the differences between the counselor and his or her clients. Prudence calls for bringing this discussion into the here-and-now by directly asking clients to discuss their thoughts and feelings about sharing personal matters with a counselor who is different from them. If concerns are expressed, a counselor should try to normalize apprehensions, and if a referral is requested and feasible, to follow through with that request. Given the fact that many Arab American clients enter community-based drug treatment as a result of legal consequences (noted earlier by Arfken et al., 2009), their options for referral may be limited by the nature of the setting. Nevertheless, taking the time to discuss differences is an important part of bridging gaps.

After addressing dissimilarities, it is important to find some areas of commonality in order to help establish clients' trust and confidence in their counselor (Abi-Hashem, 2008). Some addiction counselors use their own recovery status or experiences with alcohol and drug use as a means to connect with clients (e.g., "I understand what you must be going through, because when I was in your shoes …"). The current authors suggest avoiding this as a means of bonding with Arab American clients, as their respect for the counselor (another crucial element to the bonding process) may be diminished by such a disclosure. Instead, find other ways to connect such as sharing (a) personal heritage stories; (b) the challenges associated with making significant changes; or (c) a time when the counselor tried something new and unfamiliar. Ultimately, when counseling Arab American clients, it is important to remember the significant differences that can easily separate counselors from their clients and be prepared to navigate these differences so that trust can flourish.

Finally, whereas counselors must maintain their professional demeanor, Abi-Hashem (2008) notes the need for clinicians to balance their professionalism with a demonstrated personal ease and unconventionality when connecting with Arab American clients.

For addiction counselors, this involves the cultivation of a less rigid posture. Doing so can be challenging for novice counselors who are still learning to balance empathy with professional distance (i.e., not becoming invested in clients' problems to the extent that it causes personal distress). Counselors should treat their Arab American clients warmly and genuinely with a mixture of flexibility, friendliness, and spontaneity (all of which admittedly can be challenging when working within the field of addiction counseling). One overt sign indicating clients feel comfortable with their counselors is when they bring tokens of appreciation or gifts and/or when they invite their counselors to their home for a meal. Obviously, addiction counselors must follow the code of ethics that govern their profession regarding the acceptance of gifts and avoiding dual relationships. At the same time, counselors can do this in ways that do not damage the relationships that they worked so diligently to establish.

Appropriate Approaches and Techniques

Once trust has been established, the culturally competent counselor must be mindful of the approaches and techniques that she or he uses with Arab American clients, and how these differ from working with clients in the cultural majority. Abi-Hashem (2008) notes the importance of being intentional with the use of questions, silence, attendance to nonverbal behaviors, use of suggestions and interpretations, and the avoidance of generalizations. When using questions (even from the outset during the intake process), counselors should be patient with their clients and inquire gently. Pressuring Arab American clients with rapid-fire questions (which can become the norm in addiction counseling) can increase the distance that was so diligently circumvented earlier in the relationship. Next, the competent counselor should become very comfortable with therapeutic silence. While many addiction counselors are sensitive to the variety of resistances that addicted clients exhibit (e.g., defensiveness, evasiveness, unnecessary repetitions, indirect answers to questions), they must not misinterpret such behaviors in their Arabian clients. Rather, patience will again be rewarded with information if counselors remember Arabian clients' preferences for politeness, slow disclosures, repetitions of information, indirectness, low expressiveness, and/or minimal eye contact.

In addition to appreciating silence and the different presentation styles of Arab American clients, counselors should be ready to learn from the variety of nonverbal behaviors exhibited by their clients. Again, with patience, therapists can learn from an assortment of common phrases, gestures, and signals as to how their clients share personal emotions and thoughts (Abi-Hashem, 2008). This is particularly important given the timing necessary to provide feedback to clients. Arab American clients often seek direct advice from their health care providers and prefer an instant cure (Dwairy, 2006). Therefore, addiction counselors must be culturally sensitive in offering such feedback and interpretations and also should be clear with any offered advice, suggestions, or instructions.

The final consideration in using approaches and techniques with Arab American clients is to be particularly careful to avoid any generalizations. Whereas this may seem like it should go without saying, many messages regarding the Arabian cultures can become unwittingly ingrained into American counselors' minds, particularly given the events of September 11, 2001 (or 9/11), and associated tragedies. Imagine the damage yielded by comments such as, "You Arabs …" "the Middle East is filled with fanatics," or "Arabian women are too passive and should avoid being dominated by their men." Should such comments be inadvertently spoken by a counselor, a quick and heartfelt apology may be able to repair some of the damage. The authors recommend counselors to be honest with clients whenever a rift has occurred in the relationship, owning their portions of the rift, not making excuses, and making a commitment to being different from that point forward.

Moving into the Therapeutic Realm

Having gained rapport with culturally sensitive approaches, Abi-Hashem (2008) makes several suggestions for helping to move Arab American clients into the therapeutic realm (i.e., when "digging deep"). First, it is crucial to proceed with sensitivity when exploring the impact of clients' cultural influences on the struggles that bring them into counseling, such as their faith, values, norms, beliefs, customs, and traditions. In the area of addiction counseling, the authors cannot overemphasize the importance of sensitivity when it comes to exploring clients' cultural influences given the combined nature of the shame/disgrace that clients feel (e.g., for Muslims, the use of alcohol is a damnable offense), the familial stigmas imposed, and the societal biases and discriminations experienced. Addiction counselors have the additional struggle of having to "lean into" the natural resistance that many addicted clients exhibit when faced with the need for change. Therefore, counselors need to balance their recognition and appreciation of clients' situations and difficulties while remaining true to the needed work of addressing the maladaptive behaviors, which contributed to their arriving in drug treatment in the first place.

According to Amer and Hovey (2007) and Azaiza and colleagues (2008), many precipitants contribute to substance use for Arab Americans. Examples include:

- Acculturation
- Marginalization
- Unstable family lives
- Increased exposure, availability, and opportunity to use substances
- Trauma
  - *Civil unrest*
  - *War and/or disaster*
  - *Discrimination and/or violence*
- Grief
  - *Loss of a loved one*

- *Losses attributed to leaving the home country*
- Bereavement

Abi-Hashem (2008) noted the importance of exploring clients' issues related to the aforementioned precipitants (including trauma, grief, and loss) and for American counselors to be prepared to explore areas (e.g., war atrocities) that they have never been exposed to. Addiction counselors would then wisely apply the necessary and appropriate interventions that would address the impact of these issues on clients' substance use. To ignore the impact of such significant events during addiction treatment would be similar to affixing a bandage (e.g., "Today, I will present this psycho-educational lesson on how to manage relapse warning signs") to an amputated limb (i.e., a client's exposure to war atrocities). As a result, clients will likely continue to numb emotional trauma with alcohol and other drugs until it has been addressed therapeutically.

General Caveats

To conclude this section on treatment recommendations and therapeutic considerations, Abi-Hashem (2008) offers three general caveats that will help American counselors to connect with their Arab American clients. First, clients feel honored when counselors remember and respect the private information that has been shared with them. Addiction counselors must, therefore, be diligent to take the extra time to review case notes before engaging with their clients (thus avoiding the "one-approach-fits-all" style common to addiction treatment). Next, counselors are encouraged to engage fully in the connection process, and thus allow them to grow and transform as a result of enriching cultural encounters. This can be particularly important for addiction counselors who often find themselves burned out by what they interpret to be the same types of clients, day in and day out. Finally, Arab American clients appreciate the efforts made by their counselors. Offering oneself as a person who cares will be met with positivity and gratefulness on the part of clients.

In summary, counselors working with Arab American clients must be cognizant of potential biases and outright discrimination. Whereas prejudice and discrimination existed prior to the 9/11 attacks, negative feelings and actions against Arab Americans has increased significantly since 2001 (Padela & Heisler, 2010). Counselors are not immune to reacting to their feelings about those events and must be very careful about imposing their beliefs onto their Arab American clients. Counselors who are diligent in circumnavigating their own biases and helping their clients through their stigmas and barriers will be well on their way to helping Arab American clients live a healthy and drug-free life.

Reflection Questions

Increasing self-awareness is paramount for providing culturally competent care for Arab American clients. Use the following questions as a guide to discuss in small groups of three to four people.

1. Share three common stereotypes/myths that you have heard about Arab Americans.
2. Reflect on your attitudes and beliefs about Arab Americans. Consider how media has shaped your beliefs and/or assumptions (e.g., images of terrorism, 9/11, depictions of Arab Americans worshipping, coverage of war in the Middle East) and how they may affect your effectiveness in working with these clients.

3. Consider the patriarchal structure and adherence to strict gender roles in many Arab American families. Discuss your assumptions about women and oppression, sharing similarities and differences between your upbringing and values compared to your perception of Arab American values related to gender roles.
4. Given some of the aforementioned cultural challenges (both those of Arab Americans and those of non-Arabian counselors), share some of your concerns about helping clients navigate addiction treatment and recovery.

REFERENCES

Abi-Hashem, N. (2008). Arab Americans: Understanding their challenges, needs, and struggles. In A. J. Marsella, J. L. Johnson, P. Watson, & J. Gryczynski (Eds.), *Ethnocultural perspectives on disaster and trauma: Foundations, issues, and applications* (pp. 115–173). New York: Springer Science + Business Media. doi:10.1007/978-0-387-73285-5_5

Abou-Saleh, M. T., Ghubash, R., & Daradkeh, T. K. (2001). Al Ain community psychiatric survey 1: Prevalence and sociodemographic correlates. *Social Psychiatry and Psychiatric Epidemiology, 36*, 20–28.

Al-Issa, A. (1990). Culture and mental illness in Algeria. *International Journal of Social Psychiatry, 36*, 230–240.

Al-Krenawi, A., & Graham, J. R. (2000). Culturally sensitive social work practice with Arab clients in mental health settings. *Health Social Work, 25*, 9–22.

Amer, M., & Hovey, J. D. (2007). Sociodemographic differences in acculturation and mental health for a sample of 2nd-generation/early immigrant Arab Americans. *Journal of Immigrant and Minority Health, 9*, 335–347.

American-Arab Anti-Discrimination Committee. (n.d.). *Facts about Arabs and the Arab world*. Retrieved June 16, 2013, from http://www.adc.org/index.php?id_248 Arab American Institute (n.d.). *The U. S. Census and Arab Americans*. Retrieved June 16, 2013, from http://www.aaiusa.org/census

Arfken, C. L., Kubiak, S. P., & Farrag, M. (2009). Acculturation and polysubstance abuse in Arab American treatment clients. *Transcultural Psychiatry, 46*, 608–622. doi: 10.1177/1363461509351364

Azaiza, F., Bar-Hamburger, R., & Moran, M. (2008). Psychoactive substance use among Arab adolescents in Israel. *Journal of Social Work Practice in the Addictions, 89*(1), 21–43. http://dx.doi.org/10.1080/15332560802108613

Dayton, T. (2005). The use of psychodrama in dealing with grief and addiction-related loss and trauma. *Journal of Group Psychotherapy: Psychodrama & Sociometry, 58*, 15–34. doi:10.3200/JGPP.58.1.15-34

Dwairy, M. A. (2006). *Counseling and psychotherapy with Arabs and Muslims: A culturally sensitive approach*. New York: Teachers College Press.

Erickson, C. D., & Al-Timimi, N. R. (2001). Providing mental health services to Arab Americans: Recommendations and considerations. *Cultural Diversity and Ethnic Minority Psychology, 7(4)*, 308–327.

Ewing, J. A. (1984). Detecting alcoholism. *Journal of the American Medical Association, 252*, 1905–1907.

Karam, E. G., Yabroudi, P. F., & Melhem, N. M. (2002). Comorbidity of substance abuse and other psychiatric disorders in acute general psychiatric admissions: A study from Lebanon. *Comprehensive Psychiatry, 43*, 463–468. doi:10.1053/comp.2002.35910

Khoury, L., Tang, Y. L., Bradley, B., Cubells, J. F., & Ressler, K. J. (2010). Substance use, childhood traumatic experience, and posttraumatic stress disorder in an urban civilian population. *Depression and Anxiety, 27*, 1077–1086. doi:10.1002/da.20751

Michalak, L., Trocki, K., & Bond, J. (2007). Religion and alcohol in the U.S. National Alcohol Survey: How important is religion for abstention and drinking? *Drug and Alcohol Dependence, 87*, 268–280. Retrieved http://dx.doi.org/10.1016/j.drugalcdep.2006.07.013

Moradi, B., & Hasan, N. T. (2004). Arab American persons reported experiences of discrimination and mental health: The mediating role of personal control. *Journal of Counseling Psychology, 51 (4)*, 418–428.

Padela, A. I., & Heisler, M. (2010). The association of perceived abuse and discrimination after September 11, 2001, with psychological distress, level of happiness, and health status among Arab Americans. *American Journal of Public Health, 100*, 284–291.

United States Census Bureau (2010). *Statistical abstract of the United States.* Washington, DC.

CHAPTER 7

ASIAN AMERICANS AND PACIFIC ISLANDERS

By Tiffany Lee and Giao Tran

OVERVIEW

By the year 2050, there will be more than 40.6 million Asians living in the United States, comprising 9.2 percent of the total population (United States Census, 2008). "Asian" refers to a person having origins in the Indian subcontinent, Far East, or Southeast Asia. There are many countries included in this population, and the cultures and religions are very diverse. For instance, people from India, Pakistan, China, Japan, Korea, Malaysia, Cambodia, the Philippine Islands, Thailand, and Vietnam are all considered Asian. Their religion may be Hinduism, Islam, Sikhism, or Buddhism. Geographically, 46 percent of the Asian population live in the western United States, with 32 percent living in California. As far as ethnic groups, the largest Asian group identified is Chinese, followed by Filipino and Asian Indian (U.S. Census, 2012). In addition to Asians, this chapter will also provide information regarding Native Hawaiians and other Pacific Islanders (i.e., those who identify as being from Hawaii, Guam, Samoa, or other Pacific Islands). Overall, 1.2 million people, or 0.4 percent of the U.S. population, identified as Native Hawaiian and other Pacific Islander in 2010. More than half (56 percent) of this population, or 685,000 people, reported being Native Hawaiian and other Pacific Islander in combination with one or more other races. This particular multiracial group grew by 40 percent from 2000 to 2010 (U.S. Census, 2012).

For the purposes of this chapter, the authors will address Asians and Native Hawaiians and other Pacific Islanders separately, when necessary. However, when referring to these two populations as a group, the authors will use the acronym AAPI. The AAPI population is a heterogeneous group that is comprised of at least 20 different ethnic subgroups (Fong & Tsuang, 2007). As stated throughout this text, there are many cultural differences that exist within racial/ethnic populations. Therefore, the information presented in this chapter is generalized and will not be true for everyone who identifies as Asian, Native Hawaiian, or other Pacific Islander. Moreover, people have *intersectionality* of multiple identities (e.g., female, lesbian, foreign born). Some of these identities cause a person of color to experience additional stress due to the oppression and discrimination associated with being a part of another marginalized group (Gopaldas, 2013). Thus, the various identities (and the developmental status associated with these identities) must be taken into account when providing counseling services.

STATISTICS

According to the U.S. Census Bureau in 2010, there were 14.7 million people who identified as Asian living in America, constituting 4.8 percent of the total population (U.S. Census, 2012). Taking into account those who identified as Asian and another race, this number totaled 17.3 million people, or 5.6 percent. Over the ten years between 2000 and 2010, the Asian population grew faster than any other racial group in the United States. More specifically, the number of people who self-identified Asian as their only race increased by 43 percent, which was four times the rate of increase in the total population. Further, biracial (or multiracial) individuals who identified as Asian and another race grew even faster. From 2000 to 2010, the Asian multiracial population grew by about one million people, which constituted a 60 percent increase (U.S. Census, 2012).

In 2011, the median household income for the Asian population was $67,885 (U.S. Census, 2013). Asian groups varied greatly in their household income. For instance, Asian Indians had a median income of $92,418 in 2011, while Bangladeshi had an income of $45,185. The poverty rate was 12.8 percent, and 15.4 percent had no health insurance. In regard to the prevalence of higher education among Asian Americans, 50 percent of Asians 25 years and older reported a bachelor's degree or higher (as compared to 28.5 percent of all Americans in this age group). In addition, 20.7 percent had a graduate degree (as compared to 10.6 percent of all Americans).

Substance Use

Historically, studies have found Asians have the lowest rates of substance use, substance-related diagnoses, and treatment admissions. The National Survey on Drug Use and Health (NSDUH) has published data on alcohol and other drug use rates from 2002 to 2012 (the results are displayed below in Figure 7.1) (SAMHSA, 2013a). As shown, Asians have consistently reported the lowest rates of past-month use as compared to other racial/ethnic groups.

In addition to substance use rates, co-occurring disorders among Asian Americans also appear to be lower than in other racial/ethnic groups. In 2012, the percentage of adults (aged 18 or older) with a comorbid mental illness and substance use disorder in the past year was 1.1 percent among Asians, 3.3 percent among blacks, 3.4 percent among Hispanics, 3.8 percent among whites, 4.3 percent among persons reporting two or more races, and 14.0 percent among American Indians or Alaska Natives (SAMHSA, 2013a).

When comparing Asian Americans to the national average, researchers have found vast differences in percentage rates related to past-month alcohol use, binge alcohol use, and illicit drug use. The national averages were considerably higher. For instance, 39.8 percent of Asian Americans reported alcohol consumption in the last month, compared to alcohol use rate of 55.2 percent in the general population. Binge drinking patterns among Asians were also shown to be lower than the national average (24.5 percent versus 13.2 percent, respectively). In addition, past-month illicit drug use was over two and a half times higher in the general population. The national average was 7.9 percent and prevalence among Asians was 3.4 percent (SAMHSA, 2010).

Researchers have also examined the variations of substance use among numerous Asian subgroups. Past-month binge alcohol use ranged from a high of 25.9 percent among Korean adults to a low of 8.4 percent among Chinese adults (SAMHSA, 2010). Moreover, Japanese Americans reported the highest

Asian Americans and Pacific Islanders | 93

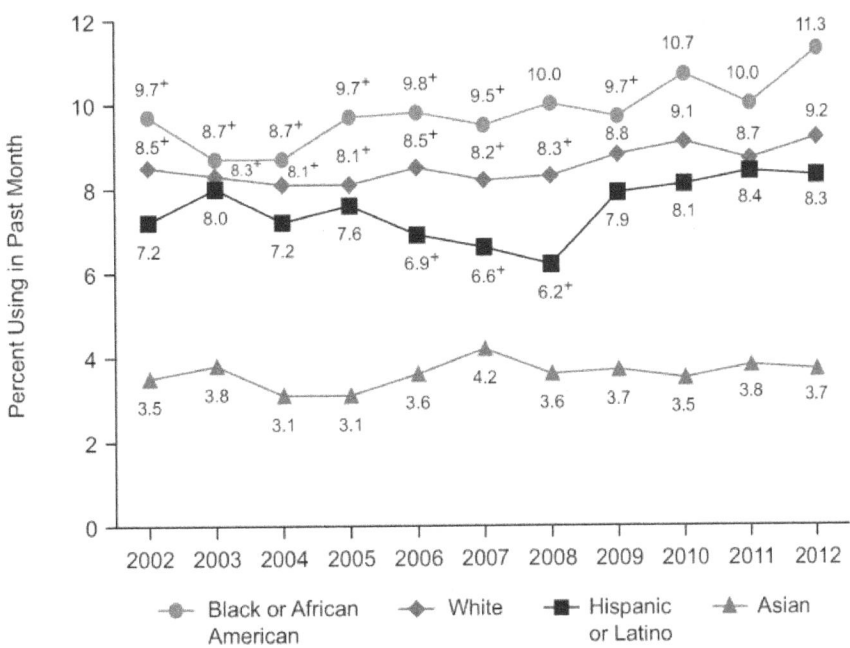

Figure 7.1: Percent of Past-Month Illicit Drug Use among Racial/Ethnic Groups. Taken from SAMHSA (2013a). *Results from the 2012 National Survey on Drug Use and Health: Summary of National Findings.* **Rockville, MD: SAMHSA.**

Source: SAMHSA / Public Domain.

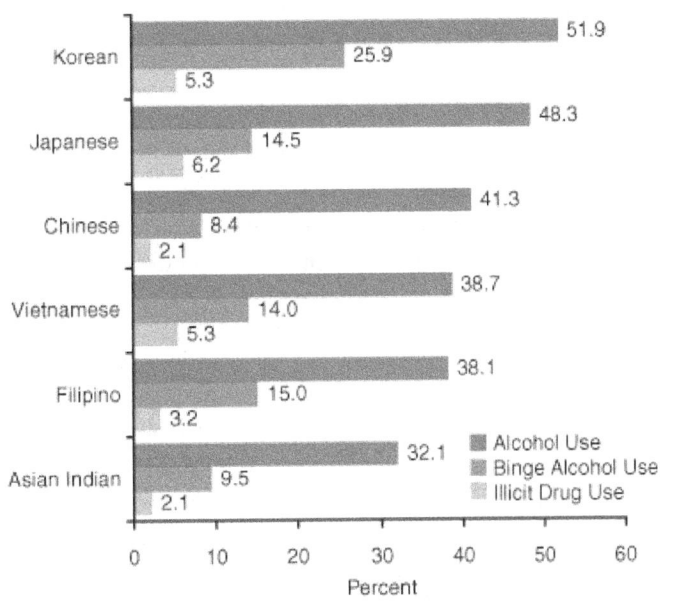

Figure 7.2: Differences in Alcohol and Illicit Drug Use among Asian Groups.

Source: SAMHSA / Public Domain.

illicit drug use rates, and Chinese and Asian Indians demonstrated the lowest rates (6.2 percent and 2.1 percent, respectively). Figure 7.2 below illustrates substance use disparities between Korean, Japanese, Chinese, Vietnamese, Filipino, and Asian Indian adults.

A recent SAMHSA (2010) report also suggests different rates of substance use by U.S.-born Asian adults and foreign-born Asian adults. U.S.-born Asians reported binge drinking frequency twice as high as foreign-born Asians (22 percent versus 11 percent). Furthermore, past-month illicit drug use among U.S.-born Asian adults was nearly triple the rate of foreign-born Asian adults (7.3 percent versus 2.5 percent).

According to NSDUH, AAPIs were less likely to need substance abuse treatment than other racial/ethnic groups (4.9 percent and 9.5 percent, respectively) (SAMHSA, 2013b). Of those entering treatment, researchers have shown AAPIs have significantly more stable living conditions, lower levels of alcohol and drug severity problems, and less lifetime criminal involvement (Niv, Wong, & Hser, 2007). AAPIs also reported more negative attitudes toward treatment and rated treatment as significantly less important than other racial/ethnic groups.

When investigating the primary drug of choice among those who enter treatment, Treatment Episode Data Set (TEDS) showed that methamphetamine was the primary substance of abuse in 20 percent of the treatment admissions by AAPIs. In contrast, only 5.9 percent of other racial/ethnic groups reported methamphetamine as the drug of choice (SAMHSA, 2012). In other words, methamphetamine was three times more likely to be identified as the primary drug used when entering treatment by AAPIs than other populations. (Among AAPIs, it should be noted methamphetamine use is particularly high among Pacific Islanders.)

As far as treatment readmissions, AAPIs who have attended treatment have demonstrated lower rates of subsequent treatment attempts (Yu & Warner, 2013). Researchers have suggested the reasons could be: (1) treatment was helpful and no additional interventions were needed for sustaining recovery; (2) treatment was not helpful due to linguistic and cultural issues with services; or (3) the preference was to use personal networks versus formal treatment programs.

In summary, the previous sections presented information on the subgroups of AAPIs, including countries of origin, population rates, education attainment and income, and the prevalence of substance use. Before discussing issues specific to substance use and abuse for this particular population, the authors provide a brief introduction into the racism and oppression that the AAPIs have faced over the past century, including how racism against this population influenced drug legislation.

Racism and Oppression

Historically, AAPIs have experienced many different forms of racism, discrimination, and oppression, including economic exploitation, harassment, and violence. The National Asian Pacific American Legal Consortium reported 243 incidents against AAPIs (generally South Asian Americans) occurred in the three months following September 11, 2001. As of January 2002, the Intergroup Clearinghouse reports there have been more than 1,700 cases of discrimination against Arab Americans, Muslim Americans, Sikh Americans, and South Asian Americans. In addition to individual acts of racism by the general public, the U.S. government also has a history of racist acts. For example, in 1942, after the attack on Pearl Harbor, President Franklin D. Roosevelt signed Executive Order 9066, which forced more than 110,000 Japanese people living on the Pacific Coast to leave their homes and businesses and move into "relocation centers" (or internment camps) in desolate areas of the western and southern United States. This relocation mandate was based on the assumption that Japanese Americans would be loyal to the emperor of Japan and could not be trusted (as cited by Kim & Park, 2013). In addition to the imposed physical containment and isolation, there have been laws enacted barring Asians from becoming citizens, owning land, and immigrating to the United States. Due to unsubstantiated claims that created intense fears among whites, various laws (such as the Immigration Act of 1924) were passed to perpetuate racism and the marginalization of AAPIs. Moreover, some of these laws had to do with controlling who could produce, dispense, and sell certain substances (e.g., opium).

In the late 1800s and early 1900s, there were declarations made that generated and maintained racism against Asians, in particular the Chinese who came to work on the railroad. In 1890, newspaper publisher William Randolph Hearst began a series of articles about the "yellow menace," describing how Chinese men were seducing white women with opium. There was already a dislike for the Chinese, who many feared would overrun America and cause whites to lose their jobs (called the "yellow peril"). To illustrate the extent of overt racism that existed during that time, see the picture below created by Joseph Keppler in 1878. The images in Figure 7.3 below depict Chinese laborers smoking opium and eating rats, as compared to a cozy domestic scene of an American family home with a sign that reads, "God Bless Our Home" near its entrance. This type of propaganda and the various tenuous allegations (against the Chinese and African Americans) influenced the passing of the Harrison Narcotics Tax Act of 1914. This law was the government's attempt to provide more control over drug use by requiring those who produce, manufacture, import, dispense, and sell opium and coca leaves (and their derivatives) to register and pay a tax.

Even half a century after the Harrison Act passed, there were still blatantly racist laws in the U.S. legislation. For instance, statues existed that prohibited marriage between AAPIs and whites. Not until 1967,

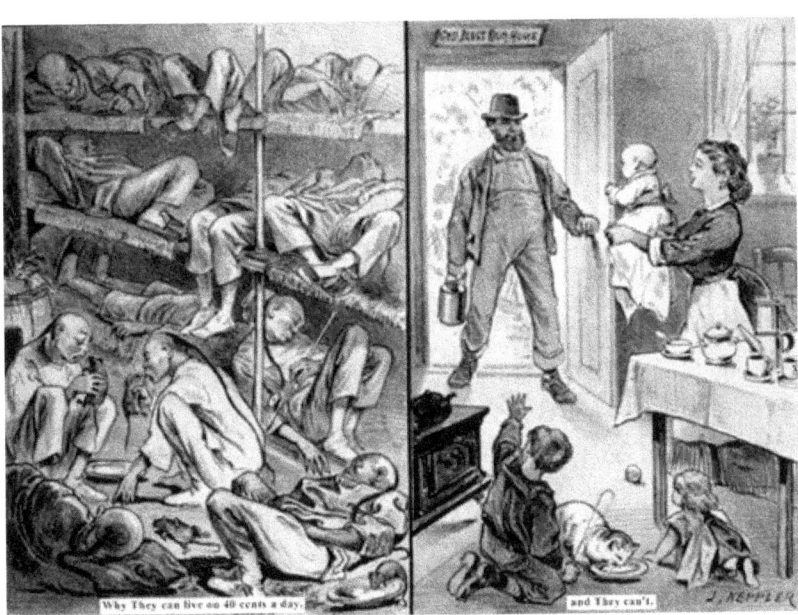

Figure 7.3: *Why They can live on 40 cents a day … and They can't.* **A racist illustration contrasting an American family and Chinese laborers.** (Retrieved from http://www.sciencephoto.com/media/268549/view or http://www.docstoc.com/docs/109549584/Political-Cartoon-Documents-4-6).

Source: Courtesy of Joseph Keppler.

with the Supreme Court's ruling in *Loving v. Virginia*, were interracial marriages and interracial sex legal in many states. Later in the 20th century, however, there were events that occurred which recognized and celebrated AAPIs. In 1978, for example, President Jimmy Carter spoke of the significant role AAPIs have played in American society with contributions to the sciences, arts, industry, government, and commerce. Legislation was passed establishing Asian/Pacific American Heritage Week. The first ten days of May were chosen to coincide with two important milestones in Asian/Pacific Islander American history: (1) the arrival of the first Japanese immigrants (May 7, 1843); and (2) the contributions of Chinese workers who helped build the transcontinental railroad (completed May 10, 1869). In 1992, Congress expanded the observance to a month-long celebration.

While progress has been made, racism, prejudice, and discrimination still exist for people of color. One has to remember that not even 60 years ago, a white and Asian could not marry one another. Currently, the overt, blatant, violent acts of racism of yesteryear have been replaced with the covert, subtle acts of racism (i.e., microaggressions) that occur for many AAPIs on a daily basis. A common example of a microaggression would be asking a U.S.-born Asian American, "Where are you from?" or "What are you?" In summary, the history of racism and the current state of oppression and marginalization of this population must be taken into account when counseling AAPIs and their families. The issues raised in this section may have an impact on substance use among AAPIs, and there are other concerns that could impact whether someone in this population uses or chooses not to use alcohol and other drugs. The next section will discuss the substance abuse issues specific to this population, including the risk and preventive factors and the barriers to treatment.

SUBSTANCE ABUSE ISSUES

Certain factors exist among individuals, as well as groups of individuals, that impact the likelihood of using substances, in addition to the probability of seeking help for addiction problems. For example, some individuals may be more at risk for substance abuse due to exposure to drug-using peers or the chronic stress associated with discrimination and oppression. On the other hand, some people have religious views or engage in activities that increase their desire to abstain from drug use and prevent substance misuse. This section will address the risk and preventive factors that apply to some AAPIs.

Risk and Preventive Factors

One aspect that may inhibit chemical misuse is biological in nature. For example, a person may not enjoy drinking alcohol because of the negative effects experienced during and after use; AAPIs (in particular East Asians) often have this ethanol sensitivity. This sensitivity results from a deficiency in the aldehyde dehydrogenase isozyme (ALDH2), which breaks down alcohol. Due to this shortage in ALDH2, a person can: (a) become flush or blotchy on the face and body; (b) have an increase in heart rate; (c) become nauseous and vomit; and/or (d) have more severe hangover effects. This is commonly called "flushing syndrome" and is frequently seen in those of Chinese, Japanese, and Korean descent. Furthermore, research asserts that those who consume alcohol and have this ALDH2 deficiency are at higher risk for esophageal cancer (National Institutes of Health, 2009).

Chemical use at an early age tends to increase the likelihood of developing a substance use disorder later on in life. One preventive factor for Asian Americans is the lower rates of use as a young adult (i.e., those aged 18 to 25 years) than the average young adult in the United States. For instance, the national average of illicit drug use among young adults is more than twice that of young Asian adults (19.7 percent versus 9.1 percent) (SAMHSA, 2010). Disparities between young Asian adults and the national average were also found in alcohol use (48.5 percent versus 61.1 percent) and binge alcohol use (25.7 percent versus 41.6 percent).

In addition to young adults, researchers have also investigated substance use in AAPI youth (i.e., younger than 18 years old). While rates among AAPIs as a group appear to be lower than youth of other racial/ethnic groups, investigations have actually found Native Hawaiian youth have higher rates of drug use when comparing youth of other racial/ethnic groups, particularly Native Hawaiians who live in rural areas (Von Wormer & Davis, 2013). When examining differences between AAPI youth and AAPI adults, substance use is more prevalent in AAPI youth than in older generations of AAPIs. These disparities have been said to be due to acculturation of youth (Le, Goebert, & Wallen, 2009).

Other studies have investigated whether substance use rates are different among Asian youth who identify as mono-racial and those youth who identify as multiracial; some results yielded great variance in use rates. For instance, one study found Chinese and Vietnamese American multiracial adolescents were four times more likely to use substances than Chinese and Vietnamese mono-racial adolescents (Price, Risk, Wong, & Klingle, 2002).

Asian adolescents in one qualitative study indicated a risk factor for use is the lack of communication by their parents about substance use. Fang, Barnes-Ceeney, and Lee (2011) reported Asian American parents rarely spoke to their children about alcohol and drugs and if they did, little was communicated. With all this being said, one strong preventive factor for substance use among AAPI adolescents is a strong relationship between parent and youth. To this end, AAPIs tend to perceive a higher negative response from parents and friends toward substance use and expect larger costs and fewer benefits from use (as cited in Luk, Emery, Karyadi, Patock-Peckham, & King, 2013). Also, if one tends to have family members or peers that do not use, one is less likely to learn about and engage in substance use. Researchers indicate AAPI youth are less influenced by social factors (i.e., Social Learning Theory) because they are not exposed as often. In general, Asians are likely to have less contact with friends and actually have more contact with their family members than their white counterparts. Researchers have shown, however, that the more exposure an Asian American adolescent has with peers, the more likely substance use can be initiated and maintained (Au & Donaldson, 2000).

One study of 329 Cambodian, Chinese, Laotian/Mien, and Vietnamese youth supported the notion of social influence as a protective factor. The researchers asked how many of the participants' friends engaged in alcohol and other drug use. Forty-five percent of the youth in the study indicated none of their friends drank alcohol, while 28 percent stated a few drank alcohol. For marijuana use, 60 percent said none and 20 percent reported a few. Lastly, with regard to "hard" drug use, 91 percent of the youth reported none and 6 percent stated a few. One other noteworthy point is that the rates of substance use among Chinese youth were the lowest in this investigation. These results support the SAMHSA (2013a) data (referenced previously in this chapter) that also indicated the lowest rates of drug use among Chinese American adults compared to other Asian Americans in the study.

The existence of a co-occurring mental health disorder can also increase the likelihood of substance use. AAPIs are shown to have lower incidences of psychological concerns, serious thoughts of suicide, and use of mental health treatment. In 2012, the prevalence of mental illness was: 13.9 percent among Asians; 16.3 percent among Hispanics; 18.6 percent among blacks; 19.3 percent among whites; 20.7 percent among persons reporting two or more races; and 28.3 percent among American Indians or Alaska Natives. (Note: The data on Native Hawaiians or other Pacific Islanders was not reported.) (SAMHSA, 2013a). In addition to mental illness, SAMHSA also reported on the rates of suicidal thoughts in the past year and found the lowest rates among Native Hawaiians or other Pacific Islanders (1.5 percent), with Asians having the second lowest rates (3.3 percent). The highest rates were among American Indians or Alaska Natives (5.9 percent). Lastly, among racial/ethnic groups, the rates of past-year mental health service use among adults aged 18 or older in 2012 were 4.4 percent for Asians; 5.3 percent for Native Hawaiians or other Pacific Islanders; 7.1 percent for Hispanics; 10.2 percent for blacks; 14.2 percent for persons reporting two or more races; 15.4 percent for American Indians or Alaska Natives; and 17.8 percent for whites (SAMHSA, 2013a).

To summarize, there are many preventive factors for AAPIs such as having adverse biological reactions to alcohol, lower rates of substance use as a young adult, and lower incidents of mental health concerns. These factors may account for the lower prevalence of substance use disorders among AAPIs compared to other racial/ethnic groups. With this being said, researchers have also suggested that AAPIs tend to underutilize mental health and substance abuse treatment services (Von Wormer & Davis, 2013). If this is the case, the occurrence of substance use problems may be higher than the numbers indicate and the problems more severe than believed. The next section will address the barriers that influence the access to, retention in, and successful outcomes of counseling and treatment programs.

Barriers

A barrier to treatment that has been identified in this population is the notion that AAPIs are the "model minority" in the United States. This ideology posits Asians are "typically well-behaved, successful, and issue-free" (Fang et al., 2011, p. 5). Fang et al.'s (2011) qualitative study indicated that, in order to live up to this stereotype, Asian Americans feel pressured to be high achievers in academics and have careers such as lawyers and doctors. These pressures could lead to substance use in an effort to relieve psychological distress, as well as be a barrier to seeking treatment. If substance use problems are recognized, the initial response by the family may be to ignore it. However, if it begins to affect the family functioning, it can bring shame. Therefore, the family may try to isolate, scold, or reject the person. Asking for help takes a lot of courage in most Asian communities because it is still considered taboo to disclose problems outside of the family. These cultural influences may reduce both the desire and the efforts among APPIs to seek treatment for substance use or mental problems. Moreover, the model minority may also impact health care providers' (e.g., medical personnel and substance abuse therapists) perception of low treatment needs in this population, thus creating another external barrier to an Asian individual's attempt to seek or stay in treatment (Niv et al., 2007). Sandhu and Madathil (2013) urge clinicians and other health care providers to challenge the model minority myth because it is problematic and overgeneralized, preventing detection and treatment of increasing psychological problems among AAPIs (South Asians in particular due to increased discrimination in the United States in recent years).

Another barrier to addiction treatment is the client's presentation of the problem in need of treatment service. According to Fong and Tsuang (2007), often AAPIs tend to report mental health concerns and consequences of substance use as physical symptoms. For example, someone with depression may complain of somatic symptoms such as frequent headaches or stomachaches. AAPIs tend to view the body and mind as one; thus, AAPIs with mental health or substance use disorders may present to medical clinics first. Researchers suggest the failure to acknowledge substance use problems is not a form of denial, but rather, a lack of awareness and understanding about the signs and symptoms of addictive disorders (Fong & Tsuang, 2007). In summary, clinicians and other health care providers are advised to remember that with AAPIs, "frequent headaches might signal frequent heartaches" (Sandhu & Madathil, 2013, p. 335). As a result, emotional afflictions may be the underlying issue of their presenting physical ailments to medical professionals. In addition to physical complaints, AAPIs may also voice emotional concerns in other ways. For instance, clients may indicate karma, supernatural forces, or angry spirits are causing them conflict. Moreover, they could report discord with spiritual or religious dimensions, which results in an imbalance or a negative state of being.

ASSESSMENT AND TREATMENT RECOMMENDATIONS

As this chapter indicates, issues arise for AAPIs that impact substance use such as biological reactions to alcohol and the acculturation of AAPI youth. While rates of substance abuse treatment admissions tend to be lower in this population, therapists will have to consider these issues when assessing and treating AAPIs and their families. This section will address the recommendations specified in the literature, and the authors suggest continued advocacy in the field related to outreach and social justice.

Immigration

Asian Americans and Pacific Islander immigrants may face some very intense stressors that affect treatment. These stressors can include inadequate and crowded housing, socioeconomic difficulties, language barriers, separation from family and friends, and post-traumatic stress caused by war and life as a refugee. Situations such as these can lead to feelings of loneliness, anxiety, hostility, guilt, extreme sadness, and powerlessness. It should be noted that there can be differing issues within racial and ethnic groups, depending on when they immigrated. Vietnamese and Cambodians who came to the United States after the Vietnam war lived in urban areas and were mostly well educated; however, those Vietnamese and Cambodian immigrants who came a decade later were primarily farmers and laborers who were illiterate and experienced starvation, violence, and refugee camps prior to arriving in America (as cited in Von Wormer & Davis, 2012). Counselors are advised to also consider if their clients' family members are immigrants and how the dynamics of acculturation come into play with their clients, who are second- or third-generation AAPIs.

Acculturation

The level to which a person has adapted to the cultural norms can impact substance use. As stated previously, Asians who were born in the United States generally had higher rates of past-month substance use than those who were not born in America, regardless of age (SAMHSA, 2010). Gender differences have been seen as well. For example, AAPI men are more likely to use tobacco than their female counterparts, but AAPI women who are more acculturated to the United States are more likely to smoke than recent immigrants (Fong & Tsuang, 2007).

Intergenerational conflicts can cause stress in the client's family as one becomes more acculturated to Western values, norms, and culture. Especially for youth and young adults, issues may arise surrounding the traditional child-rearing practices of the older generations of AAPIs. Differing perspectives on discipline, dating, marriage, curfew, parental supervision, authority, gender roles, and career choice can all impact family dynamics (Chang, 2006; Chung & Bemak, 2006; Sandhu & Madathil, 2013). Many of the family members from older generations may be immigrants and/or refugees and have endured trauma, grief issues, etc., which must be considered by the therapist. In one community sample of 300 Cambodian refugee women, 22 percent indicated experiencing the death of a spouse and 53 percent reported the loss or death of other family members (Chung, 2000). Moreover, many refugee women have experienced rape, sexual abuse, violence, and the loss of a child. Consequently, having these life events can influence how they may perceive the acculturation of their children and grandchildren, which can impact the family dynamics of AAPIs.

Language

Language can be a substantial hurdle for AAPI immigrants in receiving the substance use services they need. There are over 100 native languages among different AAPI groups, and there are also regional dialects among Asians from the same country (Social Security Administration, 2014). When working with AAPIs who have limited English skills, an interpreter is likely needed. The interpreter's competency in the following domains needs to be considered: (1) technical (verbal and written proficiency in the native and English languages); (2) cultural (familiarity with AAPI and U.S. cultures, as well as the health service organizational structure); (3) interpersonal (awareness of one's values and behaviors and good interpersonal skills); (4) ethical (professional codes related to confidentiality, impartiality, proficiency, and general conflicts of interests); and (5) personal (reliability and attention to details). Lee's (1997) book chapter provides a concise and informative overview of these competency criteria and other clinically pertinent issues in the therapeutic use of interpreters for mental health services that would likely be applicable for addiction services.

Having a professional interpreter who speaks the native language (and regional dialect if needed) of the immigrant client is a rare professional luxury that most treatment centers do not have. Thus, health service providers who work with immigrant groups and do not speak the native language of their clients often find themselves in the ethical dilemma of needing to relay on a nonprofessional interpreter who is a family member, friend, neighbor, church member, or other social contact. These lay individuals are not socialized to and held by ethical codes of the helping professions. The risk for breaking confidentiality is likely higher when using a nonprofessional interpreter, and the client should be informed about any confidentiality risks involved (Gilbert, 2005). Confidentiality maintenance is further complicated when an English-speaking minor child serves as the interpreter for his or her non–English-speaking parent. In this case, a child serving as an interpreter could disrupt the hierarchical order of power within a family system. As an interpreter, a minor child could have access to health information that children are not typically privy to within an Asian family. Furthermore, the younger the child, the less she or he is able to understand the need for keeping health status information confidential and the costs of breaking confidentiality (Gilbert, 2005). Obviously, the use of family and other social contacts as interpreters present many possible conflicts of interest that need to be weighed against the benefits of having these individuals as interpreters.

Screening and Assessment Tools

There are very few substance use instruments that have been developed for an AAPI sample or translated into an Asian language. Given the substantial differences in alcohol and other drug use within the AAPI population, as well as in comparison to individuals of European descent living in the United States, there is a clear clinical need for such instruments. A review of the recent literature reveals one self-report measure that was translated from English to Korean and was developed specifically for Korean teenagers (the Asian group that has the highest level of past-month alcohol use among AAPI minorities living in the United States). Kim (2010) found that the Korean version of the revised Problem-Oriented Screening Instrument for Teenagers (POSIT) Substance Use and Abuse Scale shows good reliability and validity in students aged 7–12 in Korea. Similarly, the Alcohol Use Disorders Identification Test (AUDIT), developed by the World Health Organization, has been used with many English-speaking AAPIs living in the United States and translated into the native languages of a number of AAPI countries. Information about other alcohol and drug instruments, including their psychometric properties within Asian and Asian American groups, is also available on the websites of the National Institute on Alcohol Abuse and Alcoholism and the National Institute on Drug Abuse.

Culture

There are significant differences in the worldview, behaviors, and values between Western culture and the Asian and Pacific Islander cultures. Moreover, these differences influence how one perceives the origins of health problems, the view of medical and psychological diagnoses, and the prevention and treatment of such health problems. In addition to the diversity between Western culture and AAPI culture, there is also diversity within the AAPI population with regard to language, religion, historical events, dress, food, etc. This section will discuss some aspects of AAPI culture that apply to many in this population; however, the reader should keep in mind the tripartite model in conceptualizing an individual discussed in an earlier chapter of this text. It is important to remember each client is similar to and different from other people at three levels: universal (e.g., we are all human); group (e.g., a person identifies as South Asian); and individual (e.g., genetic predisposition and personal experiences) (Sue, 2001). These three parts make up a client's worldview and personal identity. Therefore, counselors are encouraged to take these aspects into account and have conversations with clients about their worldview, values, and culture.

Western culture values independence, autonomy, individualism, and spontaneity—and these are contradictory to most AAPI cultural values and norms. The following is a list of cultural values of many in the AAPI population:

- Politeness, humility, emotional self-control, conformity to norms, and "saving face."
- *Filial piety* is the deep respect, honor, duty, and obligation (both physically and financially) that a person has to his or her parents throughout life.
- The individual is secondary to the interests of the family as a whole. A person's success is shared with the entire family and a person's failure is also considered a failure of the family.

- Families tend to be patriarchal in nature. Men and elders are given respect and tend to make the decisions for the family. Democratic discussions and negotiations are not commonly demonstrated. Mothers are to raise their children to be respectful and not rebellious, as this is a reflection on her and the family. The eldest son has the role of greatest responsibility.
- Emotions are not usually shared because it would be demonstrative of putting the individual first.
- Physical affection may not be shown, but love is acknowledged through behaviors that benefit the family. Public demonstration of affection such as holding hands or kissing is not common.
- Education is very important and seen as one of the main ways to higher social position and obtainment of prestige.
- Parents often limit their children's free-time activities and supervise their work habits.
- Dating a person of a different racial/ethnic group is discouraged, premarital sex is strictly prohibited, and arranged marriages are the norm in many South Asian families.

These cultural values and worldviews impact the presentation, engagement, and retention in counseling services. For instance, AAPIs may be more willing to accept substance abuse screening and care from their primary care physician than from psychiatrists or addiction professionals. Often, clients will ask for medication or injections due to the belief that mental health problems are physical health issues, and they will desire a medical approach with quick symptom relief. As stated previously, the presentation of mental health concerns can present in the form of a physical health problem, and this must be considered. However, counselors are advised to also be aware that some behaviors by AAPIs are not a presentation of psychological issues. For instance, recognize that behaviors such as speaking to a dead loved one are not signs of mental health issues, but common practices within the client's culture. In addition, be knowledgeable about the client's religious and spiritual beliefs and practices. In an attempt to address disturbances in various life areas, some AAPI clients may wish to use fortune-tellers, the horoscope/astrology, palm reading, etc.

Communication may be difficult in some cases. In addition to language barriers, communication issues can arise as a result of differences in cultural norms. For instance, be aware of verbal (e.g., tone and volume) and nonverbal (e.g., eye contact and personal space) behaviors. Asians are taught to be seen and not heard around their parents, and self-control is a commonly shared value within this population. Therefore, in counseling sessions, clients may demonstrate more silence when communicating and use fewer words. Moreover, AAPI clients may rather analyze problems than share about emotions. They may prefer to speak about facts, other people, and events versus self-disclosing about personal, emotional experiences.

The aforementioned differences in cultures may make counseling less attractive to AAPIs, and thus they can be considered barriers to treatment. However, when clients do seek services, therapists must be aware of some concerns and experiences that are specific to the AAPI population. For instance, when introduced to a radically new environment with different climates, food, mannerisms, lifestyles, dating and marriage customs, and religious practices, a client can experience "culture shock" (Sandhu & Madathil, 2013, p. 325). Clinicians must attempt to understand these lived experiences and address the stressors associated with culture shock.

As stated before, AAPIs may have immigrated to the United States with a history of trauma or could potentially be the victim of trauma while living in this country. Besides the traumatic events related to prejudice, oppression, and racism by others in the United States, some AAPIs can still be at risk for experiencing violence directed at them, even from their own families. In some circumstances, a person may be a victim of "honor violence." This type of violence can include horrible acts such as emotional, physical, or sexual abuse, threats, stalking, harassment, false imprisonment, and even homicide. Honor violence may occur due to infidelity, refusal to participate in an arranged marriage, or pregnancy. In fact, some pregnant women have been killed by their fathers or brothers in order to save the face, name, and honor of their families (Sandhu & Madathil, 2013). There have been many instances of honor violence discussed in the media, as well as in scholarly literature. However, many Americans are not aware of how prevalent this type of violence is in the world and also in this country. Among the AAPI population, honor violence is most prevalent in South Asian countries (e.g., Pakistan, India, and Bangladesh) (United Nations Population Fund, 2003). One study found that between 2004 and 2007, a total of 1,957 honor killings were recorded in Pakistan alone (Nasrullah, Haqqi, & Cummings, 2009). In 2012, the Human Rights Commission of Pakistan reported there was a rise in the number of deaths and stated 947 honor killings occurred within the year (Sayah, 2012).

In the United States, honor violence occurs as well, but it is often classified as domestic violence and not viewed through a cultural lens. The media has brought attention to these horrific cases for decades. In 1989, a 16-year-old girl in Missouri was stabbed to death by her father while she was held down by her mother; the parents indicated it was due to their daughter dating a black man, attending a school dance, and getting a job (Weldon, 2010). More recently, in December 2013, another example of honor violence happened in West Haven, Connecticut. A woman was burned on her upper torso because her husband threw hot oil on her while she was sleeping. This was reportedly due to his belief that she was committing adultery.

To summarize, clinicians should be aware of the various cultural stressors that AAPIs can experience. These stressors can include everything from experiencing daily microaggressions to facing extreme harm or death for not complying with the beliefs, norms, values, and behaviors of their culture. Consideration of these cultural issues is necessary when counselors are conceptualizing presenting problems and also when they are creating treatment plans with AAPIs.

Treatment Planning

While doing counseling work with AAPIs, there are some recommendations regarding treatment planning. Due to the specific cultural issues like the ones outlined in the previous section, therapists are urged to consider the following when implementing goals and objectives with this particular population:

- Clients may not understand the idea of "talk therapy." Therefore, discuss goals of therapy, what counseling is like, and your counseling style
- Keep in mind that East and Southeast Asian Americans may tend to prefer a logical, rational, directive, and authoritative counseling style. They tend to like solution-focused therapy and have a desire to find an immediate resolution, rather than gaining insight into the source (Kim & Park, 2013)
- A psychoeducational approach with behavioral goals can be very beneficial
- Genograms, narratives and stories, and bibliotherapy are suggested (Sandhu & Madathil, 2013)

- Include family members when possible. Also, understand the families' (a) cultural worldview; (b) premigration history and experience; and (c) degree of acculturation
- Do not discard complaints of somatic symptoms
- Have knowledge of culturally appropriate and available interventions and techniques (e.g., use of meditation, yoga, acupuncture, sing/dance, use of different dietary methods like fasting and being vegetarian, use of herbal medications)
- Recognition and use of spiritual/religious healers and influences
- Recognition of the client's traditional beliefs, superstitions, and the belief in the supernatural
- The recommendation of support groups such as Alcoholics Anonymous may be met with little interest because AAPIs are concerned about shaming oneself and the family with public discussion of problems.
- When treating an Asian American male, consider discussing masculine norms, his values associated with these expectations, current coping strategies, and peer influences that may be associated with substance use (Liu & Iwamoto, 2007).
- Challenge the model minority myth, and consider this population as equally vulnerable (if not more vulnerable) to psychological distress and substance abuse issues as people from other racial/ethnic groups.

As social justice advocates, counselors must provide outreach within AAPI communities or at events where AAPIs are present (e.g., health fairs, parades). Substance abuse therapists can provide information, increase access to treatment, and reduce misconceptions surrounding substance use, misuse, and dependency. Hand out materials such as brochures and flyers in various Asian languages (e.g., Hindi, Korean, Bengali) to advertise and deliver information. Use incentives (e.g., keychains or hats) to participate in screening. Clinicians can provide a brief intervention (using motivational interviewing strategies) on site for immediate assistance; also refer to more intensive treatment when appropriate (Yu, Clark, Chandra, Dias, & Lai, 2009).

CONCLUSIONS

Asian minorities are a growing population in the United States, and are projected to increase from 4.8 percent to 9.2 percent of the total population by 2050. The U.S. AAPI population includes individuals born in or have family heritage from many AAPI countries that are quite diverse in cultures and religions. Thus, it is important for professionals working with a specific AAPI group to gain knowledge about that group's history and cultural practices when possible.

Differences exist among the various AAPI subgroups in their current substance use. Korean Americans reported the highest level of alcohol use in the past month, and Japanese Americans showed the highest level of past-month illicit drug use. Chinese Americans reported the lowest level of substance use. Among these subgroups, individuals who identified themselves as multiracial Asian American were four times more likely to use illicit substances than those who did not identify as multiracial. Additionally, differences were found between those who were native Asian Americans and those who were born in Asia, with those born in the United States reporting two to three times more substance use than foreign-born Asians.

Recognizing the diversities within the AAPI population living in the United States, the authors provide an overview of prevalence rates, cultural issues, and clinical recommendations that could serve as a springboard for treatment professionals working with AAPI individuals with alcohol and other drug-related problems.

Studies have consistently found Asians to have the lowest rates of substance use, substance-related diagnoses, co-occurring mental illnesses, psychological concerns, and treatment admissions. There is a number of factors that may protect AAPI individuals from initiating and misusing alcohol and other drugs. These factors can be biological (e.g., lower level of ALDH2 coenzymes) or cultural (e.g., close parent-child relationship and frequent communication) in nature. Researchers have also suggested that AAPIs tend to underutilize mental health and substance abuse treatment services (Von Wormer & Davis, 2013). Furthermore, AAPIs showed lower rates of subsequent treatment attempts (Yu & Warner, 2013). There are several cultural factors that suggest the presence of cultural barriers to diagnosis and treatment of substance-related problems among Asians.

The model minority myth that portrays Asians as well-adjusted, educated, and successful minorities may prevent both AAPI individuals and treatment professionals from recognizing substance use and mental health problems present in AAPIs. Given the historical and legislative oppressions that Chinese, Japanese, and other Asian groups have faced throughout many decades of U.S. history, it is not surprising that this model minority presentation would be a desirable presentation for many AAPI individuals. Many Asian cultural values have been proposed or empirically found to be barriers to an AAPI individual's willingness to acknowledge and seek treatment for substance use and mental health problems. Addiction problems may go undetected because AAPIs tend to perceive and report mental health concerns and consequences of substance use as physical symptoms such as headaches, body aches, indigestion, etc. Other cultural barriers include inhibited emotional expression, low level of disclosure about oneself and one's family, perception of addiction and mental health issues as shameful to the family, and preference for seeking help within personal networks rather than formal treatment programs. The extent to which an AAPI person adheres to these traditional Asian values also depends substantially on their level of acculturation.

The myriad of cultural considerations in the AAPI population and its many subgroups presented in this chapter suggest that culturally competent assessment and treatment of substance use–related problems in AAPI individuals require high levels of openness and commitment by professionals, as they must learn about and understand the cultural values that may run counter to traditional Western values and practices. Because cultural identity also intersect with other personal identities, it is critical for clinicians working with Asians to conceptualize their clients' substance use and misuse within an ecological framework. This framework considers multiple layers of influences on an individual's behaviors, and these influences range from personal characteristics to microsystem variables (e.g., family and other social support systems) to macrosystem variables (e.g., discrimination and normative values). Finally, the most important tool any helping professional can possess is empathetic interviewing and listening skills. By demonstrating these skills, a counselor can provide a safe environment that encourages clients to share their presenting problems honestly, ask questions openly, and express their treatment concerns as needed.

Case Study

Jon is a 19-year-old Korean American who immigrated to the United States with his parents and younger sister when he was eight years old. Jon is a freshman at an Ivy League university. His parents sent him to college with instructions that he study hard and make good grades, so that he can become a doctor and take care of them when they get older. Jon shares that this is the farthest he has ever been from home and the longest he has ever been away from his family and friends. He has made a few Korean American friends at the university and discovered that he enjoys having several beers on their nights out. "Getting drunk" on the weekends helps him relax and forget about his academic difficulty and tenuous roommate situation with another freshman from a conservative Midwestern city. Academically, he is struggling in math and science courses, courses he was told he must perform really well in to get into Harvard or other medical schools. One academic consolation for Jon is that he is excelling in English classes, especially his creative writing courses. Jon has made several visits to the university's health services center with complaints of headaches, stomachaches, feeling nervous all the time, and sleeping problems. Jon did not understand why he was referred to the mental health counselor by a primary care physician he saw at the center, but agreed to attend the first meeting.

Discussion Questions

1. What is Jon's presenting problem?
2. What are some differential diagnoses that need to be considered based on the initial case presentation?
3. What clinical symptoms and risks must be evaluated?
4. Should laboratory tests be requested to address Jon's physical complaints? Explain your answer.
5. How might the model minority myth be relevant to conceptualizing this case?
6. What are some treatment recommendations?
7. What are some cultural barriers in socializing Jon to psychological treatment, as well as retaining him in "talk therapy?"

REFERENCES

Au, J. G., & Donaldson, S. I. (2000). Social influences as explanations for substance use differences among Asian-American and European-American adolescents. *Journal of Psychoactive Drugs, 32*, 15–23.

Chang, C. C. (2006). Counseling Korean Americans. In C. C. Lee (Ed.), *Multicultural issues in counseling* (2nd ed., pp. 171–184). Alexandria, VA: American Counseling Association.

Chung, R. C.-Y. (2000). Psychosocial adjustment of Cambodian refugee women: Implications for mental health counseling. *Journal of Mental Health Counseling, 23*, 115–126.

Chung, R. C-Y., & Bemak, F. (2006). Counseling Americans of Southeast Asian descent: The impact of the refugee experience. In C. C. Lee (Ed.), *Multicultural issues in counseling* (2nd ed., pp. 151–170). Alexandria, VA: American Counseling Association.

Condie, L. B., & Koocher, G. P. (2008). Clinical management of children's incomplete understanding of confidentiality. *Journal of Child Custody, 5*(3/4), 161–191.

Conyne, R. K., & Cook, E. P. (2004). *Ecological counseling: An innovative approach to conceptualizing person-environment interaction*. Alexandria, VA: American Counseling Association.

Fong, T. W., & Tsuang, J. (2007). Asian-Americans, addictions, and barriers to treatment. *Psychiatry, 4*(11), 51–59.

Gilbert, M. J. (2005). The case against using family, friends, and minors as interpreters in health and mental health care settings in process of inquiry—communicating in a multicultural environment. From the *Curricula Enhancement Module Series*. Washington, DC: National Center for Cultural Competence, Georgetown University Center for Child and Human Development. Retrieved from http://www.nccccurricula.info/communication/D15.html

Gopaldas, A. (2013). Intersectionality 101. *Journal of Public Policy and Marketing, 32*, 90–94.

Kim, B. S., & Park, Y. S. (2013). Culturally alert counseling with East and Southeast Asian Americans. In Garrett McAuliffe and Associates, *Culturally alert counseling: A comprehensive introduction* (2nd ed., pp. 157–183). Thousand Oaks, CA: Sage Publications.

Kim, Y. (2010). Korean version of the revised Problem-Oriented Screening Instrument for Teenagers Substance Use/Abuse Scale: A validation study. *Journal of Social Service Research, 36*, 37–45.

Le, T. N., Goebert, D., & Wallen, J. (2009). Acculturation factors and substance use among Asian American youth. *Journal of Primary Prevention, 30*, 453–473. doi: 10.1007/s10935-009-0184-x

Lee, E. (1997). *Working with Asian Americans: A guide for clinicians*. New York: Guilford Press.

Liu, W. M., & Iwamoto, D. K. (2007). Conformity to masculine norms, Asian values, coping strategies, peer group influences, and substance use among Asian American men. *Psychology of Men and Masculinity, 8*, 25–39.

Luk, J. W., Emery, R. L., Karyadi, K. A., Patock-Peckham, J. A., & King, K. M. (2013). Religiosity and substance use among Asian American college students: Moderated effects of race and acculturation. *Drug and Alcohol Dependence, 130*, 142–149.

Nasrullah, M., Haqqi, S., & Cummings, K. J. (2009). The epidemiological patterns of honour killing of women in Pakistan. *European Journal of Public Health, 19*(2), 193–197.

National Institutes of Health (2009). Alcohol flush signals increased cancer risk among East Asians. Retrieved from http://www.nih.gov/news/health/mar2009/niaaa-23.htm

Niv, N., Wong, E. C., & Hser, Y. I. (2007). Asian Americans in community-based substance abuse treatment: Service needs, utilization, and outcomes. *Journal of Substance Abuse Treatment, 33*, 313–319.

Price, R. K., Risk, N. K., Wong, M. M., & Klingle, R. S. (2002). Substance use and abuse by Asian Americans and Pacific Islanders: Preliminary results from four national epidemiologic studies. *Public Health Reports, 117*, 39–50.

Sandhu, D. S., & Madathil, J. (2013). Culturally alert counseling with South Asian Americans. In Garrett McAuliffe and Associates, *Culturally alert counseling: A comprehensive introduction* (2nd ed., pp. 315–344). Thousand Oaks, CA: Sage Publications.

Sayah, R. (2012, August). "Honor" murderer boasts of triple killing. *CNN*. Retrieved from http://www.cnn.com/2012/08/20/world/asia/pakistan-honor-confession/

Social Security Administration (2014). *Asian Americans and Pacific Islanders*. Retrieved from http://www.ssa.gov/aapi/

Substance Abuse and Mental Health Services Administration (2013a). *Results from the 2012 National Survey on Drug Use and Health: Summary of National Findings*. NSDUH Series H-46, HHS Publication No. (SMA) 13-4795. Rockville, MD: Substance Abuse and Mental Health Services Administration. Retrieved from http://www.samhsa.gov/data/NSDUH/2012summnatfinddettables/NationalFindings/NSDUHresults2012.htm#ch2.7

Substance Abuse and Mental Health Services Administration (2013b). *The NSDUH report: Need for and receipt of substance use treatment among Asian Americans and Pacific Islanders*. Rockville, MD: SAMHSA. Retrieved from http://www.samhsa.gov/data/2k13/NSDUH125/sr125-aapi-tx.pdf

Substance Abuse and Mental Health Services Administration (2012). *Data spotlight: Asian and Pacific Islander treatment admissions are three times more likely to report primary methamphetamine abuse*. Retrieved from http://www.samhsa.gov/data/spotlight/Spot090APIMethUse2012.pdf

Substance Abuse and Mental Health Services Administration (2010). *The NSDUH report: Substance use among Asian adults*. Rockville, MD: SAMHSA. Retrieved from http://www.samhsa.gov/data/2k10/179/SUAsianAdults.htm

Sue, D. W. (2001). Multidimensional facets of cultural competence: A major contribution. *Counseling Psychologist, 29*, 790–821.

United Nations Population Fund (2003). Violence against women in South Asia: A regional analysis. Retrieved from http://www.unfpa.org.np/pub/vaw/VAW_REG_Analysis.pdf

United States Census Bureau (2013). *Profile America: Facts for features*. Retrieved from http://www.census.gov/newsroom/releases/pdf/cb13ff-09_asian.pdf

United States Census Bureau (2012). *The Asian population: 2010*. Retrieved from http://www.census.gov/prod/cen2010/briefs/c2010br-11.pdf

United States Census Bureau News (2008). *An older and more diverse nation by midcentury*. Retrieved from http://www.census.gov/newsroom/releases/archives/population/cb08-123.html

Von Wormer, K., & Davis, D. R. (2013). *Addiction treatment: A strengths perspective* (3rd ed.). Belmont, CA: Brooks/Cole.

Welden, B. A. (2010). Restoring lost "honor": Retrieving face and identity, removing shame, and controlling the familial cultural environment through "honor" murder. *Journal of Alternative Perspectives in Social Sciences, 2*, 380–398.

Yu, J., Clark, L. P., Chandra, L., Dias, A., Lai, T. F. (2009). Reducing cultural barriers to substance abuse treatment among Asian Americans: A case study in New York City. *Journal of Substance Abuse Treatment, 37*, 398–406.

Yu, J., & Warner, L. A. (2013). Substance abuse treatment readmission patterns of Asian Americans: Comparisons with other ethnic groups. *American Journal of Drug and Alcohol Abuse, 39*, 23–27.

CHAPTER 8

LATINO AMERICANS

By Tara Casady

The term "Latino" refers to a diverse group of people living in the United States from several different ethnicities, racial makeup, and nationalities, including both foreign-born and people born within the United States. While the term unites many varied groups based on several potential commonalities (e.g., Iberian heritage, Spanish language, and Catholic religion), there is vast heterogeneity that limits full generalization of the cultural considerations presented in this chapter. Factors such as ethnic background, type of and reasons for migration, acculturation status, socioeconomic status, social class, political ideology, and cultural heritage all impact the identification with traditional cultural beliefs (Santisteban, Vega, & Suarez-Morales, 2006; Terrell, 1993). Thus, this chapter is meant to serve as a guide for potential considerations and as a basis for further investigation within the literature or therapeutic setting. This is particularly imperative because several subgroups labeled as Latino exist within the United States and the people within these subgroups have engaged in "selective cultural adaptation." Paz (2002) defines this as a process of examining one's own value system and making decisions regarding which values have enough significance to be preserved, and which of those may be changed or altered. This adaptation process is both fluid and constantly changing. As such, becoming culturally competent and maintaining this competence requires continuing education and experience for the counselor (Paz, 2002).

In fact, it may be surprising to learn that the terms Latino and Hispanic are not synonymous, nor are they universally accepted by the very people to whom these labels apply (Gloria & Peregoy, 1996; Martínez, 2012). Neither term describes a racial group. As such, people who identify as Latino or Hispanic may also identify as one of several racial classifications (e.g., white, black, Asian, or Native American) (Ennis, Rios-Vargas, & Albert, 2011). In fact, a majority of Latinos racially identify as either white or "some other race," according to the 2010 United States Census (Humes, Jones, & Ramirez, 2011).

The terms Latino and Hispanic are often used interchangeably; however, there are etymological differences between them. In general, Latino refers to a person from a Latin American country (e.g., countries in South America, Middle America, and the Caribbean), and Hispanic refers to a person of Spanish ancestry, which may include Spain or the various countries in which Spanish conquistadors settled (Hayes-Bautista & Chapa, 1987). These two terms are primarily used within the United States, and they are usually spoken as if referring to similar concepts. However, the terms are associated with differing histories and meanings to the varied subgroups of people to which they apply.

Researchers have investigated the preferences in terminology among Latino Americans, and one study revealed that approximately half of their participants preferred to identify themselves by their family's country of origin (e.g., Colombian or Puerto Rican). In fact, only 24 percent stated that they preferred the terms Latino or Hispanic (Martínez, 2012). As such, the term Latino will be used in this chapter, as it preserves national origin and is racially neutral (Gloria & Peregoy, 1996). More specifically, Latino/Latina Americans will refer to "individuals living in the United States with ancestry from Mexico, Puerto Rico, Cuba, the Dominican Republic, and Central or South American Spanish-speaking countries" (Sue & Sue, 2013, p. 409).

Take a moment to consider the following:

Why do you think Latinos might prefer identification by their country of origin rather than terms such as "Latino" or "Hispanic?"

What has been the extent of your personal and professional interactions with the Latino population?

Although there is much diversity among Latinos, several common cultural elements tend to exist that unite this group. These elements include shared values, norms, language, self-identity, and identity ascribed by others. They provide a basis for the understanding of the Latino American experience and are worthy of consideration in the development and treatment of substance use disorders among this population. The more substance abuse counselors are aware of the common cultural elements, as well as the variation among those in the subgroups of Latinos with whom they work, the more they may provide culturally competent counseling to the individual (Organista & Muñoz, 1996). Therefore, becoming culturally competent not only involves a broad knowledge of the Latino culture, but also requires an understanding of how cultural aspects may apply (or may not apply) to the individual.

SOCIOECONOMIC DIVERSITY OF LATINO AMERICANS

According to the 2010 U.S. Census, out of the 308.7 million people in the United States, approximately 50.5 million people (or 16 percent) self-identified as Latino. In fact, Latinos accounted for more than half of the growth of the total population between 2000 and 2010 (Ennis et al., 2011). Of the total Latino population, approximately three-quarters identified as either of Mexican, Puerto Rican, or Cuban origin. More specifically, 63 percent of the total Latino population identified as Mexican.

As a substantial and growing portion of the population, it is imperative to develop a better understanding of culturally competent service delivery. In order to provide culturally competent substance abuse services, several environmental and systemic factors are worthy of consideration, as these factors have a significant impact on treatment delivery, retention, and presentation of the substance use problems (Paz, 2002). Take a moment to review Table 8.1 below to become familiar with the socioeconomic profile of Latinos, as compared to non-Latino whites within the United States.

Table 8.1: Socioeconomic Profile of Latinos and Non-Latino Whites

GROUP	PERCENT BELOW POVERTY LEVEL	PERCENT OF PERSONS WITH H.S. DIPLOMA	PERCENT OF PERSONS WITH BACHELOR'S DEGREE	PERCENT OF PERSONS WITHOUT HEALTH INSURANCE
Latinos	25.3	30	10.3	30.1
Mexican	27.1	30.4	7.7	32.6
Puerto Rican	29.1	32.6	12.2	15.7
Cuban	19.4	31	17.6	27.5
Central American	24.7	28.6	8.1	39
South American	11.7	29.6	21.9	25.6
Other Latino	20.3	26	15.7	23.3
Non-Latino Whites	9.8	30.5	22	11.1

Source: U.S. Census Bureau (2012). Current Population Survey, Annual Social and Economic Supplement.

The socioeconomic profile of Latino Americans indicates potential inequities within the United States. For instance, approximately 25 percent of Latinos report incomes that are below the poverty range, compared to 9.8 percent of non-Latino whites. In addition, Latinos account for approximately 22 percent of those receiving food stamps, compared to 9 percent of non-Latino whites (Motel & Patten, 2013). Latinos are disproportionately affected by a lack of health insurance coverage as well, further impacting available treatment options. An individual who is uninsured but wishes to attend treatment is often funded for a set amount of time, and this is frequently determined by governmental sources rather than the client and counselor (Alegría et al., 2006). Moreover, the availability of government-funded dollars may alter the types of sessions allowed (e.g., group or individual).

> Take a moment to consider the following:
>
> *How might educational attainment or familiarity with the English language affect the manner in which you explain treatment or an informed consent document? How would you address issues such as comprehension, the vocabulary spoken, or unfamiliarity with the process of therapy?*

SUBSTANCE USE STATISTICS

Latino American adults report lower rates of past-month alcohol use than the national average (46.1 percent and 55.2 percent respectively) (Substance Abuse and Mental Health Services Administration [SAMHSA], 2010). Latinos also report lower rates of past-month illicit drug use compared to the national average (6.6 percent and 7.9 percent, respectively). While these numbers indicate less substance use among Latino Americans than the national average, some other investigations have discovered findings one must also consider. For instance, Latino adults born within the United States report higher rates of past-month alcohol use, binge alcohol use, and illicit drug use, as compared to Latinos born outside of the United

States. These disparities suggest that acculturation to mainstream values within the United States may be a risk factor for the development of a substance use disorder. Another finding worth noting is the higher prevalence of alcohol-related health problems among Latinos (Blume & Resor, 2012). In addition, there are more severe and disproportionate consequences related to substance use. These consequences include the greater likelihood of (a) hepatitis B and C infection; (b) intimate partner violence; and (c) cirrhosis of the liver. These findings highlight the importance of effective substance abuse treatment for Latino Americans (Caetano, 2003).

In addition to investigating the substance use rates among the U.S. general population, data has also been collected from those who attend addiction treatment services. Researchers have found that Latinos accounted for approximately 14 percent of all Treatment Episode Data Set (TEDS) admissions (SAMHSA, 2009). Of the total treatment admissions by Latinos, approximately 41 percent identified as Mexican, 34 percent as Puerto Rican, 22 percent as other Latino, and 3 percent as Cuban (SAHMSA, 2007). For those involved in treatment, Latino clients were more likely to report alcohol or opiate abuse (Office of Applied Studies, 2005). In fact, 21 percent of Latinos who entered treatment indicated heroin as their primary substance of use versus 11.9 percent of non-Latino whites. Refer to Table 8.2 below for information regarding primary substance of abuse at the time of admission between Latinos and non-Latino whites.

However, when researchers examined the Latino subgroups separately, they noted there were differences between the subgroups regarding the primary substance of choice. For example, people that identified as Mexican were more likely to report alcohol as the drug of choice, as compared to those who identify as Puerto Rican, who were more likely to report opiates as the drug of choice. The rate of past-month binge alcohol use also varied greatly among Latino subgroups. For instance, Puerto Ricans reported the highest rates of binge drinking (28.7 percent) among Latinos, and Central or South Americans reported the lowest rates of binge drinking (20.8 percent). In addition to the differences found with regard to primary substance of choice and binge drinking rates, variation was also noted related to the prevalence of severe mental health concerns. For instance, Cubans and Puerto Ricans reported experiencing severe mental health issues and the use of illegal drugs more often than those identifying as Mexican (Guerrero, Cepeda, Duan, & Kim, 2012; Office of Applied Studies, 2005).

As stated previously, Latinos accounted for 14 percent of all treatment admissions. Researchers have suggested that Latinos are less likely to utilize substance use disorder treatment than other racial/ethnic groups. In fact, Latinos are three times less likely to utilize this type of treatment than non-Latino whites (Tighe & Saxe, 2006). There exists a qualitative difference in treatment retention and subjective experience

Table 8.2: Percentage of TEDS Admissions by Drug of Choice at Admission in 2007

	ALCOHOL ONLY	ALCOHOL & SECONDARY DRUG	HEROIN	OTHER OPIATE	SMOKED COCAINE	OTHER ROUTE-COCAINE	MARIJUANA	METH	PCP
Latino	20.8	13.8	21.4	1.5	5.1	4.9	16.7	11.6	.3
Non-Latino White	25.9	18.2	11.9	7.4	6.3	3.3	13.5	8.7	*

* Less than .05 percent

Source: Taken from SAMHSA (2009). *Treatment episode data set (TEDS). Highlights—2007.*

of treatment delivery in comparison to other populations. According to Wells, Klap, Koike, and Sherbourne (2001), Latinos are more likely to report (a) not receiving the necessary services; (b) a delay in the receipt of care; and (c) less satisfaction with care than non-Latino whites. Additionally, Latino clients are more likely to enter treatment younger and without a previous treatment history (Guerrero et al., 2012). These may be the reasons that Latino clients are more likely to drop out of treatment sooner and report not having their needs met while involved in treatment (Guerrero et al., 2012).

There could be many factors related to the lack of retention in treatment and dissatisfaction with services among the Latino community. On the other hand, there could be countless reasons why clients stay in treatment and would be pleased with services. For instance, one researcher suggests that experiencing an empathetic counselor is more likely to lead to successful outcomes than having a counselor of the same ethnicity (Amaro Arévalo, Gonzalez, Szapocznik, & Iguchi, 2006). This suggests that empathy skills may exert a more powerful influence on treatment retention than sharing the same culture of origin. Unfortunately, there is a paucity of research to explain the occurrence of differing treatment retention problems, treatment patterns, and levels of engagement with this particular population; even less is known about variations among Latino subgroups in this regard (Guerrero et al., 2012).

RISK FACTORS

Consideration must be given to the lived experiences of those in the Latino American population, and these experiences can impact access to and retention in treatment. For instance, Latinos are exposed to unique risk factors related to immigration, acculturation, discrimination, language barriers, and disruptions in social support systems (Santisteban, Muir-Malcolm, Mitrani, & Szapocznik, 2002). A person could experience one—if not all—of these factors, which may increase the likelihood of using substances and also decrease the likelihood of seeking or completing treatment.

The Latino community is largely affected by and concerned with immigration issues within the United States. Approximately one-fourth of Latino American adults are undocumented immigrants, and half of Latinos report a concern that they, a family member, or a close friend will be deported (Lopez, Taylor, Funk, & Gonzalez-Barrera, 2013; Pew Hispanic Research Center, 2007). Immigration issues represent not only a significant barrier to receiving care, but they can also result in a lack of treatment engagement by Latino clients. Counselors must attempt to address and alleviate these concerns in the beginning of treatment. During the assessment and intake process, clinicians should provide sufficient detail regarding informed consent and the limits of confidentiality. More specifically, clients must fully understand what information is shared with whom, and when a counselor is mandated to report information and break confidentiality.

Environmental factors may also be present for many Latino Americans, thus increasing chances for substance abuse issues. For instance, Latinos may reside in neighborhoods with (a) more alcohol retailers; (b) greater availability to illicit drugs; (c) higher unemployment rates; and (d) higher poverty rates (Alegría et al., 2006). These factors increase the chances of stress due to experiencing limited resources, difficulty meeting basic needs, and easier access to alcohol and other drugs. Other risk factors may include difficult acculturation experiences, social support variation, positive attitudes and beliefs about substance use, and use of unhealthy coping mechanisms (Terrell, 1993). Substance use may be a means of coping with the stress resulting from experiencing the circumstances listed above. Therefore, in order to facilitate effective substance abuse treatment, counselors may need to simultaneously address substance use *and* the client's problems with basic needs, such as inadequate food supply or unstable housing.

TREATMENT CONSIDERATIONS AND RECOMMENDATIONS

Culturally competent counseling may be thought of as the knowledge, values, and skills that are required for a counselor to demonstrate interpersonal sensitivity, as well as develop and maintain the working alliance. In order to be culturally competent, counselors do not follow a prescribed list of dos and don'ts. There are generalities made, however, related to the broader Latino culture; this is done to create a basis of understanding. These generalities are not presented to reinforce stereotypes or encourage stereotyping behavior on the part of the counselor. The following are potential commonalities among the Latino population based on research. However, counselors are cautioned and encouraged to assess their application to a client who identifies as Latino American. This is necessary, not only to avoid stereotyping the client's behavior, but also because there are ethnocultural variations between and among ethnic groups. Moreover, variation in beliefs, values, norms, and behavior occurs at an individual level as well.

> Take a moment to consider the following:
>
> *What values are commonly encouraged in the United States? What values are you aware of that commonly exist within the Latino population? How do these compare and contrast to values encouraged from your family of origin?*

Acculturation

In the United States, 63.8 percent of the Latino population are native to the United States, and 36.2 percent are foreign born (Pew Hispanic Center, 2011). Approximately one-quarter are undocumented immigrants. Many Latino Americans have family members who have lived in the country for generations. In fact, three-quarters of the native Latino population are third generation or higher. While most of the U.S. born Latinos are at least third generation, many Latinos are recent immigrants or have parents who have immigrated to the United States. Once living in the new country, these people experience a process called acculturation. Acculturation is a fluid process by which individuals learn a new culture. This may involve modifying elements of the new culture and their culture of origin (Marín & Gamba, 1996).

Acculturation has been found to be a factor in the variation of substance use rates among this population. Latino adults born in the United States have increased rates of past-month alcohol use, binge alcohol use, and illicit drug use than those not born within the United States, regardless of age. It appears that the more acculturated one becomes to mainstream American values, the more likely one is to engage in substance use. Thus, acculturation may serve as a potential risk factor for substance use disorders (Alegría et al., 2006). These variations in substance use and substance use disorder rates not only vary by acculturation status, but also by subgroup (Alegría et al., 2006). For example, investigations have revealed the substance use and abuse by Cuban Americans have been correlated with degree of acculturation, income, and educational levels (Rothe & Ruiz, 2001).

Hypotheses exist that attempt to explain the higher substance use disorder rates among Latinos born within the United States, as compared to nonnative Latinos. One theory asserts that greater stress is associated with monocultural commitment. Monocultural commitment is when a person either completely rejects or completely accepts the values of the host culture (Miville, Koonce, Darlington, & Whitlock, 2000; Terrell, 1993). Exposure to competing values concerning substance use, coupled with the psychosocial stress experienced by immigrants, may contribute to higher rates of substance use and abuse. For example, one may encounter values in the United States in which binge use of alcohol is deemed acceptable. In this way, even though one may originate from a country in which this type of use is socially unacceptable, exposure to this value and psychosocial stress may make this coping style a more attractive option to consider.

A counselor may evaluate acculturation level through consideration of several different types of information shared throughout the assessment process. The following aspects are vital pieces of information to obtain:

- Country of origin
- Length of time in country of origin
- Length of time in the United States
- Immigration status and concerns
- Familiarity with language
- Language-based media preferences (such as Univisión)
- Amount of extended family support
- Employment status
- Place of residence and who resides with client
- Personal interests/hobbies/free-time activities
  (Adapted from Sue & Sue, 2013).

One may also utilize acculturation assessment instruments; however, few seem to capture the multidimensional nature of acculturation (Marín & Gamba, 1996). (Refer to Thomson & Hoffman-Goetz, 2009, for a systematic review of acculturation instruments.) Latinos and other ethnic minorities may respond differently than European Americans on substance use measures. Many psychological assessments have utilized European American populations in order to provide normative scores without specific normative assessment on minority populations; this can lead to diagnostic misinterpretation (Blume, Resor, & Kantin, 2009). In this way, discussion of endorsements on assessment material may provide clarification and avoid misinterpretation. However, some instruments designed to detect substance use disorders have been explicitly tested with Latino populations. For example, the CAGE (Cut down, Annoyed, Guilty, and Eye Opener) has been adapted to the Spanish language and is entitled the 4m version (Díez-Martínez, Martín-Moros, & Altisent-Trota, 1991). While originally developed in Spain, it has been shown to detect both past and present alcohol use disorders in Latinos in the United States (Saltz, Lepore, Sullivan, Amaro, & Samet, 1999). The SOCRATES is a measure to assess a client's stage of change regarding substance use and has also been adapted into the Spanish language (Miller & Tonigan, 1996). Finally, the Alcohol, Smoking and Substance Involvement Screening Test (ASSIST) has been tested with a wide variety of populations and has also been adapted into Spanish (WHO ASSIST Working Group, 2002).

POINTS FOR PRACTICE

Given the variation in acculturation among Latino individuals and the limited evidence regarding how to effectively address issues of acculturation, the author recommends the following points for practice. These are suggestions that are useful to consider when developing a case conceptualization and forming the therapeutic alliance:

- If acculturative stress is found to contribute to substance use and abuse, it may be beneficial to increase skills which manage the expectations of both cultures, including the country of origin and mainstream U.S. culture. In addition, a counselor may utilize "values clarification" exercises and discuss the pros and cons of behaving in accordance with the values of each culture.

- A counselor should exercise caution when managing differences in values, as value systems from the country of origin may have both positive and negative influences on the well-being of people who have emigrated. Investigating these contextual factors is advisable so that the development of services optimizes the positive influence of both an individual's past and present cultural systems (Alegría, 2006).

- Explain the treatment consent and limits of confidentiality. If possible, ask clients if they would prefer to read a Spanish translation of the treatment consent document, if their first language is Spanish. If not, carefully explain each component of the treatment consent and the limits to confidentiality. Check for comprehension, or inquire about questions throughout the explanation process. Always be very clear about the situations in which a therapist may break confidentiality and the situations in which this is unwarranted. Also, explain how the counselor and the clinic protect client information and confidentiality (e.g., locked records room).

- Inquire about the preference for a male or female counselor.

- If available, ask about a preference for a Spanish-speaking therapist.

- Explain the process of therapy. Clients should understand the purpose of a first session, the number and types of sessions required, and how treatment decisions are made. Providing this explanation can enhance the therapeutic alliance by demystifying the process and purpose of therapy. Also, a counselor is given the opportunity to establish trust before asking probing questions that require the client to communicate sensitive information about substance use and other problems of concern (Sue & Sue, 2013).

- Carefully assess for the history of environmental, social, economic, political, and personal stressors that influence substance use and abuse (Gloria & Peregoy, 1996).

- Gain an understanding of informal support systems that exist within the community. This may include spiritual or church sources and Spanish-speaking community organizations.

- Work within the client's cultural system, rather than trying to change the individual to fit the dominant system. By doing so, validation and respect for the client's worldview is demonstrated, and this may increase treatment retention and successful outcomes.

Value-Driven Concepts Related to Interpersonal Relationships

The development and maintenance of harmonious interpersonal relationships is a central value in Latino culture (Sue & Sue, 2013). Within this overarching value are the concepts of *familismo*, *simpatía*, *dignidad*, *respeto*, *personalismo*, and *confianza*. The presentation of these concepts and the importance placed on them will vary by individual. This variation depends on the level of acculturation and identification, with both mainstream values in the United States and country of origin. Thus, it is important for a counselor to first assess the level of acculturation. It is equally imperative that a clinician become familiar with the way in which these concepts may impact problem presentation and behavior in the therapeutic context.

Familismo

Familismo, or familism, is loosely defined as a strong commitment toward the family. The family is the basis of Latino culture (Gloria & Peregoy, 1996). Family may not only include primary family members, but also the extended family, close friends, and godparents. Familismo involves an orientation to unity, respect, duty, loyalty, and tradition (Sue & Sue, 2013). The family may participate in child rearing, obedience to parents may be stressed, and there may be an emphasis on maintaining loyalty to the family. These aspects of the Latino culture are in contrast to the Anglo-Saxon values of independence and self-reliance (Rothe & Ruiz, 2001).

Despite the conflicting beliefs and values, the strong familial support has been shown to function as a protective factor against the development of substance use disorders. In fact, the family serves as a first resource for advice and support, while seeking outside help may be discouraged. The family is an important support network, can serve as a positive influence, and can provide valuable resources to the client. This dedication to the family may also be relied upon in treatment when discussing positive reasons for behavior change. For example, maintaining a positive and productive role in one's family may provide the motivation for difficult behavior change. This requires a counselor to have an understanding of the familismo and how it may present for a client, given that many treatments for substance use disorders focus on one's personal reasons for change (in the tradition of Anglo-Saxon values of independence and self-reliance) (Center for Substance Abuse Treatment, 2009).

Substance abuse may be stigmatized and shameful within the family and community; thus, presenting for substance abuse treatment may be a difficult endeavor to begin. A client may have exhausted all the help from family and friends once he or she presents for treatment services. Given this possibility, it is beneficial for the counselor to inquire about the efforts made to manage problems with substance use prior to seeking professional services. While obligation to the family unit may function as a positive influence, it may also function as a source of stress, especially when the client's use has resulted in a negative impact on the family.

POINTS FOR PRACTICE

The importance of familismo should be evaluated so a counselor can determine the appropriate reason or purpose for certain client behaviors, as well as the behaviors by the client's family members. For instance, a counselor may erroneously interpret behavior consistent with familismo as "enabling" behaviors. If a Latino's family members supply substances or provide help in obtaining or using substances, it may be interpreted as enabling. In addition, a counselor may also consider the reliance on and closeness between a Latino's family members as poor boundaries or entrenchment. However, these behaviors may be culture bound and should be evaluated in terms of the cultural context.

- Consider the incorporation of family members in order to facilitate recovery success. The family may be useful in terms of positively reinforcing abstinence or the reduction of use and/or harmful behaviors. In addition, consult with family members throughout treatment (Terrell, 1993). Family members may provide additional information relevant to the case conceptualization and provide assistance in integrating recovery skills into the client's life.
- Avoid misconstruing shame as resistance in the therapeutic setting (Gloria & Peregoy, 1996). Assess and consider other supporting reasons for behavior beyond resistance or lack of motivation in treatment. For instance, the protection of the family unit and members is central to many Latinos. Therefore, clients may be hesitant to disclose substance-abusing behavior. A client might interpret substance-abusing behavior as shameful and may be perceived as disgracing the family unit (Gloria & Peregoy, 1996). As such, fully admitting the extent of use, how substances were obtained, or methods of financially supporting use may not be fully disclosed in beginning sessions.

Simpatía, Dignidad, Respeto, Personalismo, and Confianza

More traditionally oriented Latinos underutilize services due to the differing cultural norms that present in the therapeutic context, such as a perceived lack of warmth when encountering counseling services (US DHHS, 2001). Therefore, familiarity with Latino values concerning interpersonal interactions (e.g., *simpatía* and *dignidad*) may increase a counselor's ability to form and maintain a positive working alliance.

Simpatía is a preference for behaviors that promote smooth and pleasant social interactions (Gloria & Peregoy, 1996). A person who demonstrates simpatía strives to maintain harmony within his or her interpersonal relationships. It is the ability to connect with a client by demonstrating empathy, sincerity, and warmth. He or she behaves with *dignidad* and *respeto* toward others. *Dignidad* has been defined as the ability or skill to support the dignity or worth of the individual, while *respeto* is the ability of the clinician to appropriately demonstrate respect toward the client (Paz, 2002). These values are loosely defined; as such, it is particularly important to engage in continuing education and experience in order to fluently demonstrate these behaviors in session.

Personalismo refers to the innate personal worth of a human being, regardless of gender or social class. Personalismo emphasizes the importance of personal knowledge, politeness, and respect in interpersonal relations (Bracero, 1998). Self-disclosure of a counselor's substance use or abuse history may be requested by a Latino client, as there is a stronger affiliation with individuals and others' personal history. In this way, counselors may be evaluated on more of a personal level, rather than according to their occupational status or educational level. Personalismo is also the ability to establish individual rapport with the client and encompasses a preference for personal interactions, as opposed to impersonal interactions (Paz, 2002). A personal connection might feel uncomfortable to many counselors because of the training paradigm to which they have been taught. However, establishing personalismo is a necessary component to interactions with Latino clients. Moreover, it aids in developing a therapeutic alliance, which increases the likelihood that clients return for future sessions (Gloria & Peregoy, 1996).

The last concept to be addressed is *confianza*. Confianza is the ability to establish and maintain client trust. It is the standard by which all social relationships are built, be they personal, professional, or familial. This is a special form of intimacy based on careful management of trust and confidence (Bracero, 1998). Confianza may enter into a session as questions regarding the therapist's personal history, including his or her own substance use history. This style of communication may be culture bound and is not necessarily indicative of boundary breaking or avoidance of topics. A counselor should formulate responses in order to address inquiries of personal self-disclosure in session and the type of information the therapist is willing to release to clients.

POINTS FOR PRACTICE

It is often necessary for substance-abuse counselors to be comfortable discussing their substance use history. One therapist may have a history that is free from substance use and substance-using environments, while another clinician may have a long history of severe dependency. In terms of counseling with Latinos, this self-disclosure may assist in the development of a working alliance and establishing the counselor's legitimacy. The counselor should formulate potential responses to this type of questioning that both address client concerns and cultural interpersonal needs. These responses should also be within the counselor's own boundaries of disclosure.

- Be aware of how behavior is interpreted. Behavior that may be labeled as "enabling" or "being in denial" by Western standards may be actions that are in accordance with the above listed Latino values. One example of this may be when a person tolerates substance use from a partner so as to avoid straining or hurting the relationship. In this instance, a counselor may articulate recognition of these values and discuss ways in which family members may support non-using behavior in a culturally appropriate manner so as to maintain simpatía.

- Recognize that personalismo may present as more informal interactions as the working alliance is developed. Counselors may be more used to the maintenance of more formal interactions throughout treatment. It is possible that a counselor may be invited to family gatherings, or gifts may be presented to the therapist as a sign of gratitude for services. This is not necessarily indicative of lack of boundaries. A counselor should be familiar with not only clinic and ethical guidelines for receiving gifts, but should also consider the conditions in which it may be appropriate to receive gifts from a client.

- Determine when it is appropriate to receive hugs or touch from a client. Again, attempts to hug a counselor may not be indicative of a lack of boundaries or inappropriate behavior on the client's part, but may be culture-bound behavior. Discuss conditions under which this may acceptable or unacceptable with supervisors and colleagues. Also, understand one's own personal comfort level with touch and personal space. A counselor should be sensitive to culture-bound behavior, but must also balance personal comfort level and clinic policies.

> Take a moment to consider the following:
>
> *How might you maintain a client's best interest and respect for his or her values when it conflicts with your own?*
>
> *How might you manage the following situation?*
>
> *A 40-year-old married Mexican American client of your opposite gender presents for treatment regarding alcohol use. Following several sessions, the client has experienced success with alcohol use cessation and improved family conditions. The client presents you with a small, inexpensive gift and reports it is in thanks for your services. Do you accept the gift? Why? How do you discuss your acceptance or nonacceptance with the client? How do you apply the values of simpatía and personalismo to the interaction?*

Gender Roles

There are two types of gender role values associated with the sexes in Latino culture. Individual demonstration of the gender role values can vary with acculturation, as well as economic factors (Gloria & Peregoy, 1996). *Machismo* is the expectation that the males in the family are strong, dominant, and head of the household. While described at times with a negative connotation, machismo refers to how one provides for and protects the family and also pertains to the importance of remaining in control of oneself. In contrast, *marianismo* (relating to the Virgin Mary) is the expectation that women demonstrate self-sacrifice, nurturance, and strength in adversity. Moreover, there is an expectation that women are to be submissive to men (Sue & Sue, 2013). Similarly, while there may be negative connotations that remain related to these two concepts, females are viewed as spiritually stronger than males and may have a powerful influence on the family, even if exerted covertly. In addition, special status exists, as well as respect, for women as mothers and matriarchs of the family (Center for Substance Abuse Treatment, 2009). These gender roles, if fully understood by the counselor, may also serve as important motivators in treatment. While different roles and expectations are assigned differentially in some cases to males and females, there is also an emphasis on perseverance, survival, and respect for these roles (Center for Substance Abuse Treatment, 2009). Adherence to these roles may encourage nonuse, as well as encourage values-consistent behavior (Gloria & Peregoy, 1996).

Latina women may experience strong cultural sanctions against substance use, and this could create barriers to their desire to seek treatment as a result of stigma and shame (Terrell, 1993). The influential role of male partners during drug use initiation and continuance of use may be based on the expectation that women behave in accordance with a male partner's expectations (in the tradition of marianismo). It is important to consider the possibility of aversions to disclosing substance-using behavior in which the social community has deemed shameful. Culturally sanctioned gender roles may function to more severely punish substance-abusing behavior among females (Amaro, 2006). In this way, it may be necessary to build the working alliance and demonstrate a nonjudgmental stance during disclosures. Additionally, traditional marianismo and machismo also may function as protective factors for females. Immigration to the United States is associated with increased opportunities for drug use among both sexes, but the risk is greater for females than males (Alegría, Strathdee, & Pantin, 2012). Therefore, these two values may be preventive due to the ideology behind traditional gender roles within the Latino community.

POINTS FOR PRACTICE

Counselors may encounter gender role conflicts either within session or as the client reports difficulties. Counselors who value equality in relationships must be aware of how this bias impacts responding to client reports and treatment formulation. In other words, a counselor should be careful to avoid imposing one's own value regarding the dynamics of interpersonal relationships to the client. Cultural competence requires respect and consideration for values that may differ heavily from those of the counselor (Sue & Sue, 2013). Instead of imposing one's own values, try to help clients to problem-solve within their own cultural framework and weigh the pros and cons of different options.

- Carefully assess for comorbid mental health problems, sexual abuse, and physical abuse among Latina women. Research has shown a high prevalence between these concerns and substance use disorders in Latinas (Amaro et al., 2006). Substance-abusing behavior may be an attempt to cope with negative emotions, manage PTSD symptoms, or reduce stress.
- When working with male clients who endorse machismo, it may be helpful to reframe substance-abusing behavior. Conceptualize and discuss substance-using behaviors as actions that impact his role as head of household. Appeal to the client's sense of responsibility, rather than trying to change beliefs about his role (Rothe & Ruiz, 2001). In this sense, a substance abuse counselor with differing values should focus on the client's values-consistent behavior. Therapy that bolsters the male's role and increases the ability to provide for the family would be more appropriate than confrontational therapeutic styles (Gloria & Peregoy, 1996).

> Take a moment to consider the following:
>
> *How would you describe your view of male gender roles and female gender roles? How did you come to develop your views on gender roles?*
>
> *During a first session, how might you as a counselor informally assess for level of adherence to the above traditional values? What types of questions might you ask? How might the level of adherence to these values inform your approach?*

CONCLUSION

Latino Americans are a diverse and growing population within the United States, with varying adherence to traditional values and gender roles. In order to provide effective substance-abuse services, it is imperative that counselors gain a basic understanding of Latino culture so they may evaluate and attend to behaviors in and out of session in a culturally appropriate manner. This is especially important given the varied adherence to traditional values. Knowledge regarding culture-bound behavior and values also arms a counselor with additional methods for building a strong working alliance, bolstering motivators for treatment, and identifying the sources of substance-using behavior.

REFERENCES

Amaro, H., Arévalo, S., Gonzalez, G., Szapocznik, J., & Iguchi, M. Y. (2006). Needs and scientific opportunities for research on substance abuse treatment among Hispanic adults. *Drug and Alcohol Dependence, 84*(s), s64–s75.

Alegría, M., Strathdee, S. A., & Pantin, H. (2012). Substance risk, prevention treatments and the role of the environment and cultural context in addressing Latinos and other ethnic/racial populations. *Drug and Alcohol Dependence, 125*(s), s2–s3.

Alegría, M., Page, J. B., Hansen, H., Cauce, A. M., Robles, R., Blanco, C., …. (2006). Improving drug treatment services for Hispanics: Research gaps and scientific opportunities. *Drug and Alcohol Dependence, 84*(s), S76–S84.

Bracero, W. (1998). Intimidades: Confianza, gender, and hierarchy in the construction of Latino-Latina therapeutic relationships. *Cultural Diversity and Mental Health, 4*(4), 264–277.

Blume, A. W., Resor, M. R., & Kantin, A. V. (2009). Addiction treatment disparities: Ethnic and sexual minority populations. In P. M. Miller (Ed), *Evidenced-based addiction treatment* (pp. 311–326). New York: Elsevier, Inc.

Blume, A. W., & Resor, M. R. (2012). Harm reduction among Hispanic and Latino populations. In G. A. Marlatt, M. E. Larimer, & K. Witkiewitz (Eds.), *Harm reduction: Pragmatic strategies for managing high-risk behaviors* (pp. 272–290). New York: Guilford Press.

Caetano, R. (2003). Alcohol-related health disparities and treatment-related epidemiological findings among Whites, Blacks, and Hispanics in the United States. *Alcoholism: Clinical and Experimental Research, 27*(8), 233–241.

Center for Substance Abuse Treatment. (2009). Substance abuse treatment: Addressing the specific needs of women. Rockville (MD): Substance Abuse and Mental Health Services Administration (US). (Treatment Improvement Protocol (TIP) Series, No. 51.) Retrieved from: http://www.ncbi.nlm.nih.gov/books/NBK83240/

Díez-Martínez, S., Martín-Moros, J. M., & Altisent-Trota, R. (1991). Cuestionarios breves para la detección precoz de alcoholismo en atención primaria [Quick questionnaires for the early detection of alcoholism at primary care]. *Aten Primaria, 8*, 367–370.

Ennis, S. R., Rios-Vargas, M., & Albert, N. (2011). The Hispanic population: 2010. *U.S. Census briefs*. U.S. Department of Commerce and Economics and Statistics Administration, U.S. Census Bureau, 1–16.

Gloria, A. M., & Peregoy, J. J. (1996). Counseling Latino alcohol and other substance users/abusers. *Journal of Substance Abuse Treatment, 13*(2), 119–126.

Guerrero, E. G., Cepeda, A., Duan, L., & Kim, T. (2012). Disparities in completion of substance abuse treatment among Latino subgroups in Los Angeles County, CA. *Addictive Behaviors, 37*, 1162–1166.

Hayes-Bautista, D. E., & Chapa, J. (1987). Latino terminology: Conceptual base for standardized terminology. *American Journal of Public Health, 77(1)*, 61–68.

Humes, K. R., Jones, N. A., & Ramirez, R. R. (2011). Overview of race and Hispanic origin: 2010. *U.S. Census briefs*. U.S. Department of Commerce and Economics and Statistics Administration, U.S. Census Bureau, 1–23.

Lopez, M. H, Taylor, P., Funk, C., Gonzalez-Barrera, A. (2013). Views about unauthorized immigrants and deportation worries. *Pew Hispanic trends project*. Retrieved from http://www.pewhispanic.org/2013/12/18/3-views-about-unauthorized-immigrants-and-deportation-worries/

Marín, G., & Gamba, R. J. (1996). A new measurement of acculturation for Hispanics: The bidimensional acculturation scale for Hispanics (BAS). *Hispanic Journal of Behavioral Sciences, 18*(3), 297–316.

Martínez, J. (2012). When labels don't fit: Hispanics and their view of identity. *Pew research Hispanic trends project*. Retrieved from http://www.pewhispanic.org/2012/04/04/when-labels-dont-fit-hispanics-and-their-views-of-identity/

Miller, W. R., & Tonigan, J. S. (1996). Assessing drinkers' motivation for change: The Stages of Change Readiness and Treatment Eagerness Scale (SOCRATES), *Psychology of Addictive Behaviors, 10*(2), 81–89.

Miville, M. L., Koonce, D., Darlington, P., & Whitlock, B. (2000). Exploring the relationship between racial/cultural identity and ego identity among African Americans and Mexican Americans. *Journal of Multicultural Counseling and Development, 28*, 208–224.

Motel, S., & Patten, E. (2013, February 15). Statistical portrait of Hispanics in the United States, 2011. Retrieved from http://www.pewhispanic.org/2013/02/15/statistical-portrait-of-hispanics-in-the-united-states-2011/

Office of Applied Studies. (2005). Hispanic substance abuse treatment admissions: 2003. (DASIS Report). Rockville, MD: Office of Applied Studies, Substance Abuse and Mental Health Administration Services.

Organista, K. C., & Muñoz, R. F. (1996). Cognitive behavioral therapy with Latinos. *Cognitive and Behavioral Practice, 3*, 255–270.

Paz, J. (2002). Culturally competent substance abuse treatment with Latinos. *Journal of Human Behavior in the Social Environment, 5*(3), 123–136.

Pew Hispanic Center. (2011). *Statistical portrait of Hispanics in the United States*. Retrieved from http://www.pewhispanic.org/2012/02/21/statistical-portrait-of-the-foreign-born-population-in-the-united-states-2010/

Pew Hispanic Center. (2007). *2007 National survey of Latinos: As illegal immigration issue heats up, Hispanics feel a chill*. Retrieved from http://www.pewhispanic.org/2007/12/13/2007-national-survey-of-latinos-as-illegal-immigration-issue-heats-up-hispanics-feel-a-chill/

Rothe, E. M., & Ruiz, P. (2001). Substance abuse among Cuban Americans. In S. L. A. Straussner (Ed.), *Ethnocultural factors in substance abuse treatment* (pp. 97–110). New York: Guilford Press.

Saltz, R., Lepore, M. F., Sullivan, L. M., Amaro, H., & Samet, J. H. (1999). Alcohol abuse and dependence in Latinos living in the United States. *Archives of Internal Medicine, 159*(7), 718–724.

Santisteban, D., Vega, R. R., & Suarez-Morales, L. (2006). Utilizing dissemination findings to help understand and bridge the research and practice gap in the treatment of substance abuse disorders in Hispanic populations. *Drug and Alcohol Dependence, 84*(s), 94–101.

Santisteban, D. A., Muir-Malcolm, J. A., Mitrani, V. B., & Szapocznik, J. (2002). Integrating the study of ethnic culture and family psychology intervention science. In H. Liddle, R. Levant, D. A. Santisteban, & J. Bray, (Eds.), *Family Psychology Intervention Science*. Washington, DC: American Psychological Association Press.

Substance Abuse and Mental Health Services Administration (2009). *Treatment episode data set (TEDS). Highlights–2007. National Admissions to Substance Abuse Treatment Services*. DASIS Series: S-45, DHHS Publication No. (SMA) 09-4360, Rockville, MD.

Substance Abuse and Mental Health Services Administration, Office of Applied Studies. (June 10, 2010). *The NSDUH report: Substance use among Hispanic adults*. Rockville, MD.

Sue, D. M., & Sue, D. (2013). Counseling Latinos. In D. W. Sue & D. Sue (Eds.), *Counseling the culturally diverse* (pp. 409–424). Hoboken, NJ: John Wiley & Sons, Inc.

Terrell, D. M. (1993). Ethnocultural factors and substance abuse: Toward culturally sensitive treatment models. *Psychology of Addictive Behaviors, 7*(3), 162–167.

Thomson, M. D., & Hoffman-Goetz, L. (2009). Defining and measuring acculturation: A systematic review of public health studies with the Hispanic population in the U.S. *Social Science and Medicine, 69*(7), 983–991.

Tighe, E., & Saxe, L. (2006). Community-based substance abuse reduction and the gap between treatment need and treatment utilization: Analysis of data from the "Fighting Back" general population survey. *Journal of Drug Issues, 6*(2), 295–312.

U.S. Census Bureau. (2012). *Current Population Survey, Annual Social and Economic Supplement.* Retrieved from http://www.census.gov/2010census/data/

U.S. Department of Health and Human Services. (2001). *Mental health: Culture, race, and ethnicity—a supplement to mental health: A report of the surgeon general.* Department of Health and Human Services, Public Health Service Office of the Surgeon General, Rockville, MD.

Wells, K., Klap, R., Koike, A., & Sherbourne, C. (2001). Ethnic disparities in unmet need for alcoholism, drug abuse, and mental health care. *American Journal of Psychiatry, 158*(12), 2027–2032.

WHO ASSIST Working Group. (2002). The Alcohol, Smoking and Substance Involvement Screening Test (ASSIST): Development, reliability and feasibility. *Addiction, 97*(9), 1183–1194.

CHAPTER 9

WOMEN

An extensive literature review on substance abuse treatment and women from 1975 to 2005 found 90 percent of the articles discussing gender differences were published after 1990 (Back, Contini, & Brady, 2007). Over 20 years later, gender differences are now widely recognized within the addiction field, and there is an increased pressure placed on treatment providers to demonstrate the effectiveness of services offered to women. Attention to gender disparities and the dissemination of data regarding gender differences—or lack thereof—has been recommended by organizations such as the National Institute on Drug Abuse (NIDA; Grella, 2007) and the Institute of Medicine (Brady & Ashley, 2005). These disparities are not limited to biological characteristics (e.g., hormone levels or menstrual cycle effects) or substance use patterns, but there are vast differences in personal histories (including trauma), neurobiology, cognitive and affective responses, reasons for use, and the gender roles and cultural expectations of women in the United States. In addition, the impetus for treatment is often a referral from mental health providers or the child welfare system, while men are more likely to enter treatment due to involvement in the criminal justice system (Grella, 2009). Moreover, women experience more barriers to receiving treatment than do men and in the past were shown to be less likely to seek treatment (Green, 2006). Barriers frequently encountered by women are child care responsibilities, transportation, stigmatization, and the inability to pay for treatment. Specialized treatment programming is suggested for the treatment for females struggling with substance use issues.

Take a moment and answer the following questions:

- What percentage of women used an illicit drug in the past year?
- What percentage of women in treatment have a history of childhood sexual abuse?
- What percentage of women in treatment have contact with child welfare services? Have already lost custody of at least one child?
- What special needs and considerations should counselors have regarding women seeking addiction treatment?

The Substance Abuse and Mental Health Services Administration (SAMHSA) conducts a national survey each year, and approximately 67,500 people are interviewed about their alcohol and other drug use. Data collected in 2011 indicates approximately 6 percent of women (aged 12 or older) used an illicit drug in the last 30 days, 12 percent of women used in the past year, and 43 percent reported lifetime use (SAMHSA, 2012). In the last month, 21 percent of women indicated use of tobacco, and 47 percent used alcohol. As far as alcohol consumption, almost 16 percent of women (aged 12 or older) reported binge drinking (defined as drinking five or more drinks at the same time or within a couple of hours of each other), and a little more than 3 percent of women were considered heavy drinkers in the last month (SAMHSA, 2012). Heavy alcohol use is defined as drinking five or more drinks on the same occasion five or more days in the past 30 days. Refer to Table 9.1 below for more statistics on rates of use.

Usage rates vary between women of different races and ethnicities. In 2011, among persons aged 12 or older, the rate of current illicit drug use was lowest among Asians (3.8 percent). The rates were 8.4 percent among Hispanics/Latinos, 8.7 percent among whites, 10.0 percent among African Americans/blacks, 11.0 percent among Native Hawaiians/Other Pacific Islanders, 13.4 percent among American Indians or Alaska Natives, and 13.5 percent among persons of two or more races (SAMHSA, 2012).

Substance use, of course, does not denote the presence of a substance use disorder. What would you suspect is the percentage of women in the United States who have a substance use disorder? In 2011, the SAMHSA national survey indicated 1.7 percent of women reported abuse or dependency on an illicit

Table 9.1: Usage Rates of Illicit Drugs among Females (aged 12 and older)

DRUG	LIFETIME USE (%)	PAST-YEAR USE (%)	PAST-MONTH USE (%)
ILLICIT DRUGS	42.9	12.2	6.5
Marijuana and Hashish	37.4	8.9	4.9
Cocaine	11.1	1.0	0.4
Crack	1.9	0.1	0.1
Heroin	1.1	0.2	0.1
Hallucinogens	10.8	1.1	0.3
LSD	6.3	0.2	0.0
PCP	1.5	0.0	*
Ecstasy	4.8	0.8	0.2
Inhalants	5.5	0.5	0.2
Nonmedical Use of Psychotherapeutics	18.0	5.2	2.2
Pain Relievers	11.2	3.8	1.5
OxyContin®	1.7	0.5	0.1
Tranquilizers	7.8	2.0	0.8
Stimulants	6.7	0.9	0.3
Methamphetamine	3.4	0.3	0.1
Sedatives	2.6	0.3	0.1
ILLICIT DRUGS OTHER THAN MARIJUANA	25.6	6.4	2.6

Source: Center for Behavioral Health Statistics and Quality, National Survey on Drug Use and Health (SAMHSA, 2011).

drug in the last year, and 4.7 percent of women reported abuse or dependency on alcohol in the last year (SAMHSA, 2012). If women seek treatment services to address their abuse or dependency, often data is obtained for research purposes. For instance, SAMHSA researchers identified the primary substance of use among women by race and ethnicity when entering treatment (see Table 9.2 below). For instance, alcohol was the primary substance of abuse reported at admission by Caucasian women (35 percent) and American Indian/Alaska Native women (26 percent). Asian and Pacific Islander women reported methamphetamine most often (33 percent). African American women were more likely to cite crack/cocaine (35 percent). Hispanic/Latina women of Mexican origin reported methamphetamine as the primary drug of use (34 percent), whereas Hispanic/Latina women of Puerto Rican origin were more likely to enter treatment for heroin use (38 percent).

When people enter treatment, the severity of their substance use problems tends to be quite high and there is an impetus for seeking services. What do you think the ratio is for men in treatment versus women? Research from national studies of treatment providers indicate the proportion of female clients has increased over the past decade, but females still only constitute about one-third of the treatment population (Brady & Ashley, 2005). In 2006, of the total admissions, 20 percent were Caucasian women, 6.4 percent were African American, 2.4 percent were Hispanic, 0.9 percent were American Indian/Alaska Native, and 0.4 percent were Asian/Pacific Islander (SAMHSA, 2009).

Women are, in fact, less likely to use illicit drugs and drink less alcohol less often than men; in turn, women are less likely to develop substance-related disorders. However, when women do develop these

Table 9.2: Primary Substance of Abuse among Women Admitted for Treatment by Racial/Ethnic Group by Percentage

SUBSTANCE OF ABUSE	CAUCASIAN	AFRICAN AMERICAN	HISPANIC (MEXICAN ORIGIN)	HI-PAIIIE (PUERTO RIEAN I TRIGIN)	AMERICAN INDIAN/ ALASKA NATIVE	ASIAN/ PACIFIC ISLANDER	TWO OR MORE RACES
Alcohol	35.5	24.8	22.6	20.4	39.5	26.4	21.7
Cocaine/crack	13.3	35.0	12.0	18.4	8.0	9.2	12.0
Heroin	12.7	16.3	11.8	38.5	9.7	8.2	5.7
Other opioids	7.7	1.3	1.7	1.8	4.7	3.1	4.0
Marijuana/hashish	11.8	17.6	15.6	15.2	10.2	16.3	19.4
Methamplietamines	13.3	1.7	34.0	2.2	25.2	33.1	31.9
Benzodiazepines	1.0	0.2	0.1	0.4	0.4	0.3	0.6
Other amphetamines	0.6	0.1	0.3	0.1	0.5	0.7	0.8
Other sedatives/hypnotics	0.4	0.1	0.3	0.1	0.2	0.1	0.2
Hallucinogens	0.1	0.1	0.1	0.1	0.1	0.2	0.1
PCP	0.0*	0.4	0.5	0.3	0.1	0.2	0.2
Inhalants	0.1	0.1	0.2	0.0*	0.2	0.1	0.2
Over-the-counter (OTC) medications	0.1	0.0*	0.1	0.0*	0.1	0.1	0.1

Source: *Substance Abuse Treatment: Addressing the Specific Needs of Women.* Treatment Improvement Protocol (TIP) Series, No. 51. (Center for Substance Abuse Treatment, 2009). SAMHSA/Public Domain.

types of problems, they report experiencing a loss of control over their use in a shorter period of time (i.e., from initiation of use to dependency) and report disruption in more life areas than men do (Stevens, Andrade, & Ruiz, 2009). Moreover, women are shown to experience more health-related consequences (e.g., liver and heart damage, cancer, reproductive issues, osteoporosis, and cognitive/neurological effects) (Green, 2006; Grella, 2007; SAMHSA, 2009); one report even found death rates among female alcoholics to be much higher than those of male alcoholics (Walter, Gutierrez, Ramskogler, Hertling, Dvorak, & Lesch, 2003). The phenomenon of accelerated problems related to use is called "telescoping" (SAMHSA, 2009, p. 7), and this is more common among women than men. Therefore, when women enter treatment, they present with more severe medical, behavioral, psychological, and social problems, despite using less of the substance and for shorter periods of time (Greenfield, Back, Lawson, & Brady, 2010). In the next section, the author further discusses certain substance abuse issues specific to women.

SUBSTANCE ABUSE ISSUES

Women and men differ in reasons for the initiation of chemical use, why they continue to use, how they experience the drug, how and why they access services, the needs while in treatment, and treatment outcomes. This section will address the substance abuse issues which impact women throughout the course of their lives. The author will explore risk factors, trauma, pregnancy, barriers to treatment, and resiliency factors/protective factors before discussing treatment recommendations.

Risk Factors

Take a moment and describe a woman who is more at risk for developing a substance use disorder. What characteristics, histories, or present circumstances would play a role in an increased likelihood of substance abuse? Some risk factors differ according to the age and developmental stages of females.

Risk factors for *young girls* to initiate drug use include the following:

- Early substance use (e.g., before age 16)
- Are impulsive, sensation seekers, or risk takers
- Have parents who use, abuse, or are dependent on a substance (increases prevalence of alcohol use disorders among women by at least 50 percent)
- Have sexual or physical abuse history
- Lack strong, healthy family bonds
- Live in a chaotic, argumentative, violent household
- Lack prosocial peer supports
- Are involved with delinquent behaviors
- Not involved with religious affiliation/activities
- Have a poor self-concept
- Are exposed to drug use
- Lack coping skills (Bodinger-de Uriarte & Austin, 1991; Reed & Evans, 2009; SAMHSA, 2009).

Risk factors identified among adult women with substance abuse diagnoses have also been identified. Females are more at risk to develop substance-related problems when they: (1) have partners who use or partners who do not support their recovery; (2) experience symptoms of depression and anxiety; (3) suffer from post-traumatic stress; (4) have an eating disorder; (5) have difficulty regulating affect; (5) are single parents; (6) are unemployed; and (7) are recently separated, divorced, or widowed (Chander & McCaul, 2003; Covington, 2000; Greenfield, Back, Lawson, & Brady, 2010; Reed & Evans, 2009; SAMHSA, 2009). Moreover, the level of acculturation, discrimination, and socioeconomic status are also considered factors influencing alcohol and other drug use rates.

Trauma

Substance use can be a result of experiencing trauma and a means to self-medicate. Women with substance use disorders have a high incidence of trauma-related events. Compared to nondependent women, women who abuse substances are more likely to have a history of sexual, physical, and emotional abuse, by more perpetrators, more often, and for longer periods of time (Covington, 2000; SAMHSA, 2009). For instance, the rates of childhood sexual abuse among women seeking treatment have been as high as 80 percent (Reed & Evans, 2009). In one study, 74 percent of women enrolled in substance abuse treatment reported rape at an average age of 12 years old, and 80 percent reported physical assault at an average age of 13 years old. Initiation of drug use among these women was at an average age of 13.7 years (Stevens et al., 2009).

Women with histories of abuse are more likely to be retraumatized and revictimized again, including stranger rape, intimate partner violence, and physical assault (Hien & Scheier, 1996). What other experiences can you think of which would be defined as trauma? Trauma is not limited to the exposure of violence or a violation of one's body or mind. Events such as losing a loved one (including miscarriage or abortion), car accident, robbery/burglary, natural disasters, and catastrophic injuries or illnesses are considered traumatic (Covington, 2012; SAMHSA, 2009). In addition, intergenerational (cultural) distress or historical trauma is suffered by women of color and can result in low self-esteem, mental health issues, and substance use (Stevens et al., 2009). Researchers suggest women also survive trauma-related events, including child protective services involvement, witnessing violence, and experiencing the stigma and prejudice due to race, poverty, incarceration, or sexual orientation (Covington, 2000). Exposure to trauma may cause a woman to have suicidal ideations; have deficits in impulse control; cause emotional dysregulation; have low self-esteem; impact relationships; and create disruptions in consciousness, memory, identity, and/or perception of environment (Cormier, Dell, & Poole, 2004; Hien, 2009).

Pregnancy

Substance use while pregnant can have devastating consequences. This section will discuss the rates of use, effects to the fetus, and potential legal repercussions. The prevalence of substance use among pregnant women varies, depending on age. In 2011, current illicit drug use among pregnant women aged 15 to 44 was shown to be 5 percent. However, among pregnant women aged 15 to 17, almost 21 percent reported current illicit drug use, and only 2 percent of pregnant women aged 26 to 44 reported current illicit drug use (SAMHSA, 2012). Among pregnant women aged 15 to 44, (a) 9 percent reported current alcohol use; (b) almost 3 percent reported binge drinking, and (c) 0.4 percent reported heavy drinking. As far as tobacco use, one in six pregnant women aged 15 to 44 indicated smoking cigarettes in the past month (SAMHSA, 2012).

Alcohol use during pregnancy can cause social, emotional, and cognitive developmental problems such as hyperactivity, impulsivity, and attention, learning, and memory deficits (Ait-Daoud & Bahir, 2011). These issues fall under the category of fetal alcohol spectrum disorder (FASD). Fetal alcohol syndrome (FAS) is at the most severe end of the spectrum of fetal alcohol disorders. Some identified facial features include small eye openings, a thin upper lip, and an absence of the groove between the upper lip and nose (i.e., the philtrum). These babies tend to have a low birth weight and small head circumference (refer to the picture below). Children with FAS may be small for their age. Due to the brain damage, these children may have language and speech problems; vision and hearing issues; and problems with thinking, judgment, reasoning, and emotional regulation (Bhuvaneswar & Chang, 2009; Telethon Institute for Child Health Research, n.d.). The prevalence of FAS is estimated to be .03–1.5 cases per 1,000 births, and FASD is said to affect approximately one percent of the United States (Kilgour & Chudley, 2012). Due to the unknown amounts of alcohol that affect pregnancy, women who are pregnant or may become pregnant are advised to abstain from consuming any alcohol (including nonalcoholic beverages, as they contain a small percentage of alcohol).

Other potential consequences of prenatal substance exposure vary by the chemical used. For instance, marijuana has been suggested to cause neonatal jitteriness, a higher-pitched infant cry, potential decreases

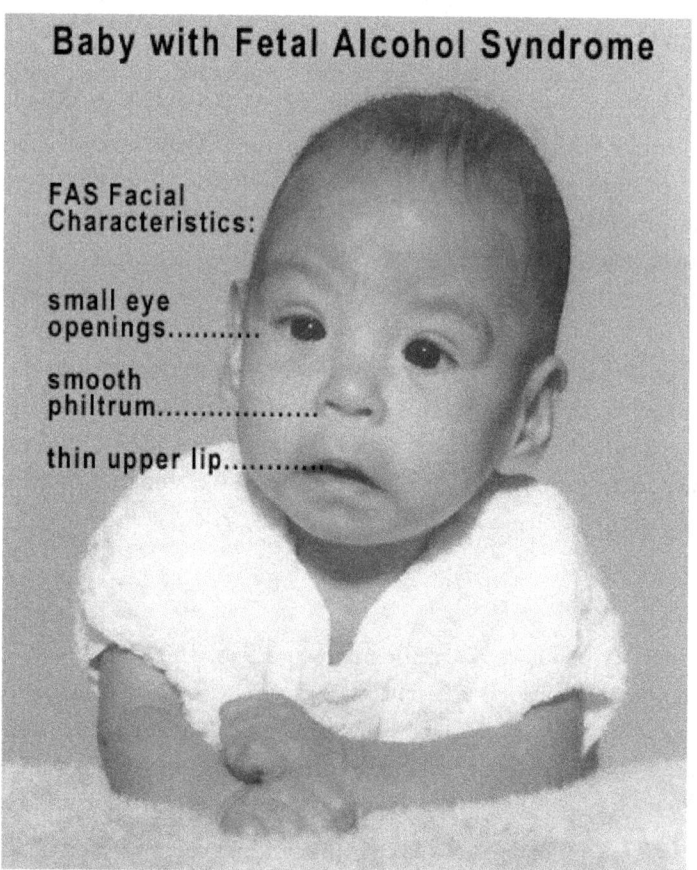

Figure 9.1: Example of Fetal Alcohol Syndrome
Source: Copyright © 2012 by Teresa Kellerman / Wikimedia Commons / CC BY-SA 3.0.

in birth weight, and motor delays (Bhuvaneswar & Chang, 2009). Cocaine use has been shown to produce cardiovascular issues, placental abruption, and attention deficiencies. Opioid use can decrease fetal heart rate and result in neonatal abstinence syndrome (NAS). NAS includes wakefulness, irritability, tremors, temperature problems, failure to thrive, disorganized suck, and potentially seizures. (Bhuvaneswar & Chang, 2009).

Of the females admitted into substance abuse treatment, four percent were known to be pregnant (SAMHSA, 2004). Pregnancy and childbearing are important factors to consider because they may represent barriers to seeking, receiving, or completing treatment. Women with substance use disorders may avoid seeking treatment for fear of losing custody of their children. In fact, as of July 2013, 17 states consider substance use during pregnancy to be child abuse under civil child-welfare statutes, and three states consider use to be grounds for civil commitment. Fourteen states require health care professionals to report suspected prenatal substance abuse, and four states require testing for prenatal drug exposure if substance use is suspected. In some communities, family treatment drug courts are put in place to monitor families with substance use issues; ten states provide pregnant women priority access to state-funded treatment programs. Refer to the Guttmacher Institute's *State Policies in Brief, Substance Abuse During Pregnancy* (2013) for a breakdown of these policies by state.

The results from prenatal drug use can be damaging to the child, substance user, and family members. For a multitude of reasons, our society must be concerned about reducing stigma and helping women eliminate alcohol and other drug use while pregnant. As for financial costs, the total lifetime cost of caring for a substance-exposed child is estimated to be between $750,000 and $1.4 million (Kalotra, 2002). However, the emotional price of losing one's parental rights is immeasurable—and ultimately, the grief over the miscarriage or death of a child is insurmountable.

Barriers to Treatment

Women face many barriers to treatment, and stigma is considered one of the most influential. Stephanie Covington (2000) points out that prior to the 1950s, it was illegal to show a woman drinking in a movie or advertisement in the United States. As our history indicates, women who use (let alone become addicted) experience stigma, or severe social disapproval, and this stigma greatly impacts the likelihood for a woman to seek treatment, access addiction services, and complete a treatment program. There are major differences between the genders in regard to how substance use is perceived. For example, excessive drinking behaviors are often glorified among males, while a woman is viewed as lacking femininity. Women internalize this stigma and feel intense guilt and shame, especially when they lack control over their use. A woman with dependency issues is often labeled as a "bad mother" and a negative image of her sexuality is generated, while the parenting skills or sexuality of a man with substance abuse issues are rarely brought up for evaluation (Greenfield & Grella, 2009).

As stated above, due to their roles as caregiver and the fear of losing custody of their children, many women do not seek treatment (Hecksher & Hesse, 2009). As cited by Grella (2009), most of the women entering into treatment are mothers of dependent children, and "at least half have had contact with child welfare … However, less than half of mothers entering treatment are living with all of their children, and up to one-third have lost their parental rights to at least one child" (p. 310). If a woman does seek substance abuse services, child-rearing responsibilities can be a barrier to treatment. Many facilities do not allow children, or there are restrictions regarding the age and number of children allowed. Moreover, women may be less motivated to participate in treatment because they may have to leave their children in the hands of another person.

Resiliency Factors/Protective Factors

Resiliency has been defined as hardiness and the ability to bounce back from adversity due to intrinsic and extrinsic protective factors (Sutherland, Cook, Stetina, & Hernandez, 2009). From a sociocultural perspective, women tend to define themselves "in relation" and are taught to be "other-focused." Thus, interpersonal and familial relationships impact resiliency. Furthermore, research shows a difference in the prevalence of addiction problems between women based on marital status. Who do you think would have the highest rates of alcohol and illicit drug abuse and dependency: a married, single, or divorced/separated woman? According to SAMHSA (2009), women (aged 18 to 49) who are married have a lower rate of substance use disorders than women of any other marital status. More specifically, 11 percent of divorced or separated women and 16 percent of single women have a substance use disorder, versus only 4 percent of married women. Therefore, the assumption is if a woman is in a stable, encouraging relationship, this can be a protective factor in treatment success. Unfortunately, women entering treatment commonly (1) are in relationships with partners who use substances; (2) have less support; and (3) experience resistance by their partners (Hecksher & Hesse, 2009; SAMHSA, 2009).

According to SAMSHA (2009), counselors should adopt a strength-based treatment approach that builds on the resources of the woman's culture, individual traits and experiences, spirituality, and family. Positive treatment outcomes (and the quality of life) can be influenced by enhancing resiliency factors (Sutherland et al., 2009). In fact, compared to men, women do typically indicate better outcomes. After six-month and five-year follow-ups, women seem to have higher rates of abstinence; demonstrate greater improvement in life areas, such as medical problems; have shorter relapse episodes; and are more likely to seek help after a relapse (Back et al., 2007).

TREATMENT RECOMMENDATIONS

As a population, women's needs in addiction treatment are fundamentally different from men's needs. Based on the substance abuse literature and the information provided previously, this section of the chapter addresses the recommendations for helpers in the social services and medical fields. More specifically, considerations regarding trauma, mental health, screening and assessment, and program planning are offered, in an effort to deliver multiculturally competent services to women struggling with substance use concerns.

Researchers indicate a high incidence of trauma is seen among both men and women who are seeking substance abuse services. As a result of these disturbing events, a co-occurring disorder commonly seen among addicted clients is post-traumatic stress disorder (PTSD). According to the *Diagnostic and Statistical Manual of Mental Disorders,* 5th Edition (*DSM-V*; American Psychiatric Association, 2013), symptoms of PTSD include:

- Nightmares, recurrent/involuntary/distressing memories, or flashbacks
- avoidance of stimuli associated with the event

- the inability to be emotionally close to others
- scanning one's environment for danger, whether physical or emotional
- being numb or feeling nothing
- an exaggerated startle response
- persistent and distorted blame of self or others
- persistent negative emotional state
- reckless or destructive behavior.

PTSD rates among substance-abusing populations are between 14 and 60 percent; up to 80 percent of individuals receiving substance abuse treatment have a lifetime history of PTSD (Hien, 2009). Current PTSD among individuals in treatment is between 30 and 59 percent (Hien, 2009). Comparing the prevalence between genders, women have a much higher incidence of this disorder. In fact, they are two to three times more likely to suffer from PTSD. As stated earlier, many women have physical and sexual abuse histories. Researchers suggest between 55 and 99 percent of women seeking treatment report a history of physical and/or sexual abuse (Greenfield et al., 2010). Substance use disorders also increase a woman's vulnerability to subsequent trauma. In addition, alcohol and other drug use can alter her judgment, decrease her ability to defend herself, and draw her into hazardous environments (SAMHSA, 2009).

As a result of the overwhelming number of women who have endured abuse, counselors are encouraged to view women in treatment as "trauma survivors." If female clients have faced trauma, what should be the goals to substance abuse treatment and trauma recovery? *Do you think counselors need to assist a woman to achieve sobriety/recovery from substance use first, and then treat the trauma?* There continues to be discussion in the behavioral health field as to the process of treatment for these two issues. In essence, there are three models to view therapeutic interventions: (1) **parallel models** incorporate simultaneous, but separate, treatment of each disorder, and each treatment is addressed by different providers/programs; (2) **sequential models** provide addiction treatment first, and are devoted to the development of coping skills and relapse prevention techniques in order to prepare clients to address the trauma at a later time; and (3) **integrated models** employ therapies to concurrently attend to both the addiction and trauma (Hien, 2009).

Trauma recovery approaches should be based on four core assumptions:

- Current dysfunctional behaviors and/or symptoms may have originated as legitimate coping responses to trauma.
- Women who experienced repeated trauma in childhood were deprived of the opportunity to develop the particular skills necessary for adult coping.
- Trauma severs fundamental connections to a person's family, a person's community, and ultimately to oneself.
- Women who have been abused repeatedly feel powerless and are unable to advocate for themselves (Harris & Anglin, 1998).

One well-known and widely used, empirically supported, integrated curriculum used with women in substance abuse therapy is *Seeking Safety: A Treatment Manual for PTSD and Substance Abuse* (Najavits, 2002). The overarching goal is to help women attain safety in relationships, thinking, behavior, and emotions.

This present-focused therapy includes 25 sessions concentrated in three domains: cognitive, behavioral, and interpersonal. The following are some examples of the session titles: PTSD: Taking Back Your Power; Honesty; Asking for Help; Setting Boundaries in Relationships; Creating Meaning; Self-Nurturing; Detaching from Emotional Pain (Grounding). One point worth noting is this curriculum has been shown to be effective for both women and men who have a trauma history, but are not suffering from PTSD (Najavits et al., 2009).

In addition to PTSD, women with substance use disorders are noted to have higher rates of depression and anxiety. Chander and McCaul (2003) state that (compared to the general population), women who are alcohol dependent are four times more likely to have an affective disorder, and they are three times more likely to have an anxiety disorder. Compared to men, women with an alcohol use disorder have higher rates of overall psychiatric comorbidity with such disorders (65 percent versus 44 percent). Moreover, the mental health concerns for women with addictions also tend to be more severe and persistent than the general population (Green, 2006). Therefore, it is vital for health service workers to appropriately screen and assess for several mental health disorders.

Screening and Assessment

Screening and assessment are often the initial contact between a woman and the treatment system. Many times, clients are referred to a treatment provider by a community agency; consequently, behavioral and medical health professionals must be aware of gender differences when an instrument is given. In addition, there are recommendations for the intake process with women, and these will also be discussed in this section. First, the author will address specific instruments and their utility.

The CAGE is a commonly used screening questionnaire that can help determine if further assessment is needed for potential alcohol problems. This tool is comprised of four questions: (1) Have you felt the need to **C**ut down on your drinking? (2) Do you feel **A**nnoyed by people complaining about your drinking? (3) Do you ever feel **G**uilty about your drinking? (4) Do you ever drink an **E**ye-opener in the morning to relieve the shakes? Two or more affirmative responses on the CAGE suggest the client is a problem drinker. One criticism of the CAGE is that it is not gender sensitive, and it is recommended clinicians use a cutoff score of 1 with women. Due to the stigma of alcohol abuse by women, especially among pregnant women, screening tools such as the CAGE may not be as effective because women may be embarrassed about disclosing their use to health care professionals (Ait-Daoud & Bashir, 2011).

Due to the likelihood of the presence of preexisting and substance-induced mental health concerns, screening and assessment becomes a crucial aspect of treatment. Some suggested screening and assessment tools include: Early Trauma Inventory, Childhood Trauma Questionnaire Assessment, PTSD checklist, Mini International Neuropsychiatric Interview (MINI), and the Beck Depression Inventory. Even without the use of formal instruments, clinicians should be screening for symptoms of post-traumatic stress (see Table 9.3 below) and depression, as well as asking about self-harm, eating disorders, and suicidal ideations/plans/intent. Moreover, according to SAMHSA (2009), women should also be screened for pregnancy considerations; immediate risks related to intoxication and withdrawal; immediate risks for present violence; past and present history of sexual victimization and interpersonal violence; and health screenings, including HIV/AIDS, hepatitis, tuberculosis, and STDs.

Table 9.3: Screening Questions for Trauma History

In your lifetime, have you suffered any of the following experiences or seen them happen to someone else?
- Child physical abuse (e.g., hitting that caused bruises or injury)
- Child sexual abuse (e.g., being molested, touched, or forced into any sexual activity)
- Child neglect (e.g., not having enough to eat, inadequate shelter)
- Domestic violence (e.g., a partner who hurt you physically)
- Crime victimization (e.g., rape, holdup)
- Serious accident (e.g., car crash, fire)
- Life-threatening illness (e.g., cancer)
- Natural disaster (e.g., hurricane, earthquake)
- War
- Captivity, incarceration, or kidnapping
- The threat of any of the events listed above
- Violence by you
- Abortion or miscarriage
- Other upsetting events (make a list)

Source: Najavits, 2002; SAMHSA, 2009

Gender-Specific Programming

Historically, addiction treatment has been based on male norms and has not accounted for the specific needs of women. A study by SAMHSA indicates many programs in the United States are still not offering special programming based on gender. Researchers found that of all substance abuse treatment facilities, six percent served women only, 37 percent offered special programs for women, and 19 percent offered special programs for pregnant women (Brady & Ashley, 2005). Furthermore, an estimated 13 percent of substance abuse treatment facilities offered child care services, and 12 percent offered prenatal services. Women-specific groups in treatment programs, as well as self-help groups (e.g., Women for Sobriety meetings), are highly recommended (Greenfield & Pirard, 2009; Stevens et al., 2009). Mixed-gender programs are less likely to be effective in providing a safe environment, thereby making women uncomfortable (especially among those with a history of victimization). In these programs, women tend to perceive men as arrogant or sexist and feel dominated or harassed in such programs (Greenfield & Pirard; Swift & Copeland, 1996).

Gender-specific programming is also important because there are gender differences concerning affective and neural responses to stressors, both qualitatively and quantitatively (Greenfield et al., 2010). For instance, with regard to cigarettes, women experience improvements in mood that men do not. This may be one reason women are not as successful at quitting as men (Stevens et al., 2009). Due to drug use, some women may be used to chaotic environments with higher levels of stress. Boredom can result; thus, engagement in high-risk, sensation-seeking, destructive behaviors may occur. Inhibitory control (e.g., the ability to not use a substance), stress reactivity (causing an urge to use), and the neural processing of behavioral reinforcers are different for men than for women (Eltron & Kilts, 2009). Moreover, women have been shown to report higher cravings when shown conditioned drug use cues (e.g., videos of drug use behavior) than do men, particularly with cocaine- and opioid-dependent females. Research also suggests women display more motivation for drug use and relapse when experiencing negative affects and interpersonal problems (Eltron & Kilts, 2009). Due to these neurobiological responses, recommendations have been put forth when providing addiction treatment to women. For example, providers can focus on stress and anxiety management, the development of coping strategies during treatment, and also employ contingency management and motivational interviewing (Grella, 2009).

Gender-specific programming must also focus on the empowerment of women (Hunter, Jason, & Keys, 2013). Empowerment is more than increasing self-esteem and self-worth. Researchers suggest addiction counselors must also address three factors of empowerment: (1) intrapersonal; (2) interactional; and (3) behavioral. During treatment, a woman's self-perceptions of control, self-efficacy, and competency (i.e., intrapersonal empowerment) should be evaluated and addressed in sessions. In addition, environmental factors must be taken into account, such as skill development and resource awareness (i.e., interactional empowerment). Empowering women to also participate in community and organizational activities and helping behavior through volunteering (i.e., behavioral empowerment) is recommended in an effort to sustain long-term recovery.

Clinicians and treatment program administrators must be committed to multicultural competency in other areas of diversity other than gender. As noted throughout this text, a person has many different identities. Women with substance use disorders are a heterogeneous population with respect to class, sexual orientation, cultural background, substances of abuse, family and parenting status, race and ethnicity, age, marital status, geographic location, and mental health status. Disparities among women of different races and ethnicities have been shown to include: homelessness, education level, health insurance, employment, and criminal justice involvement. Therefore, it is critical to (1) evaluate the effectiveness of gender-focused treatments; and (2) determine the services needed (and provided) in settings with subgroups of women who reflect the diversity of this population (Greenfield & Grella, 2009; Stevens et al., 2009).

In summary, positive treatment outcomes, including sobriety, are contingent on addressing many aspects while a women is in treatment. Gender-specific programming must be comprehensive and take a holistic approach. Issues to tackle in treatment which could impact treatment outcomes are: enhancing self-esteem and a sense of self; cultural awareness and sensitivity; establishing trusting relationships; improving physical, mental, and spiritual health; obtaining a healthy sexuality; pregnancy and parenting skills; the prevention and treatment of trauma; and developing coping and decision-making skills (Covington, 2000).

Service Needs of Women

Addiction issues must be viewed from an ecological approach that incorporates various systems. A woman is influenced by the webs of relationships within each system, and substance use has the potential to impact each of these relationships. In Figure 9.2 below, the five systems (i.e., microsystem, mesosystem, exosystem, macrosystem, and chronosystem) as defined by Bronfenbrenner (1989) are outlined. In order to adequately address substance use disorders, a woman's life must be viewed within the context of her environment at many levels.

When addiction issues are viewed through an ecological lens, it becomes apparent that treatment does not happen in a vacuum. Programs must address the multitude of service needs contained within each system. Some of these needs include: prenatal care, HIV/AIDS services, case management, family- and

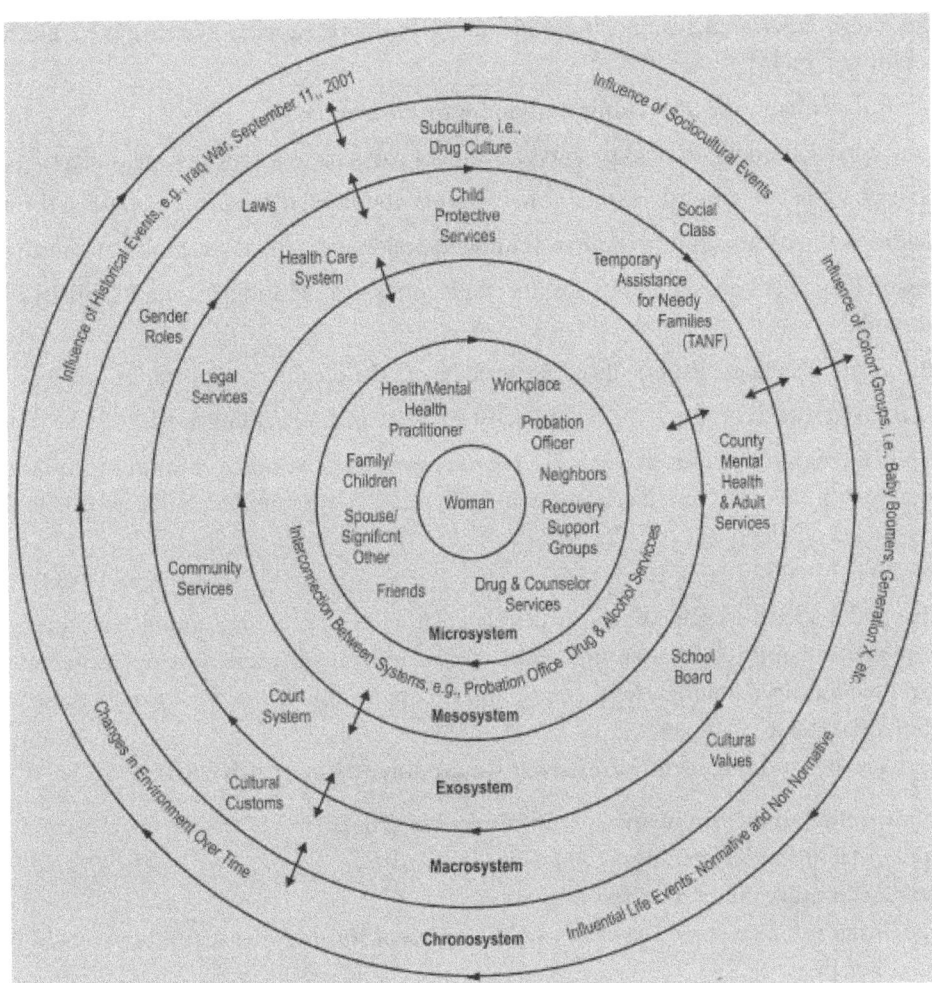

Figure 9.2: The Ecological Framework to Treat Women with Substance Use Disorders

Source: *Substance Abuse Treatment: Addressing the Specific Needs of Women.* Treatment Improvement Protocol (TIP) Series, No. 51. (SAMHSA, Center for Substance Abuse Treatment, 2009).

child-related care, legal services, educational referrals, housing assistance, and money management and budgeting. For a full listing of recommended service needs, see Appendix A.

To summarize, recommendations include treatment that:

- is gender specific and endorses a developmental perspective
- is easily assessable and attainable (e.g., no waiting lists and affordable)
- appropriately screens, assesses, and continuously monitors for mental health concerns, self-injury, suicidal ideation, eating disorders, trauma, and interpersonal violence
- takes into account the multiple identities of a woman and the implications of such identities
- is not a rigid, structured delivery style
- is non-confrontational and collaborative

- focuses on interpersonal relationships, including building support systems (i.e., use a relational model for treatment)
- addresses the enhancement of family and domestic environments
- includes behavioral couples therapy and encourages partners to attend self-help meetings
- addresses trauma concurrently and educates women about what constitutes abuse and trauma
- normalizes women's reactions to trauma. Trauma responses are normal reactions to abnormal situations
- focuses on empowerment (including intrapersonal, interactional and behavioral) and uses a strengths-based model
- is holistic and provides a variety of service needs (e.g., child care, transportation, etc.)
- uses a recovery coach or peer support specialist to assist with providing services and support
- takes on an ecological approach devoted to reducing stigma, prejudice, and misinformation directed at women with substance use disorders at an individual, programmatic, and systemic level

Exercise

A woman has many identities and these can be related to class, sexual orientation, cultural background, substances of abuse, family and parenting status, race and ethnicity, age/developmental stage, marital status, geographic location, abilities, legal status, and mental health status. Pick five of these identities to describe a potential client.

Get with a partner and discuss how treatment would differ for your two clients.

1. How do you think these two women could connect in group?
2. What potential misunderstandings could occur?
3. How could these differences manifest in group?
4. What potential risk factors and barriers would be present for this client, and how would you address these as a therapist?

REFERENCES

Ait-Daoud, N., & Bashir, M. (2011). Women and substance abuse: Health considerations and recommendations. *CNS Spectrums, 16*, 37–47. doi:10.1017/S1092852912000168

Back, S. E., Contini, R., & Brady, K. T. (2007). Substance abuse in women: Does gender matter? *Psychiatric Times, 24*, 48.

Brady, T. M., & Ashley, O. S. (Eds.). (2005). *Women in substance abuse treatment: Results from the Alcohol and Drug Services Study (ADSS)* (DHHS Publication No. SMA 04-3968, Analytic Series A-26). Rockville, MD: Substance Abuse and Mental Health Services Administration, Office of Applied Studies.

Bronfenbrenner, U. (1989). Ecological systems theory. In R. Vasta (Ed.), *Annals of child development* (pp. 187–249). Greenwich, CT: JAI Press.

Center for Substance Abuse Treatment (2009). *Substance Abuse Treatment: Addressing the Specific Needs of Women.* Treatment Improvement Protocol (TIP) Series, No. 51. HHS Publication No. (SMA) 09-4426. Rockville, MD: Substance Abuse and Mental Health Services Administration.

Chander, G., & McCaul, M. E. (2003). Co-occurring psychiatric disorders in women with addictions. *Obstetrics and Gynecology Clinics, 30*, 469–481.

Cormier, R. A., Dell, C. A., & Poole, N. (2004). Women and substance abuse problems. Retrieved June 25, 2013, from http://www.ncbi.nlm.nih.gov/pmc/articles/PMC2096682/

Covington, S. (2000). Helping women to recover: Creating gender-specific treatment for substance-abusing women and girls in community correctional settings. In M. McMahon (Ed.), *Assessment to assistance: Programs for women in community corrections* (pp. 171–233). Latham, MD: American Correctional Association.

Covington, S. (2012). Trauma services for women and girls. PowerPoint Presentation from the Family Drug Court Symposium, September 6, 2012, in Anaheim, CA.

Elton, A., & Kilts, C. D. (2009). The roles of sex differences in the drug addiction process. In K. T. Brady, S. E. Back, & S. F. Greenfield (Eds.), *Women and addiction* (pp. 147–170). New York: Guilford Press.

Green, C. A. (2006). Gender and use of substance abuse treatment services. *Alcohol Research and Health, 29*, 55–62.

Greenfield, S. F., Beck, S. E., Lawson, K., & Brady, K. T. (2010). Substance abuse in women. *Psychiatric Clinics of North America, 33*, 339–355.

Greenfield, S. F., & Grella, C. E. (2009). What is "women-focused" treatment for substance use disorders? *Psychiatric Services, 60*(7), 880–882.

Greenfield, S. F., & Pirard, S. (2009). Gender-specific treatment for women with substance use disorders. In K. T. Brady, S. E. Back, & S. F. Greenfield (Eds.), *Women and addiction* (pp. 242–256). New York: Guilford Press.

Grella, C. E. (2007). Substance abuse treatment services for women: A review of policy initiatives and recent research. Prepared for California Department of Alcohol and Drug Programs (Contract No. 06-00137). Retrieved June 6, 2013, from http://www.adp.ca.gov/oara/pdf/SARC_white%20paper_ADP_Grella.pdf

Grella, C. E. (2009). Treatment seeking and utilization among women with substance use disorders. In K. T. Brady, S. E. Back, & S. F. Greenfield (Eds.), *Women and addiction* (pp. 242–256). New York: Guilford Press.

Guttmacher Institute (2013). Substance abuse during pregnancy. *State Policies in Brief*. Retrieved July 17, 2013, from http://www.guttmacher.org/statecenter/spibs/spib_SADP.pdf

Harris, M., & Anglin, J. (1998). *Trauma recovery and empowerment: A clinician's guide for working with women in groups*. New York: Free Press.

Hecksher, D., & Hesse, M. (2009). Women and substance use disorders. *Mens Sana Monographs, 7*, 50–62.

Hien, D. A. (2009). Trauma, posttraumatic stress disorder, and addiction among women. In K. T. Brady, S. E. Back, & S. F. Greenfield (Eds.), *Women and addiction* (pp. 242–256). New York: Guilford Press.

Hien, D. A., & Scheier, J. (1996). Short-term predictors of outcome for drug-abusing women in detox: A follow-up study. *Journal of Trauma, Injury, Infection, and Critical Care, 53* (5), 882–888.

Hunter, B. A., Jason, L. A., & Keys, C. B. (2013). Factors of empowerment for women in recovery from substance use. *American Journal of Community Psychology, 51*, 91–102.

Kalotra, C. J. (2002). *Estimated costs related to the birth of a drug and/or alcohol exposed baby*. Washington, DC: Office of Justice programs Drug Court Clearinghouse and Technical Assistance Project. Retrieved June 29, 2013, from http://www1.spa.american.edu/justice/publications/babies.pdf

Kilgour, A. R., & Chudley, A. E. (2012). Fetal alcohol spectrum disorder. In J. C. Verster, K. Brady, M. Galanter, & P. Conrod (Eds.), *Drug abuse and addiction in medical illness*. New York: Springer.

Najavits, L. M. (2002). *A woman's addiction workbook: Your guide to in-depth healing*. Oakland, CA: New Harbinger.

Najavits, L. M., Schmitz, M., Johnson, K. M., Smith, C., North, T., Hamilton, N., et al. (2009). Seeking safety therapy for men: Clinical and research experiences. In *Men and Addictions*. Hauppauge, NY: Nova Science Publishers.

Reed, S. C., & Evans, S. M. (2009). Research design and methodology in studies of women and addiction. In K. T. Brady, S. E. Back, & S. F. Greenfield (Eds.), *Women and addiction* (pp. 14–31). New York: Guilford Press.

Stevens, S. J., Andrade, R. C., & Ruiz, B. S. (2009). Women and substance abuse: Gender, age, and cultural considerations. *Journal of Ethnicity in Substance Abuse, 8,* 341–358.

Substance Abuse and Mental Health Services Administration (2012). *Results from the 2011 National Survey on Drug Use and Health: Summary of National Findings,* NSDUH Series H-44, HHS Publication No. (SMA) 12-4713. Rockville, MD.

Sutherland, J. A., Cook, L., Stetina, P., & Hernandez, C. (2009). Women in substance abuse recovery: Measures of resilience and self-differentiation. *Western Journal of Nursing Research, 31,* 905–922.

Swift, W., & Copeland, J. (1996). Treatment needs and experiences of Australian women with alcohol and other drug problems. *Drug and Alcohol Dependence, 40,* 211–219.

Telethon Institute for Child Health Research. (n.d.). Alcohol, pregnancy and FASD. Retrieved June 29, 2013, from http://alcoholpregnancy.childhealthresearch.org.au/about/fetal-alcohol-spectrum-disorders-%28fasd%29.aspx

Walter, H., Gutierrez, K., Ramskogler, K., Hertling, I., Dvorak, A., & Lesch, O. M. (2003). Gender-specific differences in alcoholism: Implications for treatment. *Archives of Women's Mental Health, 6,* 253–258.

APPENDIX A

Services Needed in Women's Substance Abuse Treatment

The following services are recommended to be provided across the continuum of care, beginning with early intervention and extending to continuing care services. Promising practices designed to treat women with substance use disorders include comprehensive and integrated clinical and community services that are ideally delivered at a one-stop location. Note: This list does not incorporate the customary services that are provided in standard substance abuse treatment, but rather services that are more reflective of women's needs.

Medical Services

- Gynecological care
- Family Planning
- Prenatal care
- Pediatric care
- HIV/AIDS services
- Treatment for infectious diseases, including viral hepatitis
- Nicotine cessation treatment services

Health Promotion

- Nutritional counseling
- Educational services about reproductive health
- Wellness programs
- Education on sleep and dental hygiene
- Education about STDs and other infectious diseases; e.g., viral hepatitis and HIV/AIDS
- Preventive health care education

Psychoeducation

- Sexuality education
- Assertiveness skills training
- Education on the effects of alcohol and other drugs on prenatal and child development
- Prenatal education

Gender-Specific Needs

- Women-only programming
- Lesbian services

Cultural and Language Needs

- Culturally appropriate programming
- Availability of interpreter services or treatment services in native language

Life Skills

- Money management and budgeting
- Stress reduction and coping skills training

Family and Child-Related Services

- Child care services, including homework assistance in conjunction with outpatient services
- Children's programming, including nurseries and preschool programs
- Family treatment services, including psychoeducation surrounding addiction and its impact on family functioning
- Couples counseling and relationship enrichment recovery groups
- Parent/child services, including developmentally age-appropriate programs for children and education for mother about child safety; parenting education; nutrition; children's substance abuse prevention curriculum; and children's mental health needs, including recreational activities, school, and other related activities

Comprehensive Case Management

- Linkages to welfare system, employment opportunities, and housing
- Integration of stipulations from child welfare, TANF, probation and parole, and other systems
- Intensive case management, including case management for children
- Transportation services
- Domestic violence, including referral to safe houses
- Legal services
- Assistance in establishing financial arrangements or accessing funding for treatment services
- Assistance in obtaining a GED or further education, career counseling, and vocational training, including job readiness training to prepare women to leave the program and support themselves and their families
- Assistance locating appropriate housing in preparation for discharge, including referral to transitional living or supervised housing

Mental Health Services

- Trauma-informed and trauma-specific services
- Eating disorder and nutrition services

- Services for other co-occurring disorders, including access to psychological and pharmacological treatments for mood and anxiety disorders
- Children's mental health services

Disability Services

- Resources for learning disability assessments
- Accommodations for specific disabilities
- Services to accommodate illiteracy

Staff and Program Development

- Strong female role models in terms of both leadership and personal recovery
- Peer support
- Adequate staffing to meet added program demands
- Staff training and gender competence in working with women
- Staff training and program development entered upon incorporating cultural and ethnic influences on parenting styles, attitudes toward discipline, children's diets, level of parenting supervision, and adherence to medical treatment
- Flexible scheduling and staff coordination
- Adequate time for parent-child bonding and interactions
- Administrative commitment to addressing the unique needs of women in treatment
- Staff training and administrative policies to support the integration of treatment services with clients on methadone maintenance
- Culturally appropriate programming that matches specific socialization and cultural practices for women

TIP 51. Substance Abuse Treatment: Addressing the Specific Needs of Women.
Source: SAMHSA, 2009.

CHAPTER 10

ADOLESCENTS AND YOUNG ADULTS

OVERVIEW

Adolescence and young adulthood are sensitive times in which substantial cognitive, emotional, physical, and neurobiological development occur. As an individual's brain continues to grow and develop, many aspects of functioning are impacted such as impulse control, decision making, and abstract thinking. Adolescence and young adulthood are also times in which people are more vulnerable to peer influence and more likely to struggle with self-esteem issues. These concerns are important to consider when conceptualizing risk factors for substance use. If one initiates substance use during these times, countless negative consequences can result, including developing a substance use disorder. In fact, researchers have shown the earlier a person begins to use substances, the more likely he or she is to develop a substance use disorder. In the following sections, this author provides information regarding statistics, substance abuse issues, and assessment and treatment considerations for adolescents and young adults. The Substance Abuse and Mental Health Services Administration (SAMHSA) defines "adolescents" as those aged 12 to 17 and "young adults" as those aged 18 to 25. For the purposes of this chapter, these two age groups are defined in the same manner and referred to as two separate populations. However, at times, the two groups will also be discussed as one population, "adolescents and young adults" (AYA), and this term will denote those aged 12 to 25. Going further, the majority of college students fall into the young adult age group; thus, the author will highlight some of the particular needs and special considerations of the college population within this chapter as well.

STATISTICS

To begin, statistics will be given regarding the AYA population, including rates of substance use, substance use disorder diagnoses, and treatment admissions. Because the AYA group encompasses individuals aged 12–25, data will be presented based on specific categories. More specifically, this section addresses: (1) middle and high school students; (2) adolescents; (3) young adults; and (4) college students.

Middle and High School Students

Since 1975, "Monitoring the Future" has been a large-scale, yearly research study that surveys 8th, 10th, and 12th graders about their alcohol and other drug use. In 2013, 41,700 students were surveyed; it was determined there was an increase in lifetime illicit drug use from 2012 to 2013 among all three groups. For instance, 50.4 percent of 12th graders have tried an illicit drug in their lifetime, which was an increase of 1.3 percent from 2012. However, alcohol use rates for all three groups decreased an average of 1.5 percent, and cigarette use decreased an average of 1.4 percent (Johnston, O'Malley, Miech, Bachman, & Schulenberg, 2014). See Table 10.1 below for greater detail regarding use of various substances among this age group.

In addition to substance use rates, 12th graders were also asked about whether they disapproved of certain drug use behaviors. Interestingly, while over 45 percent of high school seniors indicated prior marijuana use in their lifetime, 49.1 percent reported disapproval of once or twice marijuana use. In fact, 74.5 percent of 12th graders stated they disapproved of regular marijuana use (Johnston et al., 2014). Researchers also inquired about perceived harm or risk associated with certain drugs. Almost 70 percent of seniors reported the occasional use of bath salts was harmful; 38.8 percent indicated it was harmful to use Adderall; 36.2 percent stated there was harm in using synthetic marijuana; and 21.3 percent reported harm in using *Salvia divinorum*. In contrast, when asked about occasional marijuana use, 19.5 percent of 12th graders perceived it to be harmful (Johnston et al., 2014).

Adolescents

SAMHSA has gathered data regarding substance use patterns, hospital visits, substance-use disorders, and treatment admissions among those aged 12 to 17. In 2010, 10.1 percent of adolescents had used an illicit drug in the past month (SAMHSA, 2011). In fact, in the same study, investigators determined 14.3 percent of youths in this age group indicated they had been approached by someone selling drugs in the past month. As far as alcohol use, 13.6 percent of 12 to 17 year olds consumed alcohol in the past 30 days, and 7.8 percent of adolescents reported binge drinking. In addition to substance use rates, data was also examined pertaining to the rates of hospital emergency department visits by adolescents aged 12 to 17. On an average day, alcohol is involved in 187 visits by adolescents, marijuana is implicated in 165 visits, and misuse of prescription or nonprescription pain relievers is associated with 74 visits (SAMHSA, 2013).

Table 10.1: Lifetime Rates of Substance Use by 8th, 10th, and 12th Graders, in 2013

	ANY ILLICIT DRUG USE	MARIJUANA	OTHER DRUGS EXCLUDING MARIJUANA	CIGARETTES	ALCOHOL
8th	20.3 percent	16.5 percent	9.3 percent	14.8 percent	27.8 percent
10th	38.8 percent	35.8 percent	15.7 percent	25.7 percent	52.1 percent
12th	50.4 percent	45.5 percent	24.7 percent	38.1 percent	68.2 percent

Source: Monitoring the Future Study (Johnston et al., 2014). Copyright © 2014 by the Regents of the University of Michigan..

Substance use disorders were found among 7.3 percent of those aged 12 to 17, and more specifically, 4.5 percent of adolescents had an alcohol abuse or dependence diagnosis (SAMHSA, 2011). The number of youths in need of treatment for an illicit drug or alcohol use problem in 2010 was 1.8 million, or 7.5 percent of the adolescent population. This represents a reduction in those identified as in need of treatment from 2002, when 2.3 million needed treatment, or 9.1 percent of this population. Of the 1.8 million youths who needed treatment in 2010, 138,000 received treatment at a specialty facility (or approximately 7.6 percent), leaving 1.7 million who needed substance abuse services, but did not receive them.

Racial and Ethnic Differences in Use

One large study conducted from 2005 to 2008 analyzed data from 72,561 youth aged 12 to 17. Adolescents were asked about their substance use in the past year, and it was determined 47.5 percent of Native American youth had used either alcohol or another drug in the past year, as compared to 39.2 percent of whites, 36.7 percent of Hispanics, 36.4 percent of multiple races/ethnicities, 32.2 percent of African Americans, and 23.7 percent of Asian/Pacific Islanders (Wu, Woody, Yang, Pan, & Blazer, 2011).

The researchers also found white, Native American, multiple race/ethnicity, and Hispanic adolescents showed a higher likelihood of having substance-related disorders than African Americans. Native Americans had the highest prevalence of substance-related disorders (15.0 percent), followed by adolescents of multiple race/ethnicity (9.2 percent), whites (9.0 percent), Hispanics (7.7 percent), African Americans (5.0 percent), and Asians or Pacific Islanders (3.5 percent). Additionally, adolescents of multiple race/ethnicity (19.4 percent), Hispanics (16.2 percent), and white race/ethnicity (14.3 percent) had higher rates of comorbid alcohol and drug use disorders than African Americans (8.3 percent).

Young Adults

In 2010, researchers found the rate of binge drinking among young adults was 40.6 percent, with the highest rates of use among those aged 21 to 25 at 45.5 percent. In addition, approximately one out of five (21.5 percent) young adults aged 18 to 25 reportedly used an illicit drug in the previous 30 days (SAMHSA, 2011). Compared to other age groups, young adults are the biggest abusers of prescription opioid pain relievers, ADHD stimulants, and antianxiety drugs. More specifically, 13 percent of those aged 18 to 25 illicitly used prescription drugs in the past year, while only 7 percent of persons aged 12 to 17 and 4 percent of those aged 26 or older did so. In 2010, almost 3,000 young adults died from prescription drug (mainly opioid) overdoses—more than those who died from overdoses of any other drug, including heroin and cocaine combined. This number was a 250 percent increase from 1999 (2908 deaths versus 833 deaths) and was an estimated eight deaths per day (National Institute on Drug Abuse [NIDA], 2013).

Substance use disorder diagnosis rates have also been examined among adults aged 18 to 25. Researchers found almost 20 percent of the young adult population qualified for such a diagnosis in 2010. When investigating further, 15.6 percent of this population had an alcohol abuse or dependence diagnosis, specifically.

College Students

Many young adults are enrolled full time in college, and this section addresses substance use rates among these students. Compared to their peers who are not enrolled full time (i.e., part-time college students and persons not currently enrolled in college), full-time college students (aged 18 to 22) are more likely to use alcohol in the past month, binge drink, and drink heavily. Among full-time college students in 2010, 63.3 percent were current drinkers, 42.2 percent were binge drinkers, and 15.6 percent were heavy drinkers. In contrast, of those young adults not enrolled full time in college, 52.4 percent were current drinkers, 35.6 percent were binge drinkers, and 11.9 percent were heavy drinkers (SAMHSA, 2011). One well-known survey, called the CORE, gathered data in 2011 from over 50,000 students nationwide. The results were consistent with SAMHSA data collected in 2010 that were previously mentioned. The CORE found 63.4 percent of students (under the age of 21) consumed alcohol in the last 30 days, and 44.8 percent reported binge drinking in the past two weeks (CORE, 2013).

Unlike alcohol use, cigarette smoking was shown to be less prevalent among full-time college students than their peers who were not enrolled full time in college. Past month cigarette use in 2010 was reported by 24.8 percent of full-time college students, as compared to 39.9 percent for those not enrolled full time. One point worth noting was that specifically among males aged 18 to 22 who were full-time college students in 2010, cigarette use significantly declined in a period of one year, from 31.7 percent in 2009 to 27.1 percent in 2010 (SAMHSA, 2011).

In 2010, an investigation of the rate of current illicit drug use among full-time college students (aged 18 to 22) revealed that 22 percent reported current illicit drug use. This rate was noted to be similar to the rate among other persons aged 18 to 22 who were part-time college students, students in other grades or types of institutions, and nonstudents (23.5 percent). Almost one-third (32.0 percent) of college students indicated smoking marijuana in the last year, and 18.7 percent indicated use in the last 30 days. In addition, approximately 5 percent reported nonmedical use of psychotherapeutic drugs, (SAMHSA, 2011). Another study found 7.6 percent of students reported illicit use of pain medication, and 7.8 reported illicit use of stimulant medications (American College Health Association [ACHA], 2013).

In lieu of focusing strictly on substance use rates, studies reveal that a large percentage of college students report low rates or nonproblematic use patterns. In 2013, the National College Health Assessment was given to over 131,000 students at 172 postsecondary institutions. Many students reportedly never used alcohol and other drugs in the past. In fact, researchers found (a) 21 percent of students in their study had never used alcohol; (b) 69 percent had never used cigarettes; (c) 62 percent had never used marijuana; and (d) 66 percent had never used other drugs (ACHA, 2013). In contrast to popular belief, the ACHA (2013) study found that a large number of students consumed alcohol in a non–binge drinking pattern. Of the drinkers in the survey, 60 percent of students reported drinking four or fewer drinks the last time they socialized.

SUBSTANCE ABUSE ISSUES

Risk Factors

Several variables are correlated with an increased probability for substance use. These variables can be at three different levels: (1) individual; (2) community and family; and (3) societal. At an individual level, substance use can be linked to biological characteristics, developmental status, and the personal attitudes toward alcohol and other drugs. All people have certain beliefs and expectations associated with alcohol, marijuana, cocaine, pain medication, heroin, etc. Thus, some people may use alcohol, but will never try illicit drugs, while others may use marijuana, but will never try cocaine. These beliefs and expectations are created and maintained by many other factors, including community, family, and society. In turn, these factors also influence whether someone tries a drug and continues to use a drug.

As an age group, adolescents and young adults tend to have specific factors that increase the likelihood of initiation and continued use of substances. For instance, AYAs tend to have the (a) belief that "it won't happen to me" (i.e., invisibility ideology); and (b) physical ability to bounce back from substance use and its consequences. These two characteristics of AYAs tend to impede abstinence from alcohol and other drugs during this time period. Another factor to consider is the developmental process of the AYA brain. One area of the brain, the frontal lobe, goes through extensive neuromaturation during adolescence, and it is important to understand how this could impact the likelihood of substance use. The frontal lobe is associated with planning, inhibition, emotion regulation, and integration of novel stimuli. Due to an undeveloped frontal lobe, AYAs tend to display poor impulse control (Shin, Chung, & Jeon, 2013). This may influence initiation of substance use in the first place; on the other hand, drugs can impact this part of the brain and cause the user to act without thinking while intoxicated. For instance, alcohol use can greatly impact the inhibitory control and decision-making abilities of an AYA (Squeglia, Jacobus, & Tapert, 2009). In fact, research has shown that heavy drinking during adolescence can lead to decreased performance on cognitive tasks of memory, attention, spatial skills, and executive functioning (Squeglia et al., 2009).

Brain development issues also influence the engagement in other behaviors such as fighting or theft. It should be noted that these kinds of behaviors also appear to be correlated to substance use as well. For instance, one study found that youths aged 12 to 17 who engaged in fighting or other delinquent behaviors were more likely than other youths to have used illicit drugs in the past month. More specifically, in 2010, past-month illicit drug use was reported by 18.3 percent of youths who had gotten into a serious fight at school or work in the past year, compared with 8.0 percent of those who had not engaged in fighting at school or work. In addition, 39.3 percent of youth who had stolen or tried to steal something worth over $50 in the past year had reported past-month drug use, compared with 8.8 percent of those who had not attempted or engaged in such theft (SAMHSA, 2011).

In an effort to address many of the risk factors identified by researchers, the following list was created. The list includes individual, community and family, and societal risk factors:

- Early onset of use
- History of abuse or neglect
- History of trauma
- Grief issues
- Emotional or mental health issues
- Low self-esteem
- Feelings of powerlessness
- Attitudes favorable to drug use

- Sensation-seeking tendencies, impulsiveness, and underdeveloped self-regulation skills
- Peers who are users
- Peer rejection in elementary grades
- Gang involvement
- Lack of alternative activities
- Low commitment to school or dropping out of school
- Engaging in deviant or antisocial behaviors
- Experiences of racism
- LGBTQ youth
- Family members who use or have attitudes favorable to drug use
- Lack of parental monitoring
- Living in extreme economic deprivation
- Living in a community where there is more access to alcohol and other drugs (Fields, 2013; Hanson, Venturelli, & Fleckenstein, 2011; Hart & Ksir, 2013; Inaba & Cohen, 2011; Levinthal, 2014; Randolph, Russell, Tillman, & Fincham, 2010).

At the societal level, the influence that media has on alcohol and drug use is substantial. Celebrities can be seen discussing their own personal drug use, and musicians can be heard endorsing the use of marijuana, Molly (i.e., ecstasy), or "syrup" (i.e., cough medicine with codeine). One study found that on Music Television (MTV), adolescents and young adults can see alcohol use every 14 minutes; drugs are present in nearly half of music videos (alcohol in 35 percent, tobacco in 10 percent, and illicit drugs in 13 percent); and in popular music, the average teenager is exposed to nearly 85 drug references a day (as cited by Strasburger, 2010). Alcohol and other drug use is also depicted in countless movies, and many films focus on illicit drug use such as *Half Baked*, *Scarface*, *Blow*, and *Pulp Fiction*. In fact, some researchers found 22 percent of movies portrayed drug scenes (as cited by Strasburger, 2010). In addition to music and movies, primetime television also regularly displays substance use. Many of these shows are very popular in the United States (e.g., *Weeds*, *Breaking Bad*). Social media sites on the Internet are other places where pictures, videos, and written statements can be streamed instantly to family, friends, and the public. Alcohol and other drugs can be advertised on these sites, and it provides a format for individuals to glorify, shame, or degrade those who use substances. In essence, social media is another avenue used to influence an AYA's stance on alcohol and other drug use.

Preventive Factors

Despite the presence of risk factors, there are facets in one's life that can protective from initiating and maintaining alcohol and other drug use. These preventive factors include: having a commitment to school, involvement in the community, participation in extracurricular activities, having a strong spiritual/religious affiliation, associating with a prosocial peer group and role models, having a strong sense of family, feeling valued, having an internal locus of control and feelings of self-efficacy, and upholding a personal opinion on alcohol and other drug use (Fields, 2013; Inaba & Cohen, 2011; Levinthal, 2014).

Researchers investigated whether alcohol and drug use rates among youth aged 12 to 17 differed, depending on the presence of various preventive factors. For instance, the results of one study suggest religion affiliation is correlated with lower rates of illicit drug use. Of the youth who agreed or strongly agreed that religious beliefs are a very important part of life, 7.9 percent indicated illicit drug use in the past 30 days. For those who disagreed with that statement, almost double (16.6 percent) reported past-month illicit drug use. Similar differences were also found for rates of past-month binge alcohol use (6.1 percent and 12.9 percent, respectively) (SAMHSA, 2011).

The strength of family bonds, the level of parental involvement, and parental attitudes toward alcohol and other drug use appear to influence rates of use among AYAs. Rates were lower for those who believed their parents would strongly disapprove of substance use, as compared to youths who believed their parents would somewhat disapprove or neither approve nor disapprove. Among youths who perceived strong parental disapproval of their smoking one or more packs of cigarettes per day, 5.8 percent reported past-month cigarette use; however, among youths who believed their parents would not strongly disapprove, rates were almost 7 times higher (39.8 percent). Also, past-month marijuana use was almost 7.5 times more prevalent among youths who did not perceive a strong parental disapproval for trying marijuana, as compared to those who did perceive a strong disapproval (32.8 percent and 4.4 percent, respectively).

Consequences of Use

Countless negative consequences occur when adolescents and young adults use alcohol and other drugs. Due to the developmental processes that happen during this time, substance use can be very detrimental to the maturation and health of the cognitive, emotional, physical, and neurological aspects of an AYA's life. When intoxicated, the following consequences are possible: (a) impaired brain functioning; (b) traumatic brain injuries; (c) risky sexual behavior; (d) unwanted sexual contact; (e) verbal and physical altercations; (f) physical injuries; (g) fatal car accidents; (h) embarrassment due to exposure on social media sites; (i) "drunk dialing or texting"; and (j) legal trouble (Fachini, Aliane, Martinez, & Furtado, 2012; Sussman, Skara, & Ames, 2008). If an AYA drives under the influence of any drug (not just alcohol), he or she could get arrested. Counselors should note that a minor (under the age of 21) who is driving with any alcohol in his or her system (e.g., a blood alcohol content of .03) can get arrested for driving under the influence. Moreover, if AYAs are caught with an illicit drug besides marijuana (e.g., cocaine, ecstasy, Adderall, Xanax, etc.) in their possession, they can be charged with a felony. "In their possession" may include on their physical person, but may also include the very presence of the substance in their car, for example.

Researchers have investigated the consequences experienced by college students. One study found that 1,825 college students die each year from alcohol-related unintentional injuries. Alcohol is involved in 599,000 nonfatal unintentional injuries, 696,000 assaults, and 97,000 cases of sexual assault and acquaintance rape (Hingson, Zha, & Weitzman, 2009). Another study asked not only about alcohol, but also other drug use. Researchers asked college students if they experienced certain consequences related to public misconduct and personal problems in the last year due to alcohol and other drug use. Thirty-three percent of students reported some form of public misconduct (e.g., trouble with police, fighting, vandalism) in the past year, and 22.0 percent stated there were serious personal problems (e.g., suicidality, being injured, sexual assault) that were experienced in the past year. When asked specifically about driving under the influence, 24.0 percent of college men and 16.9 percent of college women stated they had done so in the last year (CORE, 2013).

To be even more specific, another college study inquired about a variety of alcohol-related negative consequences, and the following statistics were found:

35 percent did something they later regretted
30 percent forgot where they were or what they did
20 percent had unprotected sex
14 percent physically injured self
3 percent got in trouble with the police
2 percent seriously considered suicide
2 percent had sex without giving consent (ACHA, 2013)

ASSESSMENT AND TREATMENT RECOMMENDATIONS

Screening and assessing for substance abuse problems may not be an easy task due to the developmental processes which occur among adolescents and young adults. Drastic biological, psychological, cognitive, and social changes are normal for this population. Thus, signs of substance-related issues may be difficult to identify by family members, teachers, and health professionals because these signs can be very similar to the typical developmental issues which are present for most adolescents and young adults. However, some questions can help ascertain if someone in this age group may have a substance use concern. They include:

- Has the AYA been extremely moody or more upset than usual?
- Are there significant changes in the AYA's choice in friends, grades, dress, general hygiene, and responsibilities?
- Is the AYA more irresponsible about his or her commitments (e.g., work, school) or not coming home on time or disregarding rules?
- Is there a noticeable decrease in motivation, mobility, or interest (especially in things that used to hold meaning or importance)?
- Are there signs of school problems (e.g., acting out, fights, delinquency) or issues with studying, completing assignments, grades, etc.?
- Is the AYA engaging in activities that are not healthy or productive and potentially damaging?
- Is the AYA lying, stealing, or cheating?
- Has the AYA behaved in ways that have concerned or troubled neighbors, relatives, teachers, roommates, or other community members?
- Has the AYA engaged in illegal activities or deviant behaviors?
- Has the AYA displayed any physical signs of drug use (e.g., dilated or pinpoint pupils, talkativeness or extreme quietness, slurred speech, fatigue, aggressiveness, etc.)?

Adapted from Fields (2013). *Drugs in Perspective* (8th ed.).

Screening and Assessment Tools

Clinicians have many instruments to choose from when screening and assessing for substance use issues among the AYA population. The following are some tools frequently used in the field and are specific to adolescents, young adults, and/or college students.

Problem-Oriented Screening Instrument for Teenagers (POSIT)
139 yes/no questions for adolescents that identify problems and service needs in ten areas (e.g., family and peer relations, social skills, aggressive behavior, physical and mental health, substance use)

Substance Abuse Subtle Screening Inventory Adolescent Version (SASSI-A2)
100 items for adolescents that identify family and social risk factors, level of defensive responding, attitudes toward substance use, and consequences of substance misuse

Teen Addiction Severity Index (T-ASI)
154 items for adolescents that produce 170 ratings in seven domains (e.g., chemical use, school status, legal status, peer and family relationships)

Rutgers Alcohol Problem Index (RAPI)
23 items for adolescents and young adults that assess negative consequences due to problem drinking

Brief Young Adult Alcohol Consequences Questionnaire (B-YAACQ)
24 items for young adults that identify consequences in eight domains (e.g., blackout drinking, impaired control, risk behaviors, academic/occupational consequences)

College Alcohol Problems Scale (CAPS)
Eight-item scale for college students that identifies personal and social problems (e.g., "engaged in unplanned sexual activity" and "drove under the influence")

One particular instrument can be very practical when a school staff person, counselor, teacher, or medical professional wishes to briefly screen for potential alcohol and other drug use concerns among AYAs. The *CRAFFT* (Knight, Shrier, Bravender, Farrell, Vander Bilt, & Shaffer, 1999) is a six-item screening tool based on the mnemonic on the individual items and may be administered to individuals under 21 years of age. Two or more positive answers would warrant further assessment.

C	Have you ever ridden in a CAR driven by someone (including yourself) who was "high" or had been using alcohol or drugs?
R	Do you ever use alcohol or drugs to RELAX, feel better about yourself, or fit in?
A	Do you ever use alcohol/drugs while you are by yourself, ALONE?
F	Do you ever FORGET things you did while using alcohol or drugs?
F	Do your family or FRIENDS ever tell you that you should cut down on your drinking or drug use?
T	Have you gotten into TROUBLE while you were using alcohol or drugs?

After careful screening and assessment, recommendations for treatment will be made, if applicable. Placement on the continuum of care (e.g., inpatient or outpatient) will depend on the severity of the problem, recovery environment, mental and physical health concerns, continued use potential, withdrawal symptoms, etc. Once the treatment modality is chosen, the next step is treatment planning, and there are several issues that should be considered when generating goals with the AYA client.

Considerations with Treatment Planning

Due to the life span development status of AYAs, counselors must be aware of how the treatment of AYAs can differ from the treatment of adult clients. For instance, the identification and articulation of emotional states may be difficult for some AYAs. Instead of saying, "I feel depressed" or "I feel anxious," an AYA who is masking emotions might say "I feel like a beer" or "I feel like a joint" (Center for Substance Abuse Treatment [CSAT], 2012). Moreover, as stated previously in this chapter, adolescence and young adulthood are periods when many essential cognitive functions are developed. The following are a few examples of these functions: (a) abstract thinking; (b) the capacity to form hypotheses and consider possible solutions; and (c) the ability to think about the thought process itself (CSAT, 2012). Therefore, problems can arise in counseling with regard to metacognition, goal setting, and making connections between past/present events, thoughts, emotions, and behaviors. Counselors will want to assess developmental levels (cognitive, emotional, etc.) in order to determine how equipped the AYA is to accurately evaluate their substance use issues.

Values Clarification

Practitioners are encouraged to discuss the importance of certain life areas (e.g., family, friends, and school) with the AYA client. In other words, it is important for clients to discuss and clarify their values; the counselor can facilitate this process by exploring the level of connections to things like academic performance, self-esteem, social interactions, and family relationships. Some AYAs may be motivated to reduce the use of substances due to family disappointment, while others may be motivated due to experiencing events that caused embarrassment or guilt. Other AYAs may be scared of legal involvement, while another is ambivalent about having contact with police officers and judges, or being incarcerated. Values clarification is part of motivational interviewing (MI). Counselors are encouraged to use MI in an effort to tip the scales of ambivalence if the AYAs are behaving in a way that is inconsistent with their values. By doing so, motivation for change may be increased based on the client's own desires, abilities, reasons, and needs for such change (Resnicow & McMaster, 2012).

A clinician should assess the severity of use (e.g., experimental, social, or substance use disorder) and risk factors (e.g., initiated use at age 12, childhood trauma, pattern of use established, and parental substance use issues) at admission and the onset of treatment. More than likely, the clinician would have discussed these concerns with the client during intake. Often, a counselor can identify several concerns or reasons that would constitute abstinence from substances; however, AYAs may not readily identify their desires, abilities, reasons, or needs to change. In fact, despite having legal involvement, failing grades, family issues, social problems, and physical health consequences, AYAs may still deny a need to abstain from alcohol or other drug use. The use of MI will assist with identifying the client's reasons for change and the importance of these reasons (i.e., values clarification).

Abstinence versus Harm Reduction

The goals for change should be abstinence with anyone who (a) is under the age of 21; (b) has a pending case or is on probation; (c) has a substance use disorder diagnosis; and (d) has many risk factors that increase the likelihood of developing a substance use disorder. However, many AYAs who present for substance abuse treatment often do not see abstinence as even a short-term goal. Clinicians may have to explore harm reduction strategies versus abstinence at the beginning. Harm reduction can include having discussions about how to lower the frequency and amount of alcohol and/or other drug use. For instance, an AYA client may normally consume four mixed drinks and three liquor shots over three hours, three days a week. After exploring goals with a counselor, an AYA may consider consuming four beers over four hours, one day a week instead. Harm-reduction approaches also address risky behaviors (e.g., blacking out or passing out, driving under the influence, unsafe sex, getting into fights when intoxicated) and explore prevention methods pertaining to high-risk behaviors. Counselors will want to discuss behaviors that can be preventive in nature such as drinking water when consuming alcohol, eating before drinking alcohol, counting the number of drinks and time of consumption, not playing drinking games, etc.

Other Goals in Treatment

Whether the AYA has a goal of abstinence or harm reduction, clinicians should address some key issues that can arise during treatment. For instance, counselors must discuss how to cope with failure, boredom, social anxiety or isolation, unhappiness, rejection, feelings of hopelessness, and low self-esteem (SAMHSA, 2008). In addition, counselors must address a lack of purpose in life, locus of control concerns (internal versus external), feelings of low self-efficacy, and aspects of emotional intelligence. Fields (2013) discusses four abilities of emotional intelligence, which a therapist can target in treatment to assist in the sobriety of AYAs, including:

- The ability to motivate oneself and persist in the face of frustration
- The ability to control impulse and delay gratification
- The ability to regulate one's mood and keep distress from hindering the ability to think
- The ability to empathize and hope

Another goal can be to provide education to AYAs about rates of use among others in their age group. Social norming should be used in an attempt to contradict the AYA's misperceptions on peer substance use rates. Often, AYAs tend to believe the frequency and amount of alcohol and other drug use are occurring at higher rates than what they really are. Clinicians can use data to show AYA clients that the frequency and amount are, in fact, less than they perceive, and most of the time, it is substantially less than what AYAs believe. For instance, a counselor who is providing services to a college student could present the ACHA (2013) data obtained from 131,000 college students at 172 postsecondary institutions. During a session, a 20-year-old male college student may state that he believes only 5 percent of college students have never consumed alcohol. The ACHA (2013) data found 21 percent of students in their study had never used alcohol. When asked about marijuana use, he may believe 10 percent of students have never smoked the drug. A counselor could inform the student that 62 percent of students reported never smoking marijuana, and 66 percent had reported never using any other drug (ACHA, 2013). Often, college students also overestimate how much alcohol is consumed during a typical drinking instance. A clinician could inform their clients that, in fact, 60 percent of students have reported drinking four or fewer drinks the last time they socialized.

Family Approaches

According to Levinthal (2010), "A drug-free family is more than a family without drugs in their lives, it is a family that is completely different from what it has been before" (p. 412). Substance use has been called a "family disease," and family members play a role without even realizing it (Vernig, 2011). Often, substance use is a symptom of consistent, pervasive dysfunctional interactions within the family system; there may be unhealthy coping mechanisms that have developed as a result of the dysfunction. In fact, family members can take on roles in an effort to maintain function (although in an unhealthy manner). For instance, members can become the chief enabler, hero, scapegoat, lost child, or mascot (see Wegscheider-Cruse, 1989, for more information on family roles). Family members are interconnected and interdependent parts of a system, and when there is a change in one member of the family, the other members are affected (CSAT, 2008). Therefore, counselors should attempt to involve the family in treatment whenever possible (if appropriate) in an effort to assist the AYA in sustaining long-term recovery. When doing so, AYAs should determine who are considered family members, as they may include extended family or nonbiological family members.

There are several different family approaches to take when providing counseling services to an AYA, but two are highly recommended: (1) multisystemic therapy (MST); and (2) multidimensional family therapy (MDFT). MST is an individualized, intensive, home-based treatment program that focuses on family, school, neighborhood, and the social network factors that contribute to antisocial behavior. According to Chambers, Lopez, and Ernst (2013), not only has MST been shown to be effective at decreasing substance use, but it also has been shown to decrease days in out-of-home placement, violent crimes, and criminal arrests. Research has also shown that MST, in conjunction with drug court, may enhance substance use outcomes.

Another family approach suggested for AYAs who use substances is multidimensional family therapy (MDFT). MDFT is a comprehensive and multisystemic family-based, outpatient program. MDFT targets four domains: (1) the youth alone and with family and peer group; (2) the parent alone and within the family context; (3) family functioning; and (4) the interactions between family members and key social systems. Studies have shown the efficacy of MDFT in reducing substance abuse, enhancing school performance, and improving family functioning in AYAs who use illicit drugs, as well as in alcohol-only users (Chambers et al., 2013).

Many AYA programs involve experiential group therapies, wilderness experiences, and equine therapy. Counselors should be aware of the inpatient and outpatient treatment programs available in their area for AYAs and their families. Also, self-help meetings are very effective in supporting the AYA and other family members impacted by substance use. Professionals are encouraged to obtain information on meetings in their county such as:

YP AA/NA meetings – for young people
Al-Anon – for family members of alcoholics
Narcanon – for family members of drug addicts
ACA – Adult Children of Alcoholics
Alateen – for teenagers of alcoholics

CODA – Codependents Anonymous

BASICS Approach

When college students present for treatment, often it is due to a legal incident (e.g., a minor-in possession-of-alcohol citation) or for having an alcohol-related incident on campus (e.g., alcohol in the dorm room). Counselors should be aware of the empirically supported approach called the Brief Alcohol Screening Intervention for College Students (BASICS) (Dimeff, Baer, Kivlahan, & Marlatt, 1999; Fachini et al., 2012). BASICS follows a harm-reduction approach and aims to motivate students (aged 18 to 24) to reduce alcohol use in order to decrease the negative consequences of drinking. Based on the principles of motivational interviewing, BASICS is delivered in an empathetic, nonconfrontational, and nonjudgmental manner and targets the identification of the discrepancies between the student's risky drinking behavior and his or her goals and values.

Programs have adapted BASICS to include group sessions, but normally it is delivered over the course of two one-hour interviews with a therapist. The first interview gathers information about the student's recent alcohol consumption patterns, personal beliefs about alcohol, and drinking history. The therapist also provides instructions for self-monitoring any drinking between sessions and helps the client to develop a customized feedback profile for use in the second interview. The second meeting involves social norming, a review of the student's negative consequences and risk factors, a discussion of perceived risks and benefits of drinking, and a plan for making changes to decrease or abstain from alcohol use.

Use of Media and Technology

The use of media and technology can be a tool to reach the AYA population. Information on alcohol and drug use (e.g., social norming) on social media sites can be one way to reduce substance use among youth and young adults. Moreover, cell phones with access to texting and the Internet can provide prevention information to AYAs, and most people in this age group have a cell phone. In fact, 83 percent of 17-year-olds own cell phones, and this percentage increases in young adulthood (as cited in Benotsch, Snipesa, Martin, & Bull, 2013). In particular, text-based communication is increasingly popular among AYAs, and this can be a means of delivering information about statistics, relapse prevention, etc. Currently, there are applications for cell phones that can calculate blood alcohol content (BAC) levels and can help with AYAs in recovery (e.g., "My sober life" application). Some of these applications for recovery have links to websites that list 12-step meetings in their areas (including Young People's meetings). In addition, computer programs have been used to assist in assessment and treatment (e.g., BASICS). Some universities have implemented alcohol education computer programs in an effort to provide prevention to their students, as well as gather data. For example, at Western Michigan University (WMU), incoming freshmen are required to complete an online program called AlcoholEDU prior to registering for classes. The students are educated on alcohol use (e.g., BAC levels, defining what constitutes "one standard drink") and how to reduce risky behaviors, and they are also provided data on actual use rates (i.e., social norming). In addition, students answer a survey on what their rate of alcohol consumption was prior to coming to WMU, and then they complete the survey again at other times during their enrollment at the university. This program is also made available for the parents of students and has the option of providing education for students who may be given a sanction by the university due to violating alcohol policies. In summary, it is important for counselors to be aware of the various social media sites, electronic modes of communication, and computer programs that are available in order to assist with prevention, screening/assessment, and treatment.

Special Considerations

Prescription Drug Use

As stated earlier, 7 percent of persons aged 12 to 17 and 13 percent of those aged 18 to 25 illicitly used prescription drugs in the past year (NIDA, 2013). AYAs have reported taking medication from their family members to use recreationally and have also reported bringing the medication to parties to share with others. While not much data has been published in regard to the prevalence of AYAs participating in these "pharm" parties, counselors should be aware of the potential for AYAs to be exposed to pharmaceutical medication by others at social gatherings (Graham-Knight & Karch, 2007). Besides pills, illicit use of prescription cough syrup with codeine is another concern among AYAs. The medicine can be mixed with soda (often Sprite), candy, and alcohol and then consumed (referred to as "lean," "purple drank," or "sizzurp"). Researchers in one study found 6.5 percent of college students in their investigation had consumed this cough syrup mix in their lifetime (Stogner & Miller, 2013).

Alcohol and Inhalants

Another consideration by teachers, counselors, and parents is the use of alcohol in various forms or the use of household products. For instance, students have reported soaking gummy bears in alcohol for consumption while at school. It is worth mentioning that there is currently a newer product available for AYAs that parents and professionals should be aware of: alcohol-infused whipped cream. The alcohol content is approximately 16–18 percent. Also, AYAs have inhaled computer cleaning products (called "dusting") or nitrous oxide from whipped cream canisters ("whippets"). In 2013, The Monitoring the Future study found 10.8 percent of 8th graders, 8.7 percent of 10th graders, and 6.9 percent of 12th graders have used an inhalant in their lifetime (Johnston et al., 2014). This number has been steadily decreasing since 1995, when the lifetime use rates were the highest at 21.6 percent of 8th graders, 19.0 percent of 10th graders, and 17.4 percent of 12th graders.

Cough and Cold Medicines

Approximately 5 percent of AYAs misused over-the-counter cough and cold medicines for recreational purposes in 2008. Of those AYAs who had misused these medications in the past year, 30.5 percent misused Nyquil, 18.1 percent misused Coricidin, and 17.8 percent misused a Robitussin product (SAMHSA, 2008). Many cold medications, such as Coricidin Cough and Cold Tablets ("Triple C" or "Skittles") and Robitussin ("Robo-tripping") contain dextromethorphan (DXM); when misused or taken in higher doses than medicinally recommended, the drug creates a dissociative high (NIDA, 2011). The user feels separate or detached from the environment and experiences distortions in perceptions and emotions. Abuse of this medication can lead to confusion, impaired motor function, numbness, nausea and vomiting, increased heart rate and blood pressure, seizures, coma, and respiratory depression (Banken & Foster, 2008; NIDA, 2011). Nonmedical use of DXM results in approximately 6000 emergency department (ED) visits each year, and people aged 12 to 20 account for almost 50 percent of the DXM-related ED visits (SAMHSA, 2006). Often, AYAs visiting the ED for DXM use had also consumed alcohol as well.

Salvia Divinorum and Synthetic Drugs

In addition to illicit use of prescription medications and over-the-counter medications, other drugs have been readily available to AYAs. One such drug is *Salvia divinorum* ("diviner's sage," or "magic mint"), which is usually a dried leaf and typically smoked from a pipe. It has rapid onset and duration of effect, with effects starting as soon as 30 seconds and usually gone within 10 minutes (Duerr, 2012). Users have been noted to experience uncontrollable laughter, confusion, visual hallucinations, multiple realities, and feelings of flying; they also tend to fall down and often lose the ability to speak clearly (Duerr, 2012). Perron et al. (2012) used data from the National Survey on Drug Use and Health (NSDUH) and found 6.1 percent of persons aged 18 to 25 have used *Salvia* in their lifetime. Use of *Salvia* is declining among 12th graders, with 3.4 percent of 12th graders reporting use in the past year, compared to 5.9 percent in 2011 and 4.4 percent in 2012 (Johnston et al., 2014). Researchers have also investigated use among college students and demonstrated that 4.4 percent of college students reported *Salvia* use within the last year (Lange, Reed, Croff, & Clapp, 2008).

Another drug of interest among AYAs has been synthetic marijuana, called Spice or K2, which is usually non-psychoactive dry plant matter coated with synthetic cannabinoids (e.g., sprayed with JWH-018) and was marketed and sold as "incense." Normally, this drug is smoked. The effects can last anywhere from one to six hours. According to Duerr (2012), use of these drugs can cause anxiety, agitation, seizure risk, paranoia, suicidal ideation, and psychosis in vulnerable patients. Although this drug has been banned since 2011, the American Association of Poison Control Centers (2014) reported that in the first month of 2014, there were 177 calls to the Poison Control Center due to synthetic cannabinoid use. However, there has been a decrease noted in calls over the past few years (i.e., 6,968 calls in 2011; 5,230 calls in 2012; 2,643 calls in 2013). In 2013, past-year use of Spice or K2 dropped from 11.3 percent to 7.9 percent among high school seniors (Johnston et al., 2014). Among one sample of college students, researchers found approximately 8.0 percent of participants (or one in 12 students) reported using the drug in their lifetime (Hu, Primack, Barnett, & Cook, 2011).

Synthetic stimulants, such as cathinone (referred to as "bath salts"), are based on the khat plant from Africa, which has been used for thousands of years (Duerr, 2012). Bath salts come in powder form ("Ivory Wave" or "Cloud Nine"), are marketed as plant food or jewelry cleaner, and can be taken orally, snorted, or injected. These drugs tend to give the user a high similar to cocaine or methamphetamines, and they are associated with feelings of euphoria, increased sex drive, and increased motivation. However, users may also experience confusion, agitation, aggression and violence, hallucinations, muscle spasms, dizziness, and heart palpitations. Prior to the government banning the drug in 2011, there was considerable public concern surrounding the drug due to the substantial media attention that highlighted the negative effects of bath salts. Researchers have shown the usage rates of bath salts among the AYA population are significantly lower than other drugs. For example, one study supported the assertion that the prevalence of lifetime use of the drug among college students was low and found 1.0 percent of their participants reported lifetime use (Stogner & Miller, 2013). In 2013, the Monitoring the Future project found low rates as well, with 1 percent of 8th graders, 0.9 percent of 10th graders, and 0.9 percent of 12th graders reporting bath salt use in the past 12 months (Johnston et al., 2014).

Legal Involvement and School-Imposed Sanctions

As stated earlier, often AYAs present for substance abuse treatment due to legal involvement (e.g., a minor gets a DUI for a BAC of .03) or violating school policies (e.g., a college student has alcohol in the dorms). Counselors may be in frequent contact with probation officers and university personnel as a result of mandated treatment requirements. Probation officers and university staff from the Office of Student Conduct may request reports on assessment information, diagnoses, participation, attendance, and treatment compliance. As part of a holistic approach, an integrated health care system should involve the AYA's probation officer, psychiatrist, university personnel/residence life, and family members, when appropriate. Therapists must be knowledgeable about the AYA's probation requirements (e.g., urinalysis testing, community service, number of treatment sessions, attendance at a victim impact panel, attendance at self-help meetings, electronic monitoring, etc.), as well as the AYA's special circumstances such as the opportunity for a sealed record upon completion of requirements. Many adolescents participate in juvenile drug court programs, and therapists communicate frequently with drug court teams about the client's progress. These courts are increasing in number. In fact, as of 2012, there were 458 juvenile drug courts in the United States (National Institute of Justice, 2012). In addition to the juvenile court system and probation requirements, counselors must also be aware of university policies and consequences of not completing university requirements by their college student clients. For instance, some colleges may put a hold on a student's record, which would not allow him or her to register for classes; in some cases, the student can be expelled.

Confidentiality and Duty to Warn

As stated above, there are many people who can be involved in the treatment of an AYA, and there are some special circumstances surrounding the confidentiality of a minor that a counselor should take into consideration. By law, more than half of states permit youth under the age of 18 to consent to substance abuse treatment without parental consent (CSAT, 2008). Thus, a provider can admit an adolescent on their own signature. The difficulty comes into play when either the adolescent refuses to permit communication with a parent or guardian or when a parent does not consent for treatment of their child (in the states that require such consent). Refer to CSAT (2008) for more information regarding consent to treatment considerations.

The federal privacy law (42 C.F.R. Part 2) protects any information about an AYA that has applied for or received any substance abuse–related assessment, treatment, or referral services from a program that is covered under the law. Cases in which confidentiality can be broken include medical emergencies, reporting child abuse, reporting a threat to another person (i.e., Duty to Warn), and communications among program staff (CSAT, 2008). When a client signs a release of information document for another person (e.g., probation officer, parent, school personnel, etc.), it is crucial that the release indicate the purpose of the disclosure and exactly what information is going to be disclosed (e.g., attendance, participation, diagnosis, etc.). Care should be taken when coordinating with others. For instance, the information to be discussed with the AYA's psychiatrist will be different from what will be discussed with school personnel, which would be different from a probation officer. In other words, some coordinating entities may not need to know certain information (e.g., mental health status, past history of abuse or trauma, current personal issues), but only that the AYA is attending and participating in treatment. In summary, clinicians should be knowledgeable about the laws and ethical codes regarding confidentiality. They should also be able to effectively and clearly communicate the limits of confidentiality to their AYA clients in an effort to create and maintain the therapeutic relationship, as well as increase the likelihood of honest disclosure. See CSAT (2008) for a sample of a consent form and more information about confidentiality, including Duty to Warn, child abuse and neglect, criminal activity, and court orders.

CONCLUSIONS

Approximately one out of every two high school seniors and one out of every five eighth graders have used an illicit drug in their lifetime (Johnston et al., 2014). Over 21 percent of young adults aged 18 to 25 reportedly used an illicit drug in the previous 30 days, and 22 percent of college students indicated use (SAMHSA, 2011). These numbers indicate a need for school personnel, medical professionals, and mental health clinicians to be competent in screening for potential substance use among the AYA population. In addition, these professionals must be knowledgeable about the risk and preventive factors, warning signs and symptoms, and consequences associated with alcohol and other drug use. Counselors in particular should be up to date on available assessment tools and must be aware of the considerations in treatment planning with this population. Certain challenges are characteristic of working with AYAs, including a low motivation to change. Also, the developmental issues that present for this age group can impact the ability for AYAs to (a) be insightful about their substance use problems and emotions; (b) have healthy self-regulation capabilities; and (c) engage in abstract thinking or metacognition. Counselors must consider harm-reduction methods with AYAs who are not motivated yet for abstinence. Moreover, when treating an AYA, it is important to employ family therapy approaches, if appropriate. Finally, counselors should (a) be aware of the special circumstances of the AYA, such as legal involvement and school sanctions, which require mandated treatment; (b) be cognizant of the limits of confidentiality; and (c) use available media outlets and technology with AYAs, if possible.

Case Study

Currently, you work at an outpatient treatment center and you have been providing individual counseling services to a 19-year-old Caucasian female for the past month. She was referred to you by her probation officer due to a Minor-in-Possession-of-Alcohol conviction. The client was taken to the hospital three months ago when she passed out while tailgating before a football game. She had a BAC of .32 at the hospital. Because the incident happened on campus and she lives in the dorms, she is also involved with the Office of Student Conduct. The client's mother came with the client at intake and requested that she be updated on her daughter's treatment because she has been very concerned about her daughter's alcohol use and recent hospitalization. She was not present during the intake interview, but she waited outside in the lobby. The client tells you that her mother is her best friend and you can tell her mother "anything." The client signs a release for all three parties. The client submits to random Breathalyzer tests as part of her probation, but she is not tested for illicit drugs at this time.

The client reports first drinking alcohol at age 13 and drinking regularly on the weekends in high school. During her first year of college, she continued to drink two to three days a week, up to ten drinks (beers and shots), and she would drink an average of six to seven drinks over a period of three hours. The client states she is 5' 2" and weighs 110 pounds. She reports blacking out approximately once every two weeks. The client also reports smoking marijuana, with the first use at age 13. She indicates smoking marijuana two to three days a week since the age of 16. The client reports a preference for marijuana over alcohol. She states she has a couple of friends at college who do not smoke marijuana, but most do. When asked about the consequences of substance use, the client discusses a decrease in GPA, being embarrassed about things she has done when intoxicated, and now has problems with the legal system and the college. The client maintains she stopped smoking marijuana since probation started, but will drink about once a week. The client reportedly is "not too worried" about failing the Breathalyzer tests. She also discusses being more sexually active since college, and a majority of these instances occurred under the influence of alcohol. When asked about symptoms of mental health issues, she endorsed feelings of hopelessness, constant sadness, anxiety, difficulty with concentrating, and memory issues. During the intake, she disclosed to you that she has a history of sexual abuse by a cousin that occurred at seven years old and that her father "was an alcoholic." He died when she was 13 years old, and this was very rough on her emotionally.

After her assessment, you recommended weekly individual counseling sessions and eight weekly group sessions in your clinic's "Young Adult" program with other 18- to 24-year-old clients. She has never missed an individual or group session and has fully participated in counseling. After seeing the client for three weeks, she showed you several scars on her upper arms from cutting. The cutting started after her father's death and continued until age 16; however, she has recently started again. She has not disclosed this information to anyone else. Sometimes when she comes home after drinking with her friends, she has overwhelming feelings of sadness and loneliness. When she starts to cry, she goes into the bathroom and cuts herself to "stop feeling." Yesterday, the client's mother left you a voicemail asking for an update on her daughter's progress in treatment, and tomorrow the monthly report is due to the probation officer.

Discussion Questions

1. What are the top three treatment concerns for you at this time?
2. What are some of the risk and preventive factors for this client?
3. What would be the (a) purpose; and (b) nature of the disclosures (written on a consent form) for the client's mother, probation officer, and the staff at the Office of Student Conduct? Would they be different?
4. What information will you disclose to the client's mother when you call her back? What information will you write in your reports to the probation officer and the Office of Student Conduct? What is your rationale for including this information?
5. What would be four treatment goals you would discuss with this client (e.g., abstinence or harm reduction)? What recommendations or referrals would you make for the client?

REFERENCES

American Association of Poison Control Centers. (2014). *Synthetic marijuana data*. Retrieved from https://aapcc.s3.amazonaws.com/files/library/Synthetic_Marijuana_Web_Data_ through_1.2014.pdf

American College Health Association. (2013). *National college health assessment II: Reference group executive summary spring 2013*. Hanover, MD: American College Health Association.

Banken, J. A., & Foster, H. (2008). Dextromethorphan: An emerging drug of abuse. *Annals of the New York Academy of Sciences, 1139*, 402–411.

Benotsch, E. G., Snipesa, D. J., Martin, A. M., & Bull, S. S. (2013). Sexting, substance use, and sexual risk behavior in young adults. *Journal of Adolescent Health, 52*(3), 307–313.

Center for Substance Abuse Treatment. (2012). *Screening and assessing adolescents for substance use disorders*. Treatment Improvement Protocol (TIP) Series, No. 31. HHS Publication No. (SMA) 12-4079. Rockville, MD: Substance Abuse and Mental Health Services Administration.

Center for Substance Abuse Treatment. (2008). *Treatment of adolescents with substance use disorders*. Treatment Improvement Protocol (TIP) Series, No. 32. HHS Publication No. (SMA) 08-4080. Rockville, MD: Substance Abuse and Mental Health Services Administration.

Chambers, J., Lopez, M., & Ernst, M. (2013). Epidemiology and treatment of substance use and abuse in adolescents. *Psychiatric Times, 30*(6), 38–41.

CORE. (2013, April). *2011 annual reference group: Executive findings*. Retrieved from http://core.siu.edu/_common/documents/report11.pdf

Dimeff, L. A., Baer, J. S., Kivlahan, D. R., & Marlatt, G. A. (1999). *Brief alcohol screening and intervention for college students*. New York: Guilford Press.

Duerr, H. A. (2012). From bath salts to spice and beyond—Elucidating emerging drugs of abuse. *Psychiatric Times*. Retrieved from http://www.psychiatrictimes.com/uspc2012/bath-salts-spice-and-beyond%E2%80%94elucidating-emerging-drugs-abuse

Fachini, A., Aliane, P. P., Martinez, E. Z., & Furtado, E. F. (2012). Efficacy of brief alcohol screening intervention for college students (BASICS): A meta-analysis of randomized controlled trials. *Substance Abuse Treatment, Prevention, and Policy, 7*, 40–50.

Fields, R. (2013). *Drugs in perspective* (8th ed.). New York: McGraw Hill.

Graham-Knight, D., & Karch, A. (2007). "Pharm party": Prescription drug use among teens. *American Journal of Nursing, 107*(12), 79.

Hanson, G. R., Venturelli, P. J., & Fleckenstein, A. E. (2011). *Drugs and society* (11th ed.). Sudbury, MA: Jones and Bartlett Publishers.

Hart, C. L., & Ksir, C. (2013). *Drugs, society and human behavior* (15th ed.). New York: McGraw Hill.

Hingson, R. W., Zha, W., & Weitzman, E. R. (2009). Magnitude of and trends in alcohol-related mortality and morbidity among U.S. college students aged 18–24: 1998 to 2005. *Journal of Studies on Alcohol and Drugs, 6*, 12–20.

Hu, X., Primack, B. A., Barnett, T. E., & Cook, R. L. (2011). College students and use of K2: An emerging drug of abuse in young persons. *Substance Abuse Treatment Prevention Policy, 6*, 16–20.

Inaba, D. S., & Cohen, W. E. (2011). *Uppers, downers, all arounders* (7th ed.). Medford, OR: CNS Productions.

Johnston, L. D., O'Malley, P. M., Miech, R. A., Bachman, J. G., & Schulenberg, J. E. (2014). *Monitoring the future national results on drug use: 1975–2013: Overview, key findings on adolescent drug use*. Ann Arbor: Institute for Social Research, University of Michigan.

Knight, J. R., Shrier, L. A., Bravender, T. D., Farrell, M., Vander Bilt, J., & Shaffer, H. J. (1999). A new brief screen for adolescent substance abuse. *Archives of Pediatric and Adolescent Medicine, 153*(6), 591–596.

Lange, J. E., Reed, M. B., Croff, J. M., & Clapp, J. D. (2008). College student use of salvia divinorum. *Drug and Alcohol Dependence, 94*(1–3), 263–266.

Levinthal, C. F. (2014). *Drugs, behavior, and modern society* (8th ed.). Boston: Pearson Education.

National Institute on Drug Abuse. (2013). *Abuse of prescription (Rx) drugs affects young adults most*. Retrieved from http://www.drugabuse.gov/related-topics/trends-statistics/infographics/abuse-prescription-rx-drugs-affects-young-adults-most

National Institute on Drug Abuse. (2011). *Facts on Dextromethorphan (DXM)*. Retrieved from http://teens.drugabuse.gov/sites/default/files/peerx/pdf/PEERx_Toolkit_FactSheets_DXM.pdf

National Institute of Justice. (2012). *Drug courts*. Office of Justice Programs. Retrieved from http://www.nij.gov/topics/courts/drug-courts/Pages/welcome.aspx

Perron, B., Ahmedani, B., Vaughn, M., Glass, J., Abdon, A., & Wu, L. (2012). Use of salvia divinorum in a nationally representative sample. *American Journal of Drug and Alcohol Abuse, 38*, 108–113.

Randolph, K. A., Russell, D., Tillman, K. H., & Fincham, F. D. (2010). Positive influences on the negative consequences of drinking among youth. *Youth and Society, 41*(4), 546–568.

Resnicow, K., & McMaster, F. (2012). Motivational interviewing: Moving from why to how with autonomy support. *International Journal of Behavioral Nutrition and Physical Activity, 9*, 19–27.

Shin, S. H., Chung, Y., & Jeon, S. M. (2013). Impulsivity and substance use in young adulthood. *American Journal on Addictions, 22*, 39–45.

Squeglia, L. M., Jacobus, J., & Tapert, S. F. (2009). The influence of substance use on adolescent brain development. *Clinical EEG and Neuroscience, 40*, 31–38.

Stogner, J. M., & Miller, B. L. (2013). Investigating the "bath salt" panic: The rarity of synthetic cathinone use among students in the United States. *Drug and Alcohol Review, 32*(5), 545–549.

Strasburger, V. C. (2010). Children, adolescents, substance abuse, and the media. *Pediatrics, 126*(4), 791–799.

Substance Abuse and Mental Health Services Administration. (2013). *Substance use by adolescents on an average day is alarming*. SAMHSA News Release. Retrieved from http://www.samhsa.gov/newsroom/advisories/1308285320.aspx

Substance Abuse and Mental Health Services Administration. (2011). *Results from the 2010 national survey on drug use and health: Summary of national findings*. NSDUH Series H-41, HHS Publication No. (SMA) 11-4658. Rockville, MD: Substance Abuse and Mental Health Services Administration. Retrieved from http://www.oas.samhsa.gov/NSDUH/2k10NSDUH/2k10Results.htm#3.1.1

Substance Abuse and Mental Health Services Administration. (2008). *The NSDUH report: Misuse of over-the-counter cough and cold medications among persons aged 12 to 25*. Rockville, MD: Substance Abuse and Mental Health Services Administration. Retrieved from http://oas.samhsa.gov/2k8/cough/cough.htm

Substance Abuse and Mental Health Services Administration. (2006). Emergency department visits involving dextromethorphan. *DAWN: Report Series, 32*, 1–4.

Sussman, S., Skara, S., & Ames, S. L. (2008). Substance abuse among adolescents. *Substance Use and Misuse, 43*(12), 1802–1828.

Vernig, P. M. (2011). Family roles in homes with alcohol-dependent parents: An evidence-based review. *Substance Use and Misuse, 46*(4), 535–542.

Wegscheider-Cruse, S. (1989). *Another chance: Hope and health for the alcoholic family* (2nd ed.). Palo Alto, CA: Science and Behavior Books.

Wu, L., Woody, G. E., Yang, C., Pan, J., & Blazer, D. G. (2011). Racial/ethnic variations in substance-related disorders among adolescents in the United States. *Archives of General Psychiatry, 68*(11), 1176–1185.

CHAPTER 11

OLDER ADULTS

By Christina Chasek

Substance use disorders in later life are often hidden problems. These disorders are rarely associated with older adults as a result of generational stereotyping and ageism. Ageism, defined by Butler (1975) as the systematic stereotyping of older generations, fosters the belief that substance abuse in older adult populations is not a problem because older adults deserve to be happy with the time they have left. There is also the perception that older adults do not abuse substances as a result of the lack of any large generational cohort of older adults using or abusing alcohol or illicit drugs. However, this is about to change as the baby boom generation enters into older adulthood.

The baby boom cohort, referring to persons born in the United States after World War II between 1946 and 1964, is the largest generational cohort on record to enter into older adulthood. Estimates indicate that as the baby boom generation ages, the number of adults aged 50 or older will reach 97 million by 2020. It is also estimated that the number of adults aged 50 or older with substance abuse problems will increase from 2.8 million to 5.7 million by 2020, making substance abuse among older adults one of the fastest-growing health problems in the United States (Beynon, 2009; Gfroerer, Penne, Pemberton, & Folsom, 2003; Han, Gfroerer, Colliver, & Penne, 2009; Wu & Blazer, 2011). This large increase in the number of older adults using substances will create a demand not only for specialized substance abuse treatment relevant to the older adult population, but also professionals who are able to provide such treatment.

The older adult population includes two distinct categories, defined by age: (1) adults from ages 50 to 64 (i.e., older adult); and (2) adults ages 65 and over (i.e., elderly). For the purposes of this chapter, the term "older adult" is used to refer to both categories, unless stated otherwise. Examining the substance use trends in these two groups reveals some alarming statistics. Overall, alcohol is the most frequently reported substance of abuse for persons over the age of 50; prescription drugs are the next most frequently abused drug, followed by illicit drugs (Bogunovic, 2012). Results from the 2012 National Survey on Drug Use and Health (Substance Abuse Mental Health Service Administration [SAMHSA], 2013) found the following rates of alcohol use in the older adult population in the previous-month time frame:

- Among 50 to 54 year olds, 58.5 percent were alcohol users, 22.7 percent were binge alcohol users, and 6.6 percent were heavy alcohol users.

- Among 55 to 59 year olds, 53.2 percent were alcohol users, 16.7 percent were binge alcohol users, and 5.0 percent were heavy alcohol users.
- Among 60 to 64 year olds, 53.1 percent were alcohol users, 14.3 percent were binge alcohol users, and 4.3 percent were heavy alcohol users.
- Among persons aged 65 or older, 41.2 percent were alcohol users, 8.2 percent were binge alcohol users, and 2.0 percent were heavy alcohol users.

The Centers for Disease Control and Prevention also found that in the older adult population, the rates of binge drinking by age were alarmingly high (Kanny, Lie, & Brewer, 2012). While binge drinking is more commonly associated with young adults aged 18 to 34 years, binge drinkers aged 65 years and older report binge drinking more often, an average of five to six times a month. This was the highest frequency of binge drinking by age reported in the survey.

These statistics are even more disturbing, given they are based on the national guidelines for alcohol consumption identified for the average-aged adult (rather than the levels of alcohol use identified for the older adult). The alcohol consumption guidelines indicated for the average-aged adult constitutes higher-risk drinking for older adults due to the older person's decreased ability to metabolize alcohol and other drugs as a result of the aging process (Hunter, Lubman, & Barratt, 2011). Two nationally recognized organizations, the American Geriatrics Society and the National Institute of Alcohol Abuse and Alcoholism (NIAAA), have modified and defined the limits of alcohol use for older adults. The American Geriatric Society's guidelines indicate that two or more drinks a day within the past 30 days is considered at-risk drinking for older adults. The NIAAA has further defined at-risk drinking for men and women aged 65 or over as more than one drink a day (American Geriatrics Society, 2003; NIAAA, 2013; Wang & Andrade, 2013). Furthermore, these guidelines indicate that older adults should be drinking no more than seven standard drinks per week, half the amount recommended for younger-aged adults.

In addition to the concerns related to alcohol use, the National Institute on Drug Abuse (NIDA, 2005) reports prescription drug use is significantly increasing among the older adult population. Even though they make up only 13 percent of the total population, older adults account for 34 percent of all drugs prescribed in the United States and over 30 percent of all of the over-the-counter medications sold (Bogunovic, 2012; Kalapatapu & Sullivan, 2010; NIDA, 2005). Older adults are often given multiple prescriptions based on legitimate medical needs; however, this can lead to unintentional misuse. In fact, Maxwell (2011) reports emergency room visits by older adults resulting from the misuse of prescribed narcotic pain medication has increased by 254 percent from 2004 to 2009. Researchers further predict that the number of older adults who use psychoactive medication without a prescription will increase by 190 percent by the year 2020, indicating that 2.7 million older adults will need treatment for the abuse of prescription drugs. The predicted increase in the number of older adults abusing prescription medications has become a national concern. As a result, heavy emphasis has been placed on providing effective substance abuse treatment for the older adult population, particularly related to prescription drug abuse.

With the aging of the baby boom generation, it is not just prescription drug abuse that is an issue; it is also illicit drug abuse. Research indicates that among adults aged 50 to 64, the rate of current illicit drug use has grown significantly during the past decade. For example, the 2012 National Survey on Drug Use and Health (SAMHSA, 2013) found that the rate of illicit drug use for adults aged 50 to 54 increased from 3.4 percent in 2002 to 7.2 percent in 2012. Among those aged 55 to 59, the rate of current illicit drug use rose from 1.9 percent in 2002 to 6.6 percent in 2012; and among those aged 60 to 64, the rate increased from 1.1 percent in 2002 to 3.6 percent in 2012. The substantial escalation in illicit drug use within the older adult population has been attributed to the greater number of aging baby boomers, as this generation has tended to use more psychoactive drugs than previous generations (Han et al., 2009; Wu & Blazer, 2011).

SUBSTANCE ABUSE ISSUES

Etiology

There are many views regarding the etiology of addiction and substance abuse, and these perspectives often have competing descriptions of addiction. For example, addiction can be described as a biological disease with genetic origins, or it can also be viewed as maladaptive behaviors with psychological and spiritual components. These competing models of addiction, however, have converged together in a composite biopsychosocial-spiritual model of addiction that has been widely adopted in the substance abuse treatment field. The biopsychosocial-spiritual model of addiction recognizes and takes into account the interacting influences of addiction that can be used to understand the patterns of substance use and abuse in the older adult population (Center for Substance Abuse Treatment [CSAT], 1999a; Doweiko, 2011; Hester & Miller, 2003; Kinney, 2011; Thombs, 2006; Wilbourne & Miller, 2002).

In the biopsychosocial-spiritual model of addiction, substance use and abuse by older adults is seen as a result of biological, psychological, cognitive, and behavioral issues converging with the common developmental issues older adults face. With this definition in mind, older adult substance abusers can be categorized into two distinct groups: early-onset substance abusers and late-onset substance abusers.

In early-onset substance abuse, older adults have developed a substance abuse problem before the age of 65, essentially bringing the substance abuse problem into old age with them. Early-onset substance abusers are more likely to have been in substance treatment before and to have more serious consequences for their substance use over their lifetime (e.g., health issues, financial problems, legal problems, and impaired cognition). They are also less likely to have a solid support system in place. In addition to the developmental challenges facing the older adult population, they are also battling a substance abuse problem. It is estimated that early-onset substance abusers make up two-thirds of the total population of older adult substance abusers (Bogunovic, 2012; Fingerhood, 2000).

In contrast to early-onset substance abuse, late-onset substance abuse is defined as beginning after the age of 60. These older adults often enter treatment in a state of crisis, are more likely to report feeling depressed, and deny having a substance abuse problem. They are, however, more likely to have a support system in place. In late-onset substance abuse, the developmental issues that arise in later adulthood are seen as triggers for substance use. These triggers include health issues, loneliness, grief, loss of esteem through retirement, financial issues, loss of mobility, and chronic pain. The abuse of substances likely has developed as a mechanism for coping with these difficult developmental issues (Bogunovic, 2012; Fingerhood, 2000; Kalapatapu & Sullivan, 2010; Segal, Qualls, & Smyer, 2011; Wu & Blazer, 2011).

Risk Factors

There are several risk factors associated with substance use among older adults due to the aging process. In the natural aging process, the brain changes in a variety of ways that is developmentally determined. The effects of many illicit and prescription drugs on the aging brain is unknown. However, given the age-related changes in the neurotransmitter systems that mediate the effects of drugs in the brain, even moderate drug use can present greater risks for the older adult (Benyon, 2009; Brown University, 2008; Dowling, Weiss, & Condon, 2008; Wu & Blazer, 2011).

Physical changes in the aging body also play a role in the risk factors of substance abuse in the older adult population. Due to changes in body composition and decreased digestive and liver functions, ingesting alcohol can cause more damage to the central nervous system, vital organs, and other body functions in older adults than in younger adults (Bogunovic, 2012; Breslow, Faden, & Smothers, 2003; Caputo et al., 2012). Moreover, there are also risks associated with reductions in lean body mass and total body water in older adults. Reductions in body mass and water content (as well as decreased kidney functioning) increase the levels of drug serums in older adults who misuse substances, causing significant effects from even a moderate amount of drug use (Beynon, 2009; Wang & Andrade, 2013).

In addition to physical changes in the aging body, there are other risk factors to consider regarding substance use in the aging population. For example, the incidence of hip fractures in the elderly increases with substance use. These bone fractures can be attributed to the number of falls that occur when the older adult is intoxicated. Moreover, bone density tends to decrease when older adults abuse substances, leading to broken bones with even minor falls. There are also risks related to the interaction of alcohol and other drugs and the prescription medications that older adults take. In fact, alcohol-medication interactions are especially common among the elderly, increasing the risk of negative health effects and potentially influencing the effectiveness of the medications.

Substance use often occurs when a person has a mental health concern, increasing the risk of co-occurring disorders when the older adult misuses substances. Although found in the general population, depressive disorders are actually more common among the elderly than among younger people and tend to co-occur with alcohol misuse. Among persons older than 65, those with alcohol use disorders are approximately three times more likely to exhibit a major depressive disorder than are those without alcohol use disorders (Simoni-Wastila & Yang, 2006; Wang & Andrade, 2013).

A unique risk factor among the older adult population is the prescription of medication for legitimate medical needs. Older adults are often given multiple prescriptions based on their complex health needs. At any given time, older adults are prescribed five or more prescriptions and take one or more over-the-counter medications for their medical issues (Qato et al., 2008). Older adults may misunderstand the proper instructions for taking these medications or even disregard the instructions in their search for pain relief. This often leads to unintentional misuse or abuse of the medications in an attempt to alleviate and treat legitimate medical issues. Other risk factors for prescription drug abuse in the older adult population include social isolation, poor health, chronic medical problems, and previous substance use or mental health issues (Simoni-Wastila & Yang, 2006; Wang & Andrade, 2013).

Another risk factor among older adults in relation to substance use is alcohol-involved traffic crashes. The elderly are the fastest growing segment of the driving population. Age, combined with substance abuse, significantly increases driving risk. For example, after consuming the equivalent amount of substances, an elderly driver with a substance use disorder is more impaired than an elderly driver without a substance use disorder and has a greater risk of a traffic accident (Simoni-Wastila & Yang, 2006).

Gender can also be considered a risk factor for substance use disorders among older adults. Older women, especially those who are socially isolated, are more at risk for prescription drug abuse than their male counterparts. Older adult women are prescribed more psychotropic and narcotic pain medication than older adult men and are at risk of misusing their medications to cope with significant developmental issues in aging. Older adult woman are also at a greater risk for economic hardships, leading to more vulnerability for substance use disorders and a faster progression of the disease (Simoni-Wastila & Yang, 2006; Kalapatapu & Sullivan, 2010; Wang & Andrade, 2013).

Barriers to Treatment

Despite the prevalence of substance use in the older adult population, there are many barriers that impact the utilization of services by the older adult population. The most significant barrier to substance abuse treatment in older adults is the fact that substance use and abuse is often under-recognized and underdiagnosed by medical and mental health professionals (Briggs, Magnus, Lassiter, Patterson, & Smith, 2011; Wu & Blazer, 2011). The caregivers and medical personnel who come into contact with older adults often do not recognize or look for substance abuse issues. They often attribute the symptoms and the complaints of older adults to age and the aging process. Increased sleep problems, memory problems, or falling are all consequences of advanced age; however, they can also be warning signs of alcohol or drug use in the older adult. Health care professionals often attribute the symptoms to dementia or Alzheimer's disease, depression, or some other common medical issue in older age rather than substance use (Han et al., 2009; Wu & Blazer, 2011). Besides caregivers and medical personnel, older adults themselves often do not recognize the symptoms of substance use disorders. This leaves older adults as a hidden and vulnerable population subject to serious health consequences as a result of their untreated substance abuse problems.

Stigma and fear associated with substance use and the elderly are other barriers to treatment and contribute to substance abuse as a hidden problem in the elderly (Wu & Blazer, 2011). There has been a perception in society that the elderly do not use or abuse substances (Beynon, 2009). The elderly themselves are often fearful to share their substance use history with others due to worries that they will be labeled "crazy" if they are diagnosed or treated for a substance abuse problem (Clay, 2007). There is also the perception as a result of ageism that the elderly are not interested in substance abuse treatment because they have a limited amount of time to enjoy their older age and they would not want to spend it in treatment (Segal et al., 2011). Older adults, their families, and society often deny the significance of substance-related problems in older age. This denial is reflected in the fact that older adults are less likely to ask for help for their substance problems and are more likely to hide their substance use problems than younger adults (Han et al., 2009; Wu & Blazer, 2011).

A final barrier to treatment for the older adult is the structure and programming of substance abuse treatment services and facilities. There are very few specialized substance abuse treatment programs that include the services necessary for the physical and medical needs of the older adult. According to the Substance Abuse and Mental Health Service Administration (2006), only seven percent of all substance abuse facilities reported having a treatment program or group specifically designed for older adults. This is a serious issue to address as the baby boomers enter into older adulthood. As stated previously, this particular generation is expected to have more substance abuse concerns than previous generations (Benyon, 2009; Han et al., 2009; Wu & Blazer, 2013).

SCREENING AND ASSESSMENT OF SUBSTANCE USE DISORDERS IN OLDER ADULTS

A significant challenge when working with the older adult population in the addiction field is confronting one's own biases and beliefs regarding the elderly and substance abuse. Counselors must recognize and address their own level of denial surrounding substance abuse by the elderly due to issues of shame, stigma, and ageism through educational endeavors and experiential activities designed to interact with this population (Bogunovic, 2012).

Another challenge in identifying the treatment needs of the older adult is the screening and assessment tools available to practitioners to use with this population. The current instruments used for substance use disorders may not be appropriate for the elderly population, including the most recent edition of the *Diagnostic and Statistical Manual* (DSM-5) developed by the American Psychological Association (2013). The DSM is used most frequently by clinicians; however, it has been criticized by some as being invalid for use with older adults (Benyon, 2009; Wang & Andrade, 2013; Wu & Blazer, 2011). There may be the need for more research regarding the changes in the Substance Use Disorders category in the DSM-5 before it can be considered a useful assessment tool for the elderly population (Beynon, 2009). The previous diagnostic manual, the DSM-IV-TR, was criticized as a poor match between the diagnostic criteria for substance abuse and dependence and the pattern of substance use in older adults. These issues continue to be a concern in the DSM-5 as a result of the lack of focus and attention on specific populations in the diagnostic criteria. For example, the diagnostic criteria (e.g., problems in the workplace or school, difficulties in social relationship/responsibilities, increasing tolerance and medical consequences, and giving up activities) are not as readily identifiable or are nonexistent in the older adult substance use population as a result of their developmental stage in life (Segal et al., 2011). To address this issue, some researchers have called for lowering the threshold to improve the validity of the DSM-5 dimensional criterion for detecting substance use disorders in the elderly population (Wang & Andrade, 2013).

There are, however, some validated and useful instruments to use with the elderly population when screening and assessing for substance use disorders and for monitoring treatment outcomes. The Addiction Severity Index (ASI), CAGE questionnaire (**C**ut down, **A**nnoyed, **G**uilty, **E**ye-opener), and the Michigan Alcoholism Screening Test-Geriatric Version (MAST-G) are all instruments that have been modified for the older adult population and have been used successfully in identifying substance use problems (Slaymaker & Owen, 2008; Wang & Andrade, 2013). The ASI captures the changes in functioning over time in substance abuse treatment for older adults, especially in the areas of substance use, family function, and psychiatric issues (Slaymaker & Owen, 2008). Despite a lack of change in the employment and legal scores, the ASI has been used successfully in research studies to measure the outcome of addiction treatment for older adults.

The CAGE questionnaire is a screening tool commonly used to identify the potential for alcohol use disorders in many different populations. This screening tool is comprised of four questions:

- Have you felt the need to **C**ut down on your drinking?
- Do you feel **A**nnoyed by people complaining about your drinking?
- Do you ever feel **G**uilty about your drinking?
- Do you ever drink an **E**ye-opener in the morning to relieve the shakes?

If the client endorses even one question on the CAGE questionnaire, there is evidence for further evaluation and assessment for alcohol use disorders (Mayfield, McLeod, & Hall, 1974). The CAGE can be easily modified for use with the older adult population with good validity. When using the CAGE, clinicians must remain aware that cognitive impairment can affect the older adult's ability to respond to the questions accurately (Mersy, 2007). To modify the CAGE for the older adult population, the clinician can change the language from "drinking" to other "drug/prescription use"; such as (1) Have you felt the need to **C**ut down on your drug/prescription use?

While the CAGE is an easy screening tool to use with older adults, the MAST-G is the most widely used and accepted screening instrument for alcohol use in the older adult population (Segal et al., 2011). The MAST-G contains 24 yes/no questions specifically developed to screen for alcohol problems in the older adult population. One affirmative answer to any of the 24 questions indicates a need for further evaluation, and a cutoff of five positive answers indicates an alcohol use disorder is present (Blow et al., 1992). (See Table 11.1 below for sample questions; the MAST-G is available for viewing on the World Wide Web.)

Regardless of the instrument used to screen or assess for substance use, the practitioner should always be cognizant of the NIAAA limitations set for alcohol use. These limitations set for older adults are different than for people of other ages. The NIAAA (2013) recommends that men aged 65 or older consume no more than one standard drink daily (defined as 12 ounces of beer, 1 ounce of hard liquor, or 5 ounces of wine) and a maximum of two drinks on any occasion. These limits are even lower for women; one standard drink per day is considered at-risk drinking. These rates are considerably lower than the recommendations for younger adults (defined as not more than 14 drinks a week for men and 7 drinks per week for women).

Determining the age of first use and the pattern of substance use across the lifespan are important when screening and assessing older adults. By obtaining this information, a clinician can distinguish between early- and late-onset substance use disorders. The identification can inform cost-effective treatment strategies, as these two groups have very different needs. Early-onset substance abusers have greater risk factors, including health dangers, given the longer period of time they have been abusing substances. Therefore,

Table 11.1: Sample Questions from the Michigan Alcoholism Screening Test-Geriatric Version (MAST-G)

SAMPLE MAST-G QUESTIONS	YES	NO
Does alcohol make you sleepy so that you often fall asleep in your chair?		
Do you hide your alcohol bottles from family members?		
Did you find that your drinking increased after someone close to you died?		
Has a doctor or nurse ever said they were worried or concerned about your drinking?		
When you feel lonely does having a drink help?		

Source: CounsellingResource Research Staff, from "Michigan Alcoholism Screening Test-Geriatric." Copyright © 2012 by CounsellingResource.

they require a more thorough and comprehensive assessment across the life span. On the other hand, late-onset substance users require more evaluation and assessment of recent patterns of substance use, recent changes in health status, and environmental factors that may have triggered the onset of substance abuse (Wu & Blazer, 2011).

A comprehensive evaluation of substance use disorders for the older adult should include numerous components. The recommended elements of such an evaluation are: (a) a clinical interview; (b) screening and assessment tools, such as the ASI, CAGE, and the MAST-G; (c) a thorough physical evaluation; (d) a medication review, including prescription drugs, over-the-counter-medications, and supplements; (e) a psychiatric assessment; (f) a social functioning assessment; and (g) collateral information from someone who knows the older adult well (Bogunovic, 2012; Simoni-Wastila & Yang, 2006; Wu & Blazer, 2011). The Consensus Panel of the Treatment Improvement Protocol has recommended that adults aged 60 and over be screened for substance use disorders as part of regular medical care (CSAT, 1998, 2005). Because older adults frequently see their primary medical caregiver for medical-related concerns, these visits are excellent opportunities to screen for and detect substance abuse problems and make referrals for a full assessment and treatment recommendations (Wu & Blazer, 2011).

TREATMENT CONSIDERATIONS AND RECOMMENDATIONS

According to the Center for Substance Abuse Treatment (1998, 2005), the following treatment approaches are recommended for older adults: Cognitive-behavioral therapy approaches; group-based approaches; individual counseling; medical and psychiatric approaches; marital and family involvement, including family therapy; and case management or community-linked services and outreach. The challenge, however, is actually *getting* the older adult into substance use treatment. Due to ageism and the other barriers discussed, the older adult is often reluctant to enter into substance abuse treatment. Bartels et al. (2004), however, found that older adults were more open to receiving mental health and substance abuse treatment when it was included as part of their primary care. An integrated primary care and substance abuse treatment model is ideal in meeting the needs of the older adult for substance abuse treatment. If the needs of older adults are to be met in the future, integrating screening and assessment for substance treatment into primary care is needed.

The need for detoxification and the management of withdrawal symptoms should be carefully evaluated prior to treatment for the older adult. This evaluation is very important, given the complications related to health concerns in their advancing years (Bogunovic, 2012). After determining the appropriate level of care related to detoxification and withdrawal issues, the least intensive treatment options should be explored first, followed by more intensive services if lower levels of treatment are not sufficient. In a review of the literature on existing treatment for older adults, Kuerbis and Sacco (2013) found that with greater treatment exposure or a higher "dosage" of treatment (regardless of level of care), older adults do better. Furthermore, they found if older adults are in treatment designed for their specific age-related issues and in treatment with their peers, they will gain far more benefits than in a generalized treatment setting.

According to the 2009 Treatment Episode Data Set (TEDS), substance abuse treatment admissions of adults aged 50 or older increased by nearly 50 percent from 2004 to 2009 (SAMHSA, 2011). Unfortunately, much of this treatment is not age specific or designed to meet the needs of the older adult population. The National Survey of Substance Abuse Treatment Services (N-SSATS) (2010) found there were fewer facilities that offered special programs or treatment for the elderly in 2009 than there were in 2004. This trend is concerning, given the large increase in the need for substance abuse treatment for the elderly, and also the fact that older adults do better in age-specific treatment (Han et al., 2009; Wang & Andrade, 2013). Experts recommend that older adults with substance abuse problems receive services that are age-specific, address the unique physical, psychological, social, and vocational changes that occur in the later stages of life and focus on the developmental needs of older adults, including grief, loss, loneliness, and medical issues (Bogunovic, 2012; CSAT, 1998; Cummings, Bride, & Rawlins-Shaw, 2006). The treatment should also include the older adult's family members to get information regarding their loved one's needs, behaviors, and complaints and to educate the family on how best to help their loved one recover (Morgan & Brosi, 2007).

Treatment plans that are developed for the older adult must include age-specific psychological, social, and health concerns goals and objectives. The intervention strategies should be nonconfrontational and supportive, as this has been found to be more effective with the older adult population (Segal et al., 2011). In addition, education—rather than confrontation—is the preferred technique to reduce denial related to substance use issues. Education about the changes in drug metabolism, the interaction of medications with substances, and the importance of compliance with medical instruction are some of the topics to include when working with older adults in treatment. Psychoeducation about the risks of substance use (e.g., excessive alcohol use, overuse of medications, mixing medications with alcohol) should also be included in the treatment for the older adult.

For the older adult population, brief intervention is recommended first, followed by intervention strategies using motivational interviewing. More intensive specialized treatment can be suggested, but only if needed (Bogunovic, 2012; CSAT, 1998, 1999b, 2005; Krahn et al., 2006; Wang & Andrade, 2013; Wu & Blazer, 2011). Schonfeld et al. (2010) developed and evaluated a brief intervention treatment for older adult substance abusers who were also suffering from depression. The brief intervention consisted of one to five sessions delivered in older adults' homes. The sessions included having older adults identify future goals for improving their quality of life and health habits, as well as education in a variety of areas. More specifically, the education provided involved information on (a) the effects of substance use on the aging body; (b) the consequences of substance use; (c) reasons to quit or cut down; (d) skills for handling risky situations; and (f) medication management. The counselors delivered the content using motivational interviewing techniques to elicit self-initiated change and to enhance the motivation for change. This treatment intervention was found to be very effective in reducing the older adults' substance use and improved the overall well-being by reducing the depression symptoms.

In addition to the brief intervention format, treatment using the 16-session curriculum developed by SAMHSA called *Substance Abuse Relapse Prevention for Older Adults: A Group Treatment Approach* was also found to be effective (CSAT, 2005; Schonfeld et al., 2010). This curriculum includes completing a functional analysis of substance use and uses cognitive-behavioral and self-management methods to address high-risk situations, including loneliness, social pressure, depression, anxiety, and anger. Schonfeld et al. (2010) found that when older adults completed the treatment curriculum, substance use decreased, and the level of functioning and well-being increased. While this curriculum is designed for use in a group format, it can be modified to be used with other older adults in an individual format as well.

Related to specialized substance use treatment, Cummings et al. (2006) found that cognitive-behavioral therapy (CBT) approaches are the most effective when treating older adults with alcohol use disorders. Cognitive-behavioral interventions should focus on strategies to help the older adult client learn new, healthier patterns of behavior to replace alcohol use. In addition, cognitive restructuring increases the awareness of the negative aspects of substance use and decreases the positive aspects of that behavior. The client should also be taught self-management techniques. These techniques would help the older adult develop new and more effective coping skills to resolve the developmental issues that led to the substance use. It is recommended that assertion training, self-monitoring, behavior contracting, reinforcement, social support development, and family involvement should be included in the CBT approach with older clients (Segal et al., 2011).

Beyond formalized treatment, participation in support group meetings such as Alcoholics Anonymous or Narcotics Anonymous can be very beneficial for the older adult. These supports are especially useful for older adults if the meetings are age matched, providing mutual support and peer bonding. This mutual support and peer bonding breaks the social isolation that is a risk factor for substance use and relapse (Bogunovic, 2012).

Counselors can engage older adults in substance abuse treatment in a variety of ways and can choose from many different formats. However, clinicians should take note of the following suggestions in an effort to enhance treatment outcomes for the older adult:

- Screening and assessing for substance abuse treatment should be integrated into primary medical care for the older adult as a way to engage the older adult in a treatment process.
- Substance abuse treatment should be age specific and tailored to the unique developmental needs of the older adult population, including age-appropriate pacing and content.
- Supportive and nonconfrontational approaches that build self-esteem should be used with older adults.
- Cognitive-behavioral approaches that are modified to take into account the older adult's cognitive ability should be used.
- A case management or community outreach component to treatment should be included for assistance with the development of skills for improving social support and social contacts.
- Treatment providers should receive specialized training in the developmental needs of older adults in order to increase effectiveness with this population.
- Treatment providers must examine their own beliefs, biases, and attitudes regarding the older adult population and treatment.

Regardless of the format of treatment used, it is imperative that treatment providers and clinicians must be prepared to meet the critical needs of the older adult population, helping to improve their quality of life in the golden years.

Exercise: Case Study–Treatment Plan Development

Lorraine is a 65-year-old woman who has been widowed twice and lives alone in her own home. She had knee replacement surgery one year ago and was put on narcotic pain medication for pain relief.

Lorraine's daughter took a leave of absence from work to care for her during her recovery. Her daughter was able to stay for six weeks, until Lorraine was able to manage her daily living activities on her own. After her daughter left, Lorraine was not able to get out much and was not able to drive anywhere by herself. Lorraine's sister was able to visit once a week; however, she only stayed for about an hour at a time. Lorraine has no other family who lives close to her, and she became bored and lonely "looking at the same four walls all day." Lorraine began to drink in the evening to reduce her boredom and help her sleep. She was advised not to drink while on the pain medication, but Lorraine thought a drink or two at night wouldn't hurt. After the pain medication dosage was reduced by her doctor, she found it difficult to manage her pain without her nightly drink. She began to drink during the day—two drinks—as well as in the evenings—two more drinks—to manage the pain and to sleep. Lorraine continued to follow up with her doctor after the surgery, and she was also seeing a physical therapist to regain mobility and to help strengthen her knee to reduce her pain. The physical pain in the knee was improving, although she continued to look forward to taking her medication and drinking. She was beginning to like how she felt during these times, as she could forget her loneliness and go to sleep. Lorraine was released from the doctor and her physical therapy 12 weeks after surgery; however, the doctor continued to prescribe the pain reliever, as she complained of continuing pain in her knee. Lorraine began to have back pain as well, and she decided to see another doctor, who specialized in back pain. She was given a prescription for a narcotic pain reliever and more physical therapy, which she avoided. Lorraine was now taking two different narcotics for pain relief and drinking daily, usually four drinks a day. She frequently slept during the day to avoid the pain, and she no longer allowed her sister to visit. She also did not go out to shop or go to the Senior Center. Lorraine's daughter phoned occasionally, but did not ask about her medication or other substance use, as her mother had not previously used any substances or consume large amounts of alcohol. Her doctors also did not ask about any substance use or other medication during her routine check-ups. The two different doctors continued to prescribe the medications to Lorraine. She began to use different pharmacies for her prescriptions to avoid the questions that might be asked. About nine months after her knee surgery, Lorraine fell during one of her drinking "episodes" and broke her hip. Her daughter came again to help her mother recover, and she was surprised to see the state her mother was in. Her daughter was very concerned about her mother and began to search for ways to help her mother return to her "usual self."

1. Write down you own biases, beliefs, and attitudes regarding substance use and the elderly that came up for you as you as read this case study. Examine these biases and beliefs. Where do they come from? How can you challenge your own biases and faulty beliefs?
2. Based on the information provided in the case study, what assessment(s) would you complete with this client? Explain why you would use these particular assessments.
3. Is Lorraine an early-onset or late-onset substance abuser? Why is this important to know?
4. Develop a treatment plan for Lorraine that includes recommendations for treatment and goals and objectives that are unique to this client. Take into account the issues and special needs of the older client as discussed in the chapter.
5. What are the barriers to treatment that Lorraine might experience that you need to plan for? How would you plan for and address these barriers in your treatment plan?

REFERENCES

American Geriatrics Society. (2003). *Clinical guidelines for alcohol use disorders in older adults.* Retrieved from http://www.americangeriatrics.org/products/ positionpapers/alcohol.shtml

American Psychiatric Association. (2013). *Diagnostic and statistical manual of mental disorders* (5th ed.). Washington, DC: Author.

Bartels, S. J., Coakley, E. H, Zubritsky, C., Ware, J. H., Miles, K. M., Arean, P. A., ... Levkoff, S. E. (2004). Improving access to geriatric mental health services: A randomized trial comparing treatment engagement with integrated versus enhanced referral care for depression, anxiety, and at-risk alcohol use. *American Journal of Psychiatry, 161*(8), 1455–1462.

Beynon, C. (2009). Drug use and ageing: Older people do take drugs. *Age and Ageing, 38*, 8–10. doi:10.1093/ageing/afn251

Blow, F. C., Brower, K. J., Schulenberg, J. E., Demo-Dananberg, L. M., Young, J. P., & Beresford, T. P. (1992). The Michigan alcoholism screening test-geriatric version (MAST-G): A new elderly-specific screening instrument. *Alcoholism: Clinical and Experimental Research, 16*, 372.

Bogunovic, O. (2012, August). Substance abuse in aging and elderly adults. *Psychiatric Times*, 39–40.

Breslow, R. A., Faden, V. B., & Smothers, B. (2003). Alcohol consumption by elderly Americans. *Journal of Studies on Alcohol, 64*, 884–892.

Briggs, W. P., Magnus, V. A., Lassiter, P., Patterson, A., & Smith, L. (2011). Substance use, misuse, and abuse among older adults: Implications for clinical mental health counselors. *Journal of Mental Health Counseling, 33*(2), 112–127.

Brown University. (2008, April). Substance abuse and the aging brain: Screening, diagnoses, and treatment. *Brown University Geriatric Psychopharmacology Update, 12*(4), 1–6.

Butler, R. (1975). *Why survive? Being old in America.* New York: Harper & Row.

Caputo, F., Vignoli, T., Leggio, L., Addolorato, G., Zoli, G., & Bernardi, M. (2012). Alcohol use disorders in the elderly: A brief overview from epidemiology to treatment options. *Experimental Gerontology, 47*, 411–416.

Center for Substance Abuse Treatment. (1999a). *Enhancing Motivation for Change in Substance Abuse Treatment.* Treatment Improvement Protocol (TIP) Series, Number 35. DHHS Pub. No. (SMA) 99-3354. Washington, DC: U.S. Government Printing Office.

Center for Substance Abuse Treatment. (1999b). *Brief Interventions and Brief Therapies for Substance Abuse: Treatment Improvement Protocol (TIP), Series 34.* Rockville, MD: Substance Abuse and Mental Health Services Administration.

Center for Substance Abuse Treatment. (2005). *Substance Abuse Relapse Prevention: A Group Treatment Approach for Older Adults.* Rockville, MD: Substance Abuse and Mental Health Services Administration.

Center for Substance Abuse Treatment. (1998). *Substance Abuse Among Older Adults: Treatment Improvement Protocol (TIP), Series 26.* Rockville, MD: Substance Abuse and Mental Health Services Administration.

Clay, R. A. (2007, January/February). Treatment for older adults: What works best? *SAMHSA News, 15*(1), 1–5.

Cummings, S. M., Bride, B., & Rawlins-Shaw, A. M. (2006). Alcohol abuse treatment for older adults: A review of recent empirical research. *Journal of Evidence-Based Social Work, 3*, 79–99. doi:10.1300/J367v03n01 05

Doweiko, H. E. (2011). *Concepts of chemical dependency* (8th ed.). United States: Brooks Cole.

Dowling, G. J., Weiss, S. R., & Condon, T. P. (2008). Drugs of abuse and the aging brain. *Neuropsychopharmocology, 33*(2), 209–218.

Fingerhood, M. (2000). Substance abuse in older people. *Journal of the American Geriatrics Society, 48*, 985–995.

Gfroerer, J. C., Penne, M., Pemberton, M., & Folsom, R. (2003). Substance abuse treatment need among older adults in 2020: The impact of the aging baby-boom cohort. *Drug and Alcohol Dependence, 69*(2), 127–135.

Han, B., Gfroerer, J. C., Colliver, J. D., & Penne, M. A. (2009). Substance use disorder among older adults in the United States in 2020. *Addiction, 104*, 88–96. doi:10.1111/j.1360-0443.2008.02411.x

Hester, R., & Miller, W. (2003). *Handbook of alcoholism treatment approaches* (3rd ed.). Boston: Allyn & Bacon.

Hunter, B., Lubman, D. I., & Barratt, M. (2011). Alcohol and drug misuse in the elderly. *Australian and New England College of Psychiatrists, 45*, 343. doi:10.3109/00048674.2010.549997

Kalapatapu, R. K., & Sullivan, M. A. (2010). Prescription use disorders in older adults. *American Journal on Addictions, 19*, 515–522. doi:10.1111/j.1521-0391.2010.00080.x

Kanny, D., Liu, Y., & Brewer, R. D. (2012). Vital signs: Binge drinking prevalence, frequency, and intensity among adults—United States, 2010. *Morbidity and Mortality Weekly Report, 61*(1), 14–19.

Kinney, J. (2011). *Loosening the grip* (10th ed.). Boston: McGraw Hill.

Krahn, D. D., Bartels, S. J., Coakley, E., Oslin, D. W., Chen, H., McIntyre, J., … Levkoff, S. E. (2006). PRISM-E: A comparison of integrated care and enhanced specialty referral models in depression outcomes. *Psychiatric Services, 57*(7), 946–953.

Kuerbis, A., & Sacco, P. (2013). A review of existing treatments for substance abuse among the elderly and recommendations for future directions. *Substance Abuse: Research & Treatment, 7*, 13–37. doi:10.4137/SART.S7865

Maxwell, J. C. (2011). The prescription drug epidemic in the United States: A perfect storm. *Drug and Alcohol Review, 30*, 264–270. doi:10.1111/k.1465-3362.2011.00291.x

Mayfield, D., McLeod, G., & Hall, P. (1974). The CAGE questionnaire: Validation of a new alcoholism screening instrument. *American Journal of Psychiatry, 131*(10), 1121–1123.

Mersy, D. J. (2007). Recognition of alcohol and substance abuse. *American Family Physician, 67*(7), 1529–1532.

Morgan, M., & Brosi, W. A. (2007). Prescription drug abuse among older adults: A family ecological case study. *Journal of Applied Gerontology, 26*, 419–432. doi:10.1177/0733464807304962

National Institute on Alcohol Abuse and Alcoholism. (2013). *Drinking guidelines for older adults*. Retrieved from http://www.niaaa.nih.gov/alcohol-health/special-populations-co-occurring-disorders/older-adults

National Institute on Drug Abuse. (2005). *Prescription drugs: Abuse and addiction. NIDA Research Report Series*. Retrieved from http://www.drugabuse.gov/sites/default/files/rrprescription.pdf

Qato, D. M., Alexander, G. C., Conti, R. B., Johnson, M., Schumm, P., Lindau, S. T. (2008). Use of prescription and over-the-counter medications and dietary supplements among older adults in the United States. *Journal of the American Medical Association, 300*(24), 2867–2878. doi:10.1001/jama.2008.892

Schonfeld, L., King-Kallimanis, B. L., Duchene, D. M., Etheridge, R. L., Herrera, J. R., Barry, K. L., Lynn, N. (2010). Screening and brief intervention for substance misuse among older adults: The Florida BRITE project. *American Journal of Public Health, 100*(1), 108–114.

Segal, D. L., Qualls, S. H., & Smyer, M. A. (2011). *Aging and mental health* (2nd ed.). United Kingdom: Wiley-Blackwell.

Simoni-Wastila, L., & Yang, H. K. (2006). Psychoactive drug abuse in older adults. *American Journal of Geriatric Pharmacotherapy, 4*(4), 380–394.

Slaymaker, V. J., & Owen, P. (2008). Alcohol and other drug dependency severity among older adults in treatment: Measuring characteristics and outcomes. *Alcoholism Treatment Quarterly, 26*(3), 259–273. doi:10.1080/07347373208020711877

Substance Abuse and Mental Health Services Administration. (2013). *Results from the 2012 National Survey on Drug Use and Health: Summary of National Findings*, NSDUH

Series H-46, HHS Publication No. (SMA) 13-4795. Rockville, MD: Substance Abuse and Mental Health Services Administration.

Substance Abuse and Mental Health Services Administration, Office of Applied Studies. (2010). *National Survey of Substance Abuse Treatment Services (N-SSATS): 2009. Data on Substance Abuse Treatment Facilities*, DASIS Series: S-54, HHS Publication No. (SMA) 10-4579, Rockville, MD: Substance Abuse and Mental Health Services Administration.

Substance Abuse and Mental Health Services Administration. (2011). *Treatment Episode Data Set (TEDS). 1999–2009. National Admissions to Substance Abuse Treatment Services*. DASIS Series: S-56, HHS Publication No. (SMA) 11-4646, Rockville, MD: Substance Abuse and Mental Health Services Administration.

Thombs, D. L. (2006). *Introduction to addictive behaviors*. New York: Guilford Press.

Wang, Y., & Andrade, L. H. (2013). Epidemiology of alcohol and drug use in the elderly. *Psychiatry, 26*, 343–438. doi:10.1097/YCO.0b013e328360eafd

Wilbourne, P. L., & Miller, W. R. (2002). Treatment for alcoholism: Older and wiser? *Alcoholism Treatment Quarterly, 20*(3/4), 41–59. doi:10.1300/J020v20n03_03

Wu, L., & Blazer, D. G. (2011). Illicit and nonmedical drug use among older adults: A review. *Journal of Aging and Health, 23*(3), 481–504. doi:10.1177/0898264310386224

CHAPTER 12

PERSONS WITH CO-OCCURRING DISORDERS

By Lauren Borges and Tiffany Lee

Substance use disorders (SUDs) rarely present in isolation, as they often co-occur with other forms of psychopathology. For the purposes of this chapter, the terms *co-occurring*, *comorbid*, and *concurrent* disorder refer to the presence of at least one SUD and at least one mental disorder at the same time. In order to constitute a co-occurring disorder, criteria for both conditions must occur independently of each other. The explicit study of SUDs and commonly comorbid psychological conditions is essential to understanding the development, maintenance, and treatment of concurrent psychopathologies. Thus, identifying the variables linking co-occurring disorders is integral to the advancement of SUD prevention and treatment.

SUDs can co-occur with a variety of psychological conditions, including mood disorders, anxiety disorders, eating disorders, personality disorders, and psychotic disorders. Often, the onset of these psychological disorders precipitates the onset of SUDs. Comorbid SUDs and psychological disorders are associated with a poorer symptom course and more negative outcomes than when SUDs or different mental health diagnoses occur in isolation. SUDs, in combination with at least one additional psychological disorder, are associated with greater risk of substance use relapse, longer treatment duration, poorer physical health, greater unemployment, heightened criminal activity, and even elevated mortality risk. This chapter will first address the prevalence of SUDs by providing some general statistics about co-occurring disorders. Then, the authors will discuss information pertaining to specific categories of psychological disorders (e.g., mood disorders, anxiety disorders, etc.). Models of comorbidity, barriers to treatment, resiliency factors, and screening and assessment methods will be presented next. The chapter will conclude with treatment considerations.

STATISTICS

In the general population, those with substance use issues commonly have mental health concerns as well. An investigation in 2012 completed by the National Survey on Drug Use and Health (NSDUH) estimated that close to 8.4 million adults in the United States have both a mental and substance use disorder (Substance Abuse and Mental Health Services Administration [SAMHSA], 2013). Figure 12.1 below illustrates the breakdown of SUDs among those with and without a mental health disorder. NSDUH also investigated the rate of co-occurring disorders of persons with various racial and ethnic backgrounds and reported the rates were: 1.1 percent among Asians, 3.3 percent among blacks, 3.4 percent among Hispanics, 3.8 percent among whites, 4.3 percent among persons reporting two or more races, and 14.0 percent among American Indians or Alaska Natives (SAMHSA, 2013).

Concerning mood disorders specifically, the National Epidemiologic Survey on Alcohol and Related Conditions (NESARC) found 41 percent of individuals with lifetime drug use disorder also met criteria for a lifetime mood disorder (Conway, Compton, Stinson, & Grant, 2006). In fact, another study analyzed the results of this survey and reported 20 percent of participants with SUDs met criteria for at least one mood disorder concurrently in a 12-month period (Grant et al., 2004). The NSDUH (2013) study examined

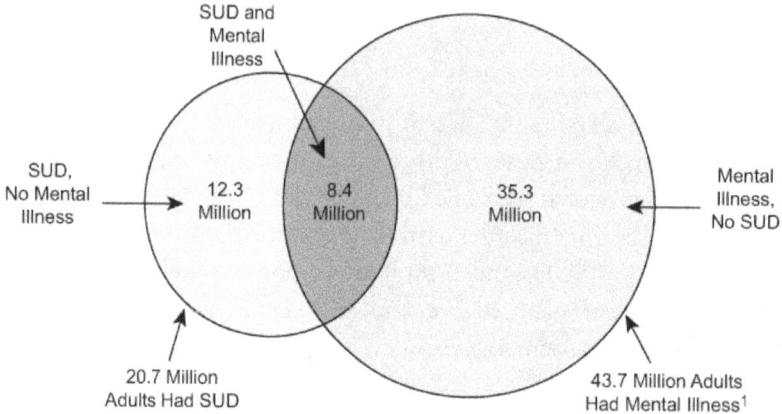

Figure 12.1: Past Year SUDs and Mental Illness among Adults Aged 18 or Older: 2012. Taken from the NSDUH data (SAMHSA, 2013).

Source: SAMHSA / Public Domain.

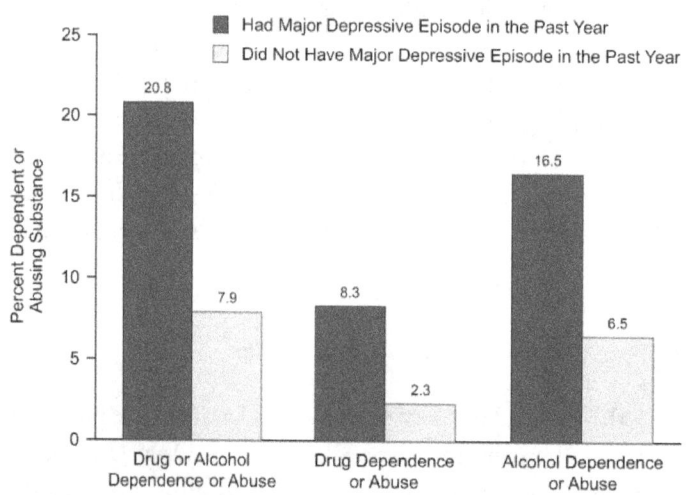

Figure 12.2: A Comparison of Dependence and Abuse Rates between those with or without a Major Depressive Episode in the Past Year.

Source: Taken from the NSDUH data (SAMHSA, 2013).

the incidence of substance abuse and dependence among those who had a major depressive episode within the last year. As expected, the rates were higher for those with such an experience (see Figure 12.2 below).

Due to the high incidence of substance use among those with mental health conditions, co-occurring mental health diagnoses are frequently observed across treatment settings. For instance, in a residential substance abuse treatment program, 55.4 percent of males and 73.7 percent of females were diagnosed with a comorbid psychiatric disorder (Chen et al., 2011). Of this sample, 32.5 percent of clients met criteria for a concurrent mood disorder, 32 percent met criteria for a comorbid anxiety disorder, 25.3 percent met criteria for co-occurring antisocial personality disorder (ASPD), 24.2 percent were diagnosed with comorbid borderline personality disorder (BPD), and 8.4 percent demonstrated concurrent psychotic symptoms (Chen et al., 2011). Moreover, 16.2 percent of males and 23.3 percent of females met criteria for three or more mental health conditions, demonstrating the prevalence of multiple co-occurring disorders (Chen et al., 2011). Outpatient treatment settings for SUDs also show similarly high rates of psychiatric comorbidity. In an outpatient sample of individuals receiving treatment for SUDs, over 50 percent met criteria for a probable mental health disorder (Watkins et al., 2004).

Large-scale epidemiological studies have also examined the prevalence of mental health disorders for those seeking substance abuse treatment services. Among treatment-seeking individuals, 40.7 percent of those with an alcohol use disorder also met criteria for an independent, concurrent mood disorder within the 12-month sampling window (Grant et al., 2004). Of the individuals in this sample seeking treatment for a drug use disorder, 60 percent also met criteria for at least one concurrent mood disorder (Grant et al., 2004). These statistics may underrepresent the prevalence of co-occurring SUDs and mental health conditions, as it has been established that many people do not get help for their SUDs or psychological concerns. The findings from the NSDUH (2013) study support this assertion, as the research indicates 53.7 percent of the 8.4 million adults with a co-occurring disorder did not receive any treatment for either

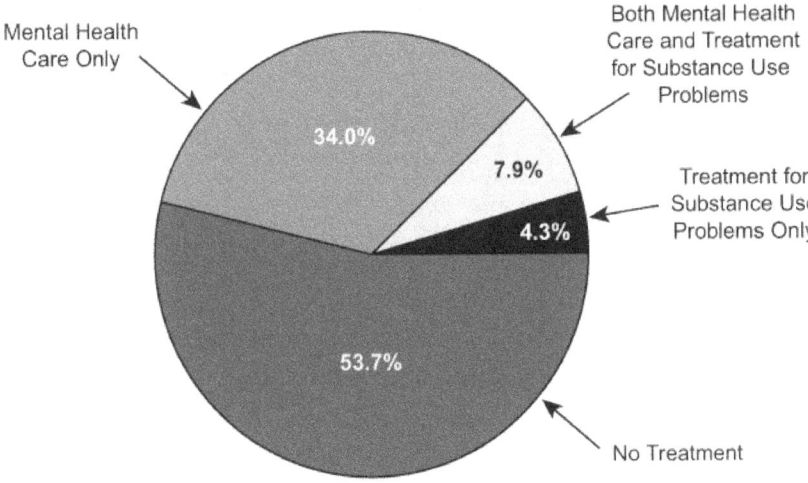

Figure 12.3: Past-Year Mental Health Care and Treatment for Substance Use Problems among Adults Aged 18 or Older with Co-Occurring Disorders.

Source: Taken from the NSDUH data (SAMHSA, 2013).

of their co-occurring disorders. Only 7.9 percent received treatment for both conditions. (Refer to Figure 12.3 below.)

The statistics provided in this section not only highlight the existence of co-occurring disorders in the general population, but also indicate the prevalence of mental health disorders among those who abuse substances. As stated earlier, mood disorders and anxiety disorders are the most prevalent co-occurring mental health disorders with SUDs. Therefore, the authors address these disorders first. Then, eating disorders, psychotic disorders, and personality disorders are discussed in the following sections. In each section, brief descriptions of the disorders are given, along with research findings.

MOOD DISORDERS

Mood disorders are common among those with SUDs, and these include major depressive disorder (MDD), dysthymia, and bipolar disorder. In a large-scale study assessing comorbid SUDs and non–substance induced mood disorders in the past 12 months, 19.7 percent of those with SUDs also met criteria for any co-occurring mood disorder. More specifically, among respondents with SUDs, 14.5 percent of respondents had a diagnosis for MDD, 3.5 percent had dysthymia, and 5 percent had mania (Grant et al., 2004). When lifetime comorbidity rates were assessed in the same study, 21.6 percent of individuals with a mood disorder also met lifetime criteria for a drug use disorder (Conway et al., 2006). Conversely, among respondents with a lifetime drug use disorder, 40.9 percent met lifetime criteria for a mood disorder (Conway et al., 2006).

The issue of differential diagnosis must be considered when evaluating individuals for co-occurring mood disorders and SUDs. Substance-induced mood disorders can occur as the result of substance use, and these disorders evoke clinically significant depression, mania, or both. To be diagnosed with a mood disorder that is substance induced, features of the mood disorder must develop during or shortly after substance intoxication or withdrawal. Conversely, non–substance induced mood disorders (also called preexisting disorders) must be present during periods of sobriety from substances.

Major Depressive Disorder

The above statistics illustrate the prevalence of depressive disorders in samples of individuals with SUDs. Depressive disorders can be broadly identified based on the presence of a sad, empty, or irritable mood. This low mood occurs in conjunction with cognitive and somatic changes that impair a person's daily life functioning. To meet diagnostic criteria for MDD, persistence of the symptoms identified above must last for a period of two weeks or more.

Among those with co-occurring SUDs and depressive disorder, MDD is found to be the most prevalent. In fact, 24 percent of people with MDD endorsed a lifetime comorbidity of SUDs (Kessler et al., 2003). Twelve-month comorbidity rates for MDD and SUDs were similar in that 19.2 percent of participants with MDD also met criteria for SUDs, and 14.5 percent of participants with SUDs met criteria for MDD (Grant et al., 2004). A sample receiving outpatient SUD treatment showed slightly higher rates of MDD (29.4 percent), which speaks to the prevalence of comorbid SUDs and MDD in a treatment setting (Davis et al., 2006). It should be noted the severity of drug use (e.g., an abuse versus a dependence diagnosis) appears to affect comorbidity rates in MDD. For example, among individuals with depression in a treatment setting, 49 percent were drug dependent, compared to 28 percent who were diagnosed with a drug abuse diagnosis (Conway et al., 2006).

Dysthymia

Dysthymia is also frequently comorbid with SUDs. Dysthymia is a depressive disorder that shares many of the same features as MDD, but is differentiated by its symptom duration. To meet diagnostic criteria for dysthymia, a depressed mood, as well as symptoms associated with this mood (e.g., low energy, poor appetite, difficulty concentrating) must be endorsed. These behaviors must be present for at least a two-year period, without breaks for more than two months at a time within those two years.

Researchers have found 27.3 percent of those with dysthymia meet criteria for a lifetime drug use disorder, whereas 11.4 percent of individuals with a drug use disorder meet criteria for lifetime dysthymia (Conway et al., 2006). When data from the same study were analyzed using 12-month comorbidity rates, of the individuals meeting criteria for SUDs, 3.5 percent qualified for dysthymia. Of those with dysthymia, 18 percent met criteria for SUDs within the past 12 months (Grant et al., 2004). As seen with MDD, dysthymia is also more common among those with a drug dependence diagnosis than those with a drug abuse diagnosis. For example, in one study, 21.4 percent of drug-dependent individuals met criteria for dysthymia, as compared with 8 percent of those who met criteria for drug abuse (Conway et al., 2006).

Bipolar Disorder

Bipolar disorder can be broadly understood as a mood disorder that is comprised of manic and often depressive episodes. An individual may experience a major depressive episode either before or after a manic episode. Manic episodes are representative of a pattern of persistently elevated, grandiose, or irritable mood and an abnormal drive toward goal-directed activity lasting at least one week. To meet diagnostic criteria for bipolar disorder, at least one manic episode must be experienced that is not better accounted for by any other disorder.

Bipolar disorder is highly comorbid in populations with SUDs. In fact, 30 percent to over 50 percent of individuals with a bipolar I diagnosis also meet lifetime criteria for SUDs (Cerullo & Strakowski, 2007). Twelve-month prevalence rates of comorbidity indicate 28 percent of people with mania also meet criteria for SUDs when compared with 5 percent of individuals with SUDs qualifying for a mania diagnosis (Grant et al., 2004). Moreover, 37.5 percent of individuals with mania have a lifetime comorbid drug use disorder (Conway et al., 2006). Increased odds of developing bipolar disorder have been more strongly associated with substance dependence, suggesting a more robust relationship between SUDs and bipolar disorder specifically (Kenneson, Funderburk, & Maisto, 2013).

ANXIETY DISORDERS

In broad terms, anxiety disorders reflect difficulties in functioning related to excessive fear and anxiety. These functional impairments are evidenced by pervasive disruptions in behavior and daily life tasks. Along with mood disorders, anxiety disorders are very prevalent among those who have substance abuse concerns. In fact, a large scale epidemiological study found 30 percent of individuals with a lifetime history of drug use disorder met lifetime criteria for at least one anxiety disorder (Conway et al., 2006). The same study also found that 18 percent of individuals with a SUD met criteria for any anxiety disorder over a 12-month period (Grant et al., 2004). Another study showed, among persons with an alcohol use disorder specifically, 33 percent of a treatment-seeking sample also met criteria for one or more anxiety disorders. Within this same survey, 43 percent of those seeking treatment for a drug use disorder also met criteria for at least one comorbid anxiety disorder (Grant et al., 2004). As evidenced earlier with the comorbidity between mood disorders and SUDs, the risk of an anxiety disorder diagnosis is greater among individuals with substance dependence than with substance abuse. While several anxiety disorders are highly comorbid with SUDs, the authors address the most prevalent below. These include generalized anxiety disorder, social phobia, specific phobia, panic disorder, obsessive-compulsive disorder, and post-traumatic stress disorder.

Generalized Anxiety Disorder

Generalized anxiety disorder (GAD) occurs when a person experiences excessive anxiety and worry about a number of events and activities; this contributes to impairment in functioning. GAD is the most commonly concurrent anxiety disorder with SUDs. In fact, SUDs affect half of those with lifetime GAD (Alegría et al., 2010). Among individuals with SUDs, 4.2 percent also met criteria for GAD in the past 12 months (Grant et al., 2004). In this same study, 19 percent of those with GAD met 12-month comorbidity criteria for a SUD (Grant et al., 2004). People with GAD and SUDs tend to fare worse in treatment than those with a single diagnosis of either disorder.

GAD symptoms tend to precede the onset of SUDs. Thus, it is highly likely that these symptoms can lead to the development and maintenance of ineffective emotion regulation behaviors like substance use (Marmorstein, 2012). Research has supported this hypothesis. For instance, when criteria are met for both GAD and SUDs, people do tend to endorse significantly higher rates of substance use to facilitate relief from anxiety symptoms (Alegría et al., 2010).

Social Phobia

Social phobia occurs when a person has fear or anxiety in social situations, which is clinically significant. These social situations specifically involve exposure to the possibility of being evaluated by others (e.g., giving a speech, having a conversation, sharing an opinion). To be considered for a diagnosis of social phobia, the fear or anxiety regarding these situations must be amplified, cause avoidance, and lead to clinically significant distress or impairment in functioning. Among individuals meeting criteria for social phobia, 22.3 percent met criteria for a lifetime drug use disorder (Conway et al., 2006). Social phobia co-occurs in 4.7 percent of individuals with SUDs in a 12-month period (Grant et al., 2004). Higher rates of SUDs are demonstrated in individuals with social phobia, as 16.1 percent of those with social phobia also demonstrate SUDs (Grant et al., 2004).

Specific Phobia

Specific phobias are characterized by significant fear or anxiety related to a certain object or situation (e.g., animals, flying, viewing blood, receiving an injection, and/or heights). Individuals meeting criteria for specific phobia must not only consistently avoid the feared event or object, but this avoidance, fear, or anxiety causes significant impairment in functioning. Specific phobias are also one of the most frequently comorbid anxiety disorders with SUDs. Among people meeting criteria for a specific phobia, 18.8 percent met lifetime criteria for a drug use disorder (Conway et al., 2006). In addition to the prevalence of co-occurring SUDs and specific phobia in a lifetime, there are also high rates within a 12-month period. For instance, 13.8 percent of people with a specific phobia also had a SUD, and 10.5 percent of people with a SUD in a 12-month period also had a specific phobia (Grant et al., 2004).

Panic Disorder

A panic disorder diagnosis entails the presence of frequent, unexpected panic attacks that reach a peak within minutes. A person's experience of these panic attacks must lead to either a significant maladaptive behavioral change related to these attacks or chronic worry about having additional panic attacks. To qualify for a panic disorder diagnosis, this experience cannot be attributed to the effects of substance use. Among individuals meeting lifetime diagnostic criteria for a drug use disorder, 23.1 percent met criteria for a comorbid panic disorder diagnosis (Conway et al., 2006). Of those with SUDs, 2.8 percent met criteria for panic disorder within the past 12 months. Participants who met criteria for panic disorder demonstrated higher 12-month comorbidity rates as 17.3 percent also met criteria for SUDs (Grant et al., 2004).

Substance use is also prevalent among people with both panic disorder and agoraphobia. Agoraphobia can be conceptualized as significant fear or anxiety related to at least two of the following situations: using public transportation, open spaces, enclosed spaces, standing in lines or crowds, or being outside of one's home alone. Among individuals with SUDs, 1.5 percent also met criteria for panic disorder with agoraphobia in the past 12 months (Grant et al., 2004). When 12-month comorbidity rates of SUDs are analyzed among those experiencing panic disorder with agoraphobia, 24.1 percent met criteria for a co-occurring SUD. Even higher rates of co-occurrence were demonstrated when lifetime symptoms of the co-occurring disorders were assessed, as 34.2 percent of individuals with panic disorder and agoraphobia met criteria for a lifetime SUD (Conway et al., 2006).

Obsessive-Compulsive Disorder (OCD)

Obsessive-compulsive disorder (OCD) refers to the clinically significant presence of obsessions and/or compulsions. Obsessions denote recurrent or persistent thoughts, urges, or images that are considered unwanted or intrusive. Compulsions are repetitive behaviors or mental acts, that a person feels compelled to engage in based on these intrusive thoughts or mental rules. While rates of OCD are low in the general population, researchers have found 24 percent of people meeting criteria for OCD also met criteria for lifetime SUDs (Ruscio, Stein, Chiu, & Kessler, 2010). More specifically, 18 percent of individuals with OCD met lifetime criteria for a drug use disorder (Mancebo, Grant, Pinto, Eisen, & Rasmussen, 2009). The comorbidity of OCD and SUDs may suggest that the behaviors consistent with OCD and SUDs facilitate emotion regulation (e.g., abusing anxiolytic drugs and engaging in behavioral compulsions provides relief from uncomfortable emotions like anxiety).

Post-traumatic Stress Disorder (PTSD)

Trauma can result from numerous experiences, including emotional, physical, and sexual abuse, as well as assault, war, natural disasters, terrorism, and interpersonal violence. A post-traumatic stress disorder

(PTSD) diagnosis (according to the DSM-IV-TR) involves exposure to a traumatic event in some capacity, experiencing intrusive recollections of this event, avoidance and/or numbing behaviors in response to this experience, and persistent hyperarousal. These symptoms must endure for over one month to qualify as a PTSD diagnosis. PTSD is one of the most researched comorbid disorders with SUDs.

In a large epidemiological study assessing lifetime rates of comorbid psychopathology, almost half of people with PTSD (46.4 percent) met criteria for SUDs (Pietrzak, Goldstein, Sothwick, & Grant, 2011). Studies examining those seeking treatment for SUDs have found 36 to 50 percent of these individuals also met criteria for lifetime PTSD (Brady, Back, & Coffey, 2004). One of the reasons the comorbidity of PTSD and SUDs has been so heavily researched is due to its prominence in veteran populations. More severe combat exposure has been well established as a risk factor for the development of PTSD. This trend also appears relevant to SUDs. For instance, severe combat exposure has been associated with 93 percent greater odds of alcohol misuse (Santiago et al., 2010).

Another population with a high prevalence of PTSD and SUDs is women. Between 55 and 99 percent of women who abuse substances have a history of trauma, compared to rates of 36 to 51 percent in the general population. However, not all those who experience trauma develop PTSD. Studies have shown PTSD rates among women who abuse substances range between 14 and 60 percent, and women who use substances are still more than twice as likely to have PTSD as men. Moreover, women with PTSD were five times more likely than women without PTSD to have substance use disorders (Center for Substance Abuse Treatment, 2009). In summary, the statistics gathered among the veteran population and among women demonstrate their vulnerability to the development of PTSD and concurrent SUDs, suggesting that screening and treatment of comorbid psychopathology is especially pertinent in these populations.

EATING DISORDERS

Eating disorders refer to significant disruptions in eating that interfere with daily life functioning. These disruptions tend to occur when a person loses control over eating behaviors. The individual may experience a clinically significant restriction of food intake, periods of eating an excessively large caloric intake in a two-hour period (i.e., binge eating), and/or the use of inappropriate compensatory behaviors to prevent weight gain (e.g., excessive exercise, laxative misuse, self-induced vomiting).

Lifetime rates for the co-occurrence of any substance use disorder and eating disorder are high. Researchers have found lifetime rates of co-occurring SUDs and bulimia nervosa, anorexia nervosa, and binge-eating disorder to be 36.8 percent, 27 percent, and 23.3 percent, respectively (Hudson, Hiripi, Pope, & Kessler, 2007). Some studies have found lifetime comorbidity rates of up to 70 percent of individuals with bulimia nervosa meeting criteria for a lifetime SUD (Pearlstein, 2002). As these co-occurring rates demonstrate, individuals with a bulimia nervosa diagnosis are more likely to have a comorbid SUD. Eating disorders and concurrent SUDs may be a particularly volatile combination related to physical health and stability. The highest mortality rates of all psychological disorders are associated with eating disorders and SUDs, making the co-occurrence of these disorders particularly deadly.

PSYCHOTIC DISORDERS

Psychotic disorders or schizophrenia spectrum disorders can be broadly viewed as unusual patterns in perception that are maladaptive. To meet criteria for a psychotic disorder, a person must experience perceptual abnormalities through the presence of symptoms like delusions, hallucinations, disorganized thinking or speech, grossly disorganized or abnormal motor behavior (e.g., catatonia), and negative symptoms (e.g., diminished emotional expression). Schizophrenia is one of the most researched psychotic disorders to co-occur with SUDs.

As many as half of all individuals with schizophrenia meet criteria for SUDs in a lifetime (Dixon, 1999). Substance use often precipitates and worsens psychotic features. In particular, cannabis use has been heavily researched over the years in relation to its link to schizophrenia. Several studies have shown cannabis use (particularly in adolescence) can substantially increase the likelihood of a person developing schizophrenia (Parakh & Basu, 2013). Many researchers now believe that using the drug while the brain is still developing boosts levels of the chemical dopamine in the brain, which can directly lead to schizophrenia.

PERSONALITY DISORDERS

Personality disorders can be conceptualized as enduring patterns of inner experiences and behaviors, which (a) significantly deviate from an individual's cultural expectations; (b) are persistent and inflexible; and (c) cause significant impairment in functioning. The *Diagnostic and Statistical Manual* has recognized three behavioral clusters, each of which subsumes distinct behavioral patterns. The pervasive presence of abnormally odd or eccentric behaviors falls under the classification of *Cluster A* personality disorders. Paranoid personality disorder, schizoid personality disorder, and schizotypal personality disorder are included in Cluster A personality disorders. *Cluster B* personality disorders are distinctly dramatic, erratic, and emotional in nature. Within Cluster B personality disorders are antisocial personality disorder (ASPD), borderline personality disorder (BPD), histrionic personality disorder, and narcissistic personality disorder (NPD). Personality disorders with anxious or fearful qualities are embodied by *Cluster C*. Avoidant personality disorder, obsessive-compulsive personality disorder, and dependent personality disorder are included within Cluster C personality disorders.

Personality disorders are highly comorbid with SUDs. In fact, almost one-fourth (22.6 percent) of individuals with a personality disorder met criteria for concurrent SUDs (Lezenweger, Lane, Loranger, & Kessler, 2007). Moreover, people with a personality disorder diagnosis are over 12 times more likely to experience a lifetime drug dependence diagnosis, compared to those without a personality disorder. High rates of comorbidity were found between SUDs and personality disorders in a large-scale study, as 30.7 percent of those with a personality disorder diagnosis met criteria for concurrent alcohol use disorder, while 10.6 percent were diagnosed with a co-occurring drug use disorder (Trull, Jahng, Tomko, Wood, & Sher, 2010).

Another large-scale epidemiological study investigated the rates of comorbid SUDs among the three clusters and found the highest prevalence was among those with Cluster B personality disorders (39.9 percent). Twelve percent of people with a Cluster C personality disorder diagnosis met criteria for concurrent SUDs, and 11.5 percent of individuals with a Cluster A personality disorder met criteria for comorbid SUDs (Lezenweger et al., 2007).

Cluster B Personality Disorders

While rates of comorbidity with SUDs are high among those with any personality disorder diagnosis, Cluster B personality disorders are associated with a particularly high vulnerability for SUDs. Known for dramatic and erratic behavioral features, Cluster B personality disorders have been heavily researched, as they are indicative of emotional dysfunction. Borderline personality disorder (BPD) is the most empirically established personality disorder concerning pervasive emotional dysfunction. Lifetime rates of alcohol dependence and drug dependence are 41.6 percent and 17.7 percent, respectively, among individuals with a diagnosis of BPD (Trull et al., 2010). Moreover, 12-month comorbidity rates of BPD and SUDs are also elevated, as 38.2 percent of people with BPD were also found to have SUDs (Lezenweger et al., 2007).

High rates of SUDs have also been found among those with antisocial personality disorder (ASPD) and narcissistic personality disorder (NPD). For example, lifetime rates of alcohol dependence and drug dependence among individuals with an ASPD diagnosis are 49.2 percent and 23.4 percent, respectively (Trull et al., 2010). A study of 12-month comorbidity rates found 40.5 percent of individuals meeting criteria for ASPD also met criteria for SUDs in the past year (Lezenweger et al., 2007). With regard to NPD, one study found lifetime rates of SUDs to be 64.2 percent among individuals with this disorder (Stinson et al., 2008). When the prevalence of NPD and SUDs were assessed for a 12-month period, rates of SUD co-occurrence were demonstrated in 40.6 percent of those with NPD (Stinson et al., 2008).

To summarize, people experiencing mental health concerns have a higher propensity to use substances. While mood disorders and anxiety disorders are shown to be the most common among those with SUDs, other psychological disorders also increase the likelihood for one to develop a substance use problem. In the next section, etiological theories as to why those with mental health issues may be using substances at higher rates than the general population are presented.

MODELS OF COMORBIDITY

Self-Medication Model

The self-medication hypothesis suggests that the presence of a psychiatric disorder aids in the development of SUDs. According to this rationale, SUDs are said to develop secondarily to a primary psychological condition, like a mood or anxiety disorder. This theory posits individuals use alcohol and other drugs that specifically cause a reduction in primary psychiatric symptoms (e.g., people with anxiety disorders abuse anxiolytic drugs due to the anxiety-reducing properties of these drugs). The self-medication hypothesis can be viewed as a behavioral model of substance abuse, in that self-medication facilitates negative reinforcement from psychiatric symptoms (Blume, Schmaling, & Marlatt, 2000).

However, the self-medication hypothesis is not without theoretical flaws. Individuals with co-occurring psychological disorders and SUDs do not always abuse substances that directly reduce psychological symptoms. For instance, people with depressive disorders often abuse depressants rather than stimulants, which can cause amplification of depressive symptoms. The self-medication hypothesis also fails to account for the development of SUDs as a primary condition to secondary mental health diagnoses (Boschloo, van den Brink, Penninx, Wall, & Hassin, 2012). While the self-medication hypothesis is attractive in its etiological account of co-occurring conditions, this model does not offer a complete conceptualization of the causes and maintenance of SUDs and comorbid psychopathology.

Emotion Regulation Model

Another way to understand the development and maintenance of SUDs and co-occurring psychopathology is to look at variables implicated across these disorders. Emotion regulation can be understood as one such variable. In its most basic form, *emotion regulation* is defined as the process through which people covertly and overtly respond to emotions. The construct of emotion regulation includes all implicit strategies (e.g., suppressing thoughts or emotions) and explicit strategies (e.g., using substances) that are used to alter one's emotional experience. Emotion regulation constitutes any strategy that is used to decrease, maintain, or increase one or more components of an emotional response (Gross & Thompson, 2007). Thoughts, emotions, and behaviors are all impacted through emotion-regulation strategies.

Individuals reporting pervasive emotion dysregulation are likely to engage in maladaptive behaviors (e.g., substance use) to regulate aversive emotions (Linehan, Bohus, & Lynch, 2007). It is said there are six core components implicated in emotion dysregulation. *Emotion dysregulation* occurs when a person has (1) a lack of emotional awareness; (2) the absence of emotional clarity; (3) nonacceptance of emotional responses; (4) problems with impulse control; (5) difficulties engaging in goal-directed behavior; and (6) limited access to emotion-regulation strategies (Gratz & Roemer, 2004). The high rates of co-occurring disorders point to the potential regulatory function of chemical use (e.g., using drugs for the purpose of altering one's emotional experience). Substances may be used to increase, decrease, or maintain an emotional response.

To treat these conditions, clinicians do not need to determine which diagnosis presented first; rather, practitioners must understand the variables linking the co-occurrence of these behaviors. For example, those with co-occurring disorders may use substances to provide relief from aversive emotions (e.g., to reduce anxiety), to change an emotional experience (e.g., to feel numb or to feel "high"), to facilitate relief from physiological discomfort, or to establish relief from withdrawal. Additionally, a person may also engage in other ineffective behaviors that maintain comorbid psychiatric conditions. For instance, someone with concurrent social phobia and a SUD likely both avoids or leaves social situations and consumes a substance to reduce anxiety. In this case, these avoidance behaviors (leaving the situation and the resulting substance use) are considered maladaptive emotion-regulation strategies that reduce emotional arousal, and at the same time result in the persistence of psychopathology.

Etiological Research

To understand the mechanisms of action associated with substance abuse, researchers have assessed the degree to which substance use has provided emotional relief or evoked a change in emotion among those who have psychological disorders. The following paragraphs address several investigations into self-medication and emotion regulation.

Depression

Research supports the regulatory function of substance use in depression. To assess the salience of self-medication in SUDs and comorbid mood disorders, one study employed questions like, "Did you EVER drink alcohol to improve your mood or make yourself feel better when you (felt sad, blue depressed, or down/didn't care about things or enjoy things) for at least two weeks?" (Bolton, Robinson, & Sareen, 2009). Bolton et al. (2009) found that 22.9 to 47 percent of individuals with mood disorders reported self-medication with substances.

Bipolar disorder

Research also suggests that people with bipolar disorder use substances to regulate emotions. One study assessed reasons for substance use among those with bipolar disorder and SUDs. Seventy-nine percent of participants with these co-occurring disorders reported using substances to "improve mood," compared to 68 percent with SUD only and 45 percent of those with bipolar disorder only (Bizzarri et al., 2007).

PTSD

Cue reactivity research has indicated emotion-regulation deficits may contribute to relapse and the maintenance of substance use in a co-occurring SUD and PTSD sample (Coffey et al., 2002). Trauma-related memories were found to evoke intense negative emotions among individuals with cocaine or alcohol dependence. In addition, participants reported an increase in substance use cravings after being shown trauma-image cues (Coffey et al., 2002).

Impulsivity among individuals with PTSD and SUDs has also been investigated as a variable associated with emotion dysregulation. In one study, clients with comorbid PTSD and SUDs were found to engage in significantly more impulsive behaviors and reported more emotion dysregulation, when compared to clients with SUDs only (Weiss, Tull, Viana, Anestis, & Gratz, 2012).

BPD

The treatment of emotion dysregulation associated with SUDs and comorbid conditions has been well established in the BPD literature. In a sample of people with co-occurring BPD and SUDs, a treatment that targeted emotion dysregulation was associated with (a) improved mood; (b) an increase in emotion regulation strategies; and (c) a decrease in substance use. This study demonstrated emotion dysregulation as a variable linking BPD and SUD symptomatology (Axelrod, Perepletchikova, Holtzman, & Sinha, 2011).

In summary, there are many etiological theories of SUDs. As for co-occurring disorders in particular, empirical evidence has supported both the self-medication and emotion-regulation models. Continued research is needed to address the causes of substance use in this population so that the most effective treatments can be provided. To appropriately service those with co-occurring disorders, scholars and clinicians must also be unrelenting in their efforts to remove the many risk factors and barriers this population faces, which negatively affect access, retention, and treatment outcomes.

RISK FACTORS AND BARRIERS TO TREATMENT

Many risk factors and barriers to treatment exist among people with co-occurring disorders. Some of these include untreated psychological issues, untreated substance use concerns, age, unemployment, and housing instability. This section addresses a few of the risk factors and barriers this population faces with regard to mental health and substance abuse services.

Research suggests the behaviors of SUDs and comorbid psychopathology mutually amplify the symptoms of the other disorder. In other words, substance use is a risk factor for relapse in mood, anxiety, and psychotic disorders. Moreover, individuals with underlying untreated mood disorders are considered to be at greater risk for substance use relapse. Relapses in substance use and/or relapse of a mood episode (or increased symptoms of a psychological disorder) increase the risk for problematic coping behaviors, which may result in suicide or overdose. One study compared people with comorbid MDD and SUDs to those with MDD and no SUDs and discovered those with comorbid disorders experienced greater symptom severity. When compared to MDD alone, dually diagnosed individuals displayed (a) an increased risk in suicidal behaviors; (b) an earlier age of onset of depression; (c) greater symptoms of depression; (d) criteria for more co-occurring anxiety disorders; and (e) an overall greater functional impairment (Davis et al., 2006). The severity of one's SUD also impacts risk for more severe psychological issues. For instance, individuals with substance dependence have higher odds of meeting criteria for a mood disorder than those with a substance abuse diagnosis. This finding suggests that higher levels of SUD psychopathology increase the risk for more symptoms of a mood disorder.

Age has also been found to be a risk factor for the development of comorbid SUDs and mental health conditions. In particular, young adults are the most vulnerable to the co-occurrence of SUDs and psychopathology. In fact, the odds of a secondary mood disorder increase in young adults after developing a primary SUD (Kenneson et al., 2013). Age has been established as a general risk factor for SUDs, anxiety disorders, and mood disorders; this suggests that young adulthood is a particularly risky time for the development of dual diagnoses (Grant et al., 2009).

Another risk factor related to co-occurring disorders is poorer physical health. Individuals meeting criteria for SUDs and concurrent mental health conditions are more likely to endorse a number of comorbid health complications. Blood-borne pathogens like hepatitis C and HIV are elevated in this population, based on an increased likelihood of engagement in impulsive sexual behaviors (e.g., having unprotected sex with an IV drug user) and hazardous drug-using behaviors (e.g., needle sharing) (Dausey & Desai, 2003). Higher rates of chronic pain have also been seen among people with comorbid SUDs and psychopathology. In an epidemiological study comparing individuals meeting criteria for PTSD and SUDs to those only meeting criteria for SUDs, participants meeting criteria for both disorders were more likely to endorse more concurrent medical conditions, suggesting poorer physical health in this population (Pietrzak et al., 2011).

In addition to the risk factors and barriers addressed above, people with comorbid psychiatric conditions and SUDs generally experience a number of stressors related to quality of life. These individuals tend to report more financial distress, job loss, lower educational levels, heightened interpersonal stressors, and legal difficulties. Moreover, co-occurring disorders are quite common among the homeless population. In a meta-analysis of several studies that assessed SUDs in homeless populations, 37.9 percent of homeless individuals were considered alcohol dependent, and 24.4 percent were drug dependent (Fazel, Khosla, Doll, & Geddes, 2008). Furthermore, in a sample of homeless individuals meeting criteria for PTSD, 92 percent of that sample met criteria for a concurrent SUD (McCauley et al., 2012). In conclusion, all of the factors addressed in this section contribute to higher rates of treatment dropout, relapse, and symptoms of psychopathology among people with co-occurring SUDs and mental health diagnoses.

RESILIENCY FACTORS

While psychopathology is typically more severe among dually diagnosed clients, a number of resiliency factors can prevent the worsening of symptoms, development of additional disorders, and reemergence of formerly treated problems. A well-established protective factor is consistent treatment for dually diagnosed individuals. The most effective treatments for co-occurring disorders are ones that include a number of different contexts for therapy (e.g., inpatient, residential, outpatient, etc.) and incorporate various therapeutic activities (e.g., individual therapy, skills groups, support groups, etc.). Moreover, frequent medication management and regular medication compliance are important protective factors for psychological stability.

A strong therapeutic alliance is also predictive of motivation and persistence in treatment. Regular attendance of individual and group therapy protects against the worsening of psychopathology, while also increasing mental health and well-being. Clients can address multiple treatment goals through individual therapy sessions and in group contexts. In addition to therapy, the establishment and maintenance of a prosocial, substance-free support network are vital to the protection against substance relapse and psychological instability. Support groups for various mental health conditions and experiences (e.g., grief support groups), as well as 12-step meetings, are encouraged. Membership in teams and clubs, taking classes, working, etc., are also ways of establishing social support. Researchers have shown that, especially for women, greater perceived social support is a factor associated with increased quality of life (Brown, Jun, Min, & Tracy, 2013).

Abstinence from alcohol and other substances is also considered a resiliency factor among this population. Reasons for acquiring and maintaining abstinence are numerous. Substance use can provoke the onset of a mood or anxiety episode, worsen psychological symptoms, and potentially add other mental health problems. Abstaining can prevent further psychological or physical degeneration that may have occurred as a result of the substance use.

SCREENING AND ASSESSMENT

Accurate screening and assessment are essential to developing and maintaining an effective treatment plan for any diagnosis. Given the high rates of comorbidity, it is recommended that those clients seeking services for psychological disorders independent of SUDs also receive screening for SUDs. Conversely, people referred to treatment for SUDs must also be screened for potentially concurrent psychopathology. Taken together, substance abuse treatment providers must practice continuous and frequent mental health screening.

Often, clinicians do not appropriately screen for conditions that co-occur with SUDs. One study found that less than 17 percent of individuals with comorbid psychiatric conditions were identified as struggling with these conditions upon entry into outpatient SUD treatment (Watkins et al., 2004). Another study suggested only 42 percent of inpatient substance use treatment facilities offer comprehensive mental health screenings as part of the intake process (Chen et al., 2011). Not receiving any treatment or delaying treatment may (a) cause existing psychopathology to worsen; (b) contribute to the development or reemergence of new psychological conditions; and/or (c) increase the likelihood of continued substance use.

Care must be taken during the screening process. Substance intoxication and withdrawal often mimic symptoms of mood, anxiety, and psychotic disorders. Therefore, it is necessary to differentiate co-occurring psychopathology from substance-induced behaviors or disorders. For instance, methamphetamine intoxication has the potential to mimic the symptoms of mania. Moreover, people with comorbid SUDs might find it hard to explain their thoughts, emotions, and behaviors during times of sobriety. Among these individuals, periods of sobriety may be limited, and/or they may not know how to describe their internal experiences to a clinician.

Counselors must also glean information concerning the presence of both current and lifetime psychopathology. It is important to understand a client's psychological history when developing a new case formulation and treatment plan. Depending on a client's motivation for change and the reason for referral into treatment, accuracy in reporting psychological symptoms during the assessment process may be an issue. Factors like legal mandates for treatment could contribute to dishonesty during the assessment process. Additionally, individuals may over-report psychopathology due to the perception that a more intense symptom picture might facilitate a better quality of care or a more desirable living situation.

The integration of medical and mental health services may help to address poor treatment adherence among individuals with SUDs and concurrent mental health conditions (Pietrzak et al., 2011). Primary care settings and homeless shelters may offer earlier access to screening and treatment processes, which would allow for more timely and efficient treatment planning. Thus, professionals in these settings must be aware of some of the complications associated with screening and assessing this population. For example, the use of medication may mask symptoms of comorbid psychopathology (e.g., benzodiazepine use may mask anxiety symptoms), which could cloud the assessment process.

Steps of Assessment for Co-Occurring Disorders

The treatment improvement protocol (TIP) by SAMHSA (2005) recommends a 12-step assessment process for those with co-occurring disorders (Appendix A). Counselors are to effectively engage the client through the use of motivational interviewing strategies, screen for comorbid mental health conditions, assign a formal diagnosis, and consider quality of life–interfering behaviors. The severity of both an individual's

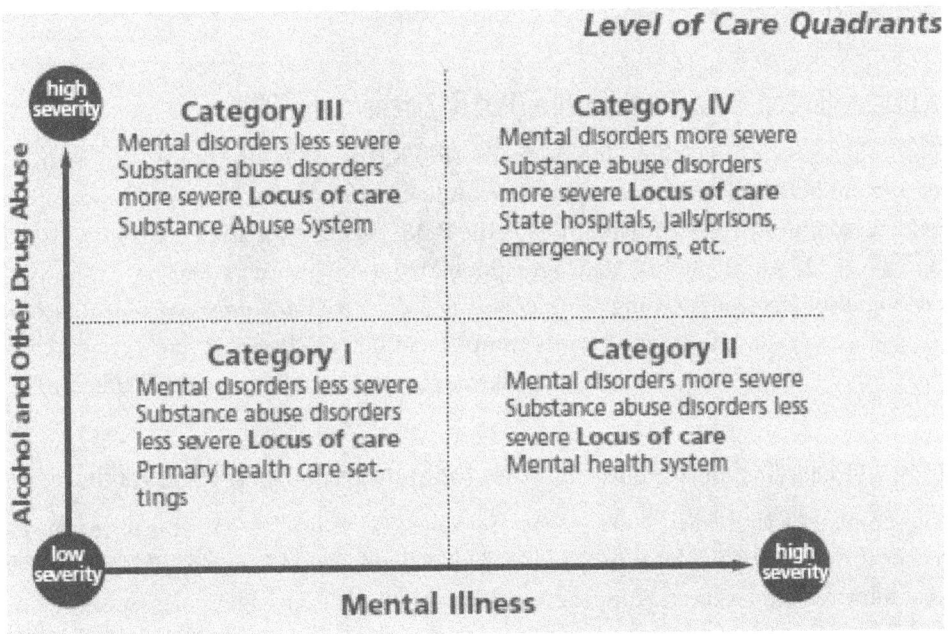

Figure 12.4: Taken from *"Treatment Improvement Protocol for Persons with Co-Occurring Disorders."*
Source: SAMHSA (2005).

SUD and co-occurring mental health condition must also be explicitly assessed. The TIP recommends the use of Figure 12.4 below in the designation of the severity of these conditions.

Measures for Comorbid SUDs and Mental Health Conditions

A number of instruments screen for either SUDs or comorbid psychopathology. More rarely, however, are screening tools available which identify the potential existence of co-occurring disorders. Screeners are not meant to serve diagnostic purposes, but rather highlight areas where a more comprehensive diagnostic assessment (e.g., Global Appraisal of Individual Needs [GAIN]) is indicated. Many of the screeners listed below can be incorporated into treatment. These measures may be repeated throughout treatment and shared with the individual to motivate continued change. All of the measures included in this chapter have been empirically validated and have demonstrated reliability and validity. Additional screeners and diagnostic assessments of SUDs, mental health conditions (e.g., depression and anxiety), comorbid SUDs and psychopathology, and variables related to the development of dual diagnoses (e.g., emotion dysregulation) are included in Appendix B.

Mini-International Neuropsychiatric Interview (MINI; Sheehan, 1998)

The Mini-International Neuropsychiatric Interview (MINI) is a 15–30 minute empirically validated diagnostic interview that assesses 20 DSM-IV mental disorders. The MINI was validated against a much longer diagnostic interview, the Structured Clinical Interview for DSM Diagnoses (SCID-I). The disorders assessed by the MINI are SUDs, mood disorders, anxiety disorders, eating disorders, psychotic disorders, and antisocial personality disorder (ASPD). The MINI quickly screens out individuals who do not meet criteria for a disorder using an ordered series of questions. Suicidal behaviors can also be assessed through the use of the MINI.

Psychiatric Diagnostic Screening Questionnaire (PDSQ; Zimmerman, 1999)

The Psychiatric Diagnostic Screening Questionnaire (PDSQ) is a 15–20 minute, 125-item screener for 13 common mental health disorders. In addition to evaluating for SUDs, the PDSQ measures symptoms of disorders that commonly co-occur with SUDs. The PDSQ screens for anxiety disorders (GAD, PTSD, panic disorder, OCD, social phobia, and agoraphobia), mood disorders (major depressive disorder), psychosis, eating disorders (binge-eating disorder and bulimia nervosa), and somatoform disorders (hypochondriasis and somatization disorder). Clients complete an initial self-report screener, which is scored. A clinician then administers follow-up interviews in areas that demonstrate a positive screening.

Global Appraisal of Individual Needs–Short Screener (GSS; Dennis, Chan, & Funk, 2006)

The Global Appraisal of Individual Needs–Short Screener (GSS) is a 20-item measure that can serve as a brief screener if the 1.5- to 2.5-hour full GAIN diagnostic interview is not feasible. The GSS takes five minutes to administer and has been empirically validated in both adult and adolescent samples. Subscales of the GSS include internalizing disorders, externalizing disorders, substance disorders, and crime/violence. The spectrum of behaviors measured by the GSS makes it appropriate to preliminarily screen for SUDs and comorbid mental health conditions. If a clinician suspects substance use and/or additional mental health concerns, more comprehensive assessment is needed to assign diagnoses or develop a treatment plan.

Patient Health Questionnaire (PHQ; Spitzer, Kroenke, & Williams, 1999)

The Patient Health Questionnaire (PHQ) is a ten-minute mental health screener that is derived from the much longer Primary Care Evaluation of Mental Disorders (PRIME-MD) interview. This screener was developed to test for mental health conditions in primary care settings. Symptoms of depression (major depressive disorder and "other depressive symptoms"), anxiety (panic disorder and "other anxiety symptoms"), somatoform disorder, substance use (alcohol use disorder), and eating disorders (bulimia nervosa and binge-eating disorder) are measured.

Behavior and Symptom Identification Scale (Basis-24; Eisen, Normand, & Belanger, 2004)

The Behavior and Symptom Identification Scale–24-item version (Basis-24) is a 10–20 minute self-report questionnaire that was developed by McLean Hospital. The Basis-24 is not only an important screening tool for treatment planning, but is a useful measure of a client's progress toward treatment goals, as it can be administered on a weekly basis. The Basis-24 measures substance use and a number of mental health symptoms with regard to the client's functioning in the past week. Scoring of the Basis-24 generates an overall score in addition to subscale scores in the areas of depression/functioning, relationships, self-harm, emotional lability, psychosis, and substance abuse, making this an ideal self-report measure for clients with co-occurring disorders. The client's environmental quality is also measured via questions asking about living situation, employment and financial status, education level, and social support.

TREATMENT RECOMMENDATIONS FOR CO-OCCURRING DISORDERS

Successful treatment plans are developed and maintained as the result of a collaboration between the client and therapist, and, if desired, the client's family. These plans must be tailored to fit the client's assessment

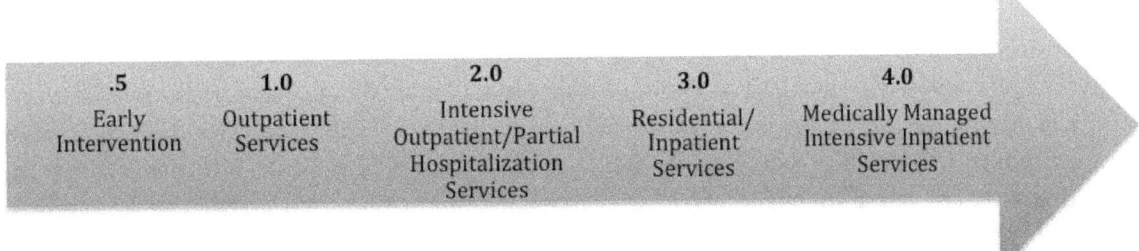

Figure 12.5: ASAM Dimensions and the Continuum of Care. Adapted from *"How the ASAM Criteria Work."*
Adapted from American Society of Addiction Medicine (n.d.) Available at http://www.asam.org/publications/the-asam-criteria

results, preferences, means, and treatment history. According to the American Society of Addiction Medicine (ASAM), there are six dimensions which help clinicians determine the most effective treatment recommendation (e.g., inpatient, intensive outpatient, or outpatient treatment). Figure 12.5 below is a snapshot of the ASAM placement criteria and the various modalities of treatment on the continuum of care. The severity levels of these dimensions (low to very high) provide an objective measure to assist practitioners with treatment planning.

ASAM Dimensions	
Dimension 1	Acute phase of intoxication and/or withdrawal potential → Assessing past and present substance use and withdrawal experiences
Dimension 2	Biomedical conditions and complications → Assessing an individual's medical health history and presence of current physical conditions
Dimension 3	Emotional, behavioral, and/or cognitive conditions and complications → Assessing an individual's thoughts, emotions, behaviors and mental health issues
Dimension 4	Readiness to change → Assessing an individual's stage of change
Dimension 5	Relapse, continued use, or continued problem potential → Assessing an individual's history of relapse, continued use, and/or continued problems
Dimension 6	Recovery/living environment → Assessing an individual's recovery/living environment and the people, places, and things that comprise that environment

CONTINUUM OF CARE

Psychiatric medications are commonly prescribed in the treatment of dual diagnoses, regardless of the treatment modality that is recommended. Medications have demonstrated efficacy in treating components of SUDs, anxiety disorders, mood disorders, and psychotic disorders. While not explicitly addressed throughout this treatment section, medication adherence and appropriate medication management are always components of treatment for clients who may need psychiatric medication. Best practice suggests that medication be combined with comprehensive psychotherapy to attain successful outcomes for mood disorders, anxiety disorders, eating disorders, personality disorders, and psychotic disorders.

The treatments identified in the next section represent some of the most researched, efficacious therapies for SUDs and comorbid mental health conditions. A multidimensional, integrated health care treatment approach may be the most helpful method for targeting co-occurring disorders. Treatment approaches must attempt to include all persons involved with the client's care. For instance, a client may be working with a substance abuse counselor, psychiatrist, probation officer, and child welfare case manager. An integrated health care system should be in place that allows all of these professionals to coordinate care and share treatment strategies together.

Treatments for Co-Occurring Disorders

The therapies discussed below are empirically supported treatments for co-occurring disorders. The following will be addressed: (1) cognitive-behavioral therapy; (2) dialectical behavior therapy; (3) acceptance and commitment therapy; (4) motivational interviewing; (5) contingency management; (6) 12-step programming; (7) relapse prevention; and (8) harm reduction. The first three modalities can be conceptualized as stand-alone treatments, and the last five approaches are considered supplemental and are to be used in conjunction with other treatments.

Cognitive Behavioral Therapy (CBT)

Cognitive behavioral therapy (CBT) addresses maladaptive thoughts, emotions, and behaviors as targets for treatment and has been established as an evidence-based treatment for co-occurring disorders. CBT practitioners target the following when treating substance abuse concerns: (a) urges to use substances; (b) where individuals are likely to use substances; (c) how to avoid triggers; and (d) coping skills.

Within CBT, clients are taught coping skills that assist them in tolerating interpersonal and emotion dysregulation via changing their problematic thoughts, emotions, and behaviors. For instance, if a person suffered from concurrent panic disorder and SUD, that individual would be taught to reevaluate problematic thoughts related to both substance abuse (e.g., "I have to have a Xanax right now") and panic (e.g., "This panic attack will kill me"). The counselor would assist in restructuring these thoughts to be more realistic or factual ("I do not need my Xanax to handle this situation, nor will I die"). Use of breathing exercises, self-soothing, and grounding skills may be taught to help relieve intense emotional distress and reduce vulnerability to relapse. CBT practitioners may incorporate in-session practices, role-plays, homework to facilitate skill generalization, and visual aids to help the client practice CBT principles.

While CBT is frequently used in mental health and substance abuse treatments, it may not be effective for many clients. As stated earlier in this chapter, some clients may lack the motivation for treatment and may not acknowledge a problem with either their mental health or substance use (i.e., precontemplation stage). CBT is to be used with those who are motivated for change and who are making attempts to be sober and stabilize their mental health issues (i.e., the action stage). Most clients, however, do not enter treatment in the action stage of change. Moreover, traditional CBT may not always be effective with this population because it may not (a) address the persistent emotion dysregulation experienced by these clients; and (b) target the underlying function of the maladaptive behaviors present among these individuals.

Dialectical Behavior Therapy (DBT)

Dialectical behavior therapy (DBT) is a treatment that was initially developed to decrease suicidal behaviors in BPD. As indicated earlier in this chapter, substance use issues are common among those with BPD. In DBT, substance use is perceived as a behavior that facilitates emotion regulation. The skills of DBT have been shown to not only be effective in treating behaviors associated with BPD, but also in the treatment of substance abuse and dependence.

DBT is comprised of weekly individual and group therapy sessions. Group therapy consists of skills training modules, which address core mindfulness, distress tolerance, emotion regulation, and interpersonal effectiveness. DBT attempts to reduce problematic behaviors commonly associated with pervasive emotion dysregulation; some examples of these behaviors include substance abuse, deliberate self-harm, suicidal ideation, binge eating, and extreme avoidance behaviors. The substance abuse treatment goals of DBT encompass: (a) decreasing substance use and behaviors associated with use; (b) reducing urges to use; (c) avoiding opportunities to use; and (d) increasing engagement in healthy behaviors (Dimeff & Linehan, 2008).

As stated before, research suggests DBT is effective in treating SUDs and comorbid psychopathology. Compared to community treatment as usual (TAU), clients with co-occurring SUDs and BPD who were treated with DBT were less likely to prematurely terminate treatment (Linehan et al., 1999). In another study comparing TAU to DBT for substance-dependent and suicidal clients, DBT was associated with significantly lower levels of self-mutilating behavior and alcohol abuse when compared to TAU (van den Bosch, Koeter, Stijnen, Verheul, & van den Brink, 2005). Research has also shown substance use decreased during the course of DBT as emotion-regulation skill use increased, thus supporting the etiological theory that substance use often reflects a person's attempt to regulate their emotions (Axelrod et al., 2011; Berking et al., 2011).

Acceptance and Commitment Therapy (ACT)

Acceptance and commitment therapy (ACT) is a treatment that focuses on helping clients engage in flexible and adaptive emotion-regulation strategies, as many clients with co-occurring disorders demonstrate psychological inflexibility. *Psychological inflexibility* is when a client (a) avoids distressing thoughts, uncomfortable emotions, or painful memories (e.g., refuses to accept or acknowledge these experiences); (b) lacks clarity of values; (c) is "stuck" in thoughts, attitudes, or beliefs (i.e., cognitive fusion); and (d) excessively ruminates on negative thoughts or painful memories.

Within an ACT paradigm, the avoidance referred to in the definition of psychological inflexibility is called *experiential avoidance*. Experiential avoidance is the attempt to distance oneself from aversive internal experiences. Substance use can aid in experiential avoidance because it often decreases negative thoughts, emotions, or bodily sensations or increases more desirable internal experiences.

While ACT can be conceptualized under the CBT treatment umbrella, components of ACT vary significantly from those of standard CBT. *Rather than restructuring the content of thoughts, ACT proposes a different method of interacting with one's thoughts.* ACT prescribes the practice of observing and accurately labeling internal experiences as what they are (e.g., to label one's thoughts as thoughts). For example, rather than buying into the thought "I am worthless," a person would notice the thought and think, "I am having the thought/judgment that I am worthless."

Research suggests ACT outperforms treatment as usual (TAU) with regard to several outcome measures. For instance, ACT has been shown to be more successful in reducing substance use and feelings of shame, as well as increasing involvement in follow-up treatment (Luoma, Kohlenberg, Hayes, & Fletcher, 2012). Another study investigated opiate use rates among participants of an intensive 12-step treatment program and compared rates to those receiving ACT. ACT was associated with a significantly greater decrease in opiate use at six-month follow-up than those in the 12-step treatment (Hayes et al., 2004).

Motivational Interviewing (MI)

Motivational interviewing (MI) is an approach that is employed to reinforce a client's movement toward behavioral change. MI places emphasis on the motivation to change rather than on how to change. The practice of MI is guided by four basic principles. First, the therapist must convey empathy. Rather than judging a client's behaviors, MI emphasizes using reflective listening strategies to display acceptance of the client's presenting behaviors. Developing discrepancies, another core component of MI, involves illuminating the distance between the client's current behaviors and the life the client would like to live. By highlighting these discrepancies, individuals become aware of the disconnection between their current behaviors and their goals and values. This awareness often moves the client in the direction of behavior change. Rolling with resistance is another core principle of MI. Rather than arguing with the client for change, the MI therapist offers new perspectives and information to move individuals toward change. The final principle of MI, supporting self-efficacy, is when the therapist reinforces the client's language that is indicative of self-confidence in changing behavior.

In addition to working from these principles, the therapist attempts to evoke, reinforce, and increase change talk from the client. Strategies like reflective listening are implemented to help support change dialogue. The more frequently a client is able to verbally advocate for change, the more likely that individual will be to actually make behavioral changes. Clients are able to change problematic behaviors through reinforcement of language that indicates any of the DARN-C change talk: a (**D**) desire to change, the (**A**) ability to change, (**R**) reasons to change, and the (**N**) need for change, which all work in tandem to generate a (**C**) commitment from the client toward change.

Motivational enhancement therapy (MET) is a treatment method using MI principles and was originally conceived as a prelude to treatment. MET is typically administered for one to four sessions. Miller and Rollnick (2004), the developers of MI, argue a few sessions of MET as a freestanding intervention is not sufficient to ameliorate most target behaviors. MI is most commonly conceptualized as a supplementary style or strategy to enhance another treatment paradigm (e.g., CBT). One session of MI at the start of treatment has been empirically demonstrated to increase treatment retention and also increase therapist perception of the client's motivation toward change (McCambridge & Strang, 2004). Program attendance patterns were shown to be better with the MI admission group than the standard preadmission session participants (Martino, Carroll, O'Malley, & Rounsaville, 2000). However, the effects of MI tend to diminish over time if MI is administered in isolation. The influence of MI appears to be much stronger when its additive effects are tested, as MI was originally developed and intended (Hettema, Steele, & Miller, 2005).

Contingency Management

Contingency management (CM) employs the principles of positive reinforcement to alter the frequency of undesirable behaviors like substance abuse. CM treatments for SUDs provide reinforcers such as vouchers or money based on negative tests for substances. To establish a CM program, a specific and reasonable behavior must be selected to increase or decrease. Following the selection of a behavior to change, a reinforcer must be chosen that can be maintained throughout treatment. A reinforcement schedule is then designed to most successfully increase or decrease the desired behavior. Next, a behavioral contract is drafted that includes the specifics of behaviors to be changed (e.g., amount of behavior change, time frame of change, specific reinforcement for a given amount of change).

CM programs have demonstrated empirical efficacy in reducing substance use and increasing health-related behaviors (e.g., medication adherence, regular exercise). CM programs have also been shown to motivate behaviors like treatment attendance, which is directly linked to a reduction of maladaptive behaviors (Ledgerwood, Alessi, Hanson, Godley, & Petry, 2008). CM should be considered a supplemental strategy to initiate change and motivation when working with dually diagnosed clients, as it does not provide the development of adaptive skills in regulating emotions or thoughts.

12-Step Programs

Programs implementing the 12-step model promote abstinence from all mood-altering substances. While standard 12-step programs only target substance abuse, 12-step programs specifically designed for dually diagnosed individuals also target concurrent mental illness. These programs (e.g., Double Trouble Recovery [DTR] and Dual Recovery Anonymous) are structured very similarly to standard 12-step programs, in that a recovering person (with dual diagnoses) chairs all meetings. These meetings offer a support-group style, and they emphasize the client's accountability to oneself, others, and a higher power. The 12 steps of DTR programs are identical to standard 12-step programs, with the exception of steps 1 and 12, since these steps were amended to include information relevant to dually diagnosed individuals (e.g., powerlessness to mental health disorders and substance abuse). The remaining 12 steps retain the same language as traditional 12-step programs.

Like CM, 12-step programs do not target the underlying function of SUDs. Research evidence does suggest, however, that 12-step programs are effective in reducing behaviors associated with SUDs and in improving self-efficacy and social support for individuals with dual diagnoses (Aase, Jason, & Robison, 2008). Factors like self-efficacy and social support are important variables across treatment paradigms; however, these variables do not directly account for the relationship between SUDs and comorbid psychopathology. These programs are not recommended to be stand-alone treatments for SUDs and co-occurring psychological conditions. In fact, Wilson and colleagues (2000) propose a conceptual model in which 12-step programs can be used with ACT. The treatment tenets of ACT (like creative hopelessness, values clarification, and control as the problem) can be understood within 12-step models.

Relapse Prevention

Individuals engaging in relapse prevention are taught to make significant lifestyle modifications that decrease urges to use substances (e.g., seeking a new career, if working as a bartender triggers alcohol use). Clients are encouraged to increase exposure to healthy activities (e.g., regular exercise) as another means of preventing relapse. One of the most important components of relapse prevention is to prepare for imminent lapses. Clients learn to identify risks to lapse, pinpoint when the lapse begins to occur, and use an array of coping skills to get back on track with regard to target behaviors.

Relapse prevention strategies can be applied to SUDs and comorbid psychopathology. For example, a man struggling with depression may have the treatment goal of going to work every day. He may experience a lapse when he does not feel like going to work and ends up sleeping in. With relapse prevention methods, he will learn to identify this behavior as a lapse and address this lapse as soon as possible (by going in to work later in the day or the next day), rather than avoiding work altogether. Even when a relapse does occur, clients are instructed to continually apply relapse prevention skills and renew a sense of commitment to treatment goals.

Harm Reduction

The last method to be addressed, harm reduction, is an approach that aims to decrease high-risk behaviors associated with substance abuse, through increasing behavioral safety. Harm reduction is not an abstinence-based strategy. Like MI, harm reduction emphasizes meeting the client at the appropriate level of commitment to change in order to maximize movement toward therapeutic goals. The purpose of harm reduction is not to ignore harmful behaviors, but to minimize the damaging effects of these behaviors. Harm reduction tends to employ individual efforts and sometimes community efforts (e.g., community needle-exchange programs). While some traditional treatment paradigms for SUDs promote abstinence-only models (e.g., 12-step programs), a harm-reduction model purports that behavior change is behavior change, regardless of complete abstinence.

If clients are able to reduce substance use, use a less dangerous substance, or use a substance in a less dangerous manner, this behavior is considered progress toward their treatment goals. Given the targets of harm reduction, this supplement to a comprehensive treatment might be particularly helpful to dually diagnosed populations with environmental and/or medical risk factors (e.g., homeless individuals, clients with HIV). Research suggests that harm reduction effectively reduces high-risk behaviors like drunk driving and needle sharing among intravenous drug users (Ritter & Cameron, 2006).

STRATEGIES FOR COUNSELING CLIENTS WITH CO-OCCURRING DISORDERS

The previous sections of this chapter review the behavioral complexities associated with SUDs and comorbid conditions. Some of the features of SUDs and concurrent psychopathology (e.g., emotionally taxing behaviors like suicidality and interpersonal ineffectiveness) can lead to burnout among mental health providers working with these individuals. Implementation of protective strategies among clinicians can reduce the risk of burnout. Self-care is an example of one such protective factor. Just as therapists educate clients to engage in self-care behaviors, establishing a healthy diet, sleep, and exercise routines are essential in reducing stress levels and vulnerability to increased stress among mental health practitioners.

Addressing ineffective therapist behaviors while practicing skillful behaviors can increase the efficacy of therapy and decrease the risk of factors like exhaustion, which contribute to burnout. Integrative treatment approaches facilitate a unified treatment front. Whether in residential or community settings, coordination of care reduces the likelihood of problematic behaviors, such as poor therapy attendance. The implementation of integrative treatment plans that are developed by and accessible to all treatment providers can not only aid in burnout reduction, but can result in a better quality of client care. A unified treatment team is essential in promoting the well-being of clients and therapists across treatment settings.

Continued research is essential in an effort to advance effective diagnostic and treatment strategies for clients with co-occurring disorders. Practitioners must persist in attempting to understand how to measure and treat relevant variables implicated in the development and maintenance of SUDs and co-occurring mental health conditions. Participation in various forms of supervision and continued education can also provide therapists with the most up-to-date and empirically supported treatment protocols. Lastly, the dissemination of training programs that target competency in evidence-based treatments for co-occurring disorders also ensures that therapists have the tools necessary to effectively treat this population.

CONCLUSION

Substance use disorders commonly co-occur with mood disorders, anxiety disorders, eating disorders, personality disorders, and psychotic disorders. From the research highlighted in this chapter, it is apparent that people with mental health conditions are more vulnerable to SUDs. Increased susceptibility to SUDs among those with a mental health condition may be attributed to self-medication and efforts to provide relief from negative emotions, physiological symptoms, or withdrawal. Assessments and treatments that evaluate and target the establishment of healthy emotion-regulation strategies may serve dually diagnosed clients most effectively. Furthermore, the use of comprehensive treatment strategies (along with an integrated health care system) will not only decrease symptoms of co-occurring disorders, but ultimately will aid in a better quality of life.

Case Study

Currently, you work at an outpatient substance abuse treatment facility. A 33-year-old unemployed, single, Caucasian female is coming to you today for a substance abuse assessment as part of her parole requirement. She has been randomly testing at the parole office since her release from prison three months ago. Last week, she tested positive for methamphetamine and marijuana. During the assessment and intake process, the client is noted to have tangential thoughts, speak loudly and quickly, be fidgety, and constantly pick at her arms and hands. When answering your questions about her mental health history, the client endorses many symptoms. She states she has had constant feelings of sadness and hopelessness, irritability, insomnia, and a lack of focus since she was a teenager. When discussing insomnia, the client stated she can go for days without sleeping, but still feel like she is "bouncing off the walls" and "going crazy." The client also reports she recently has been engaging in impulsive behaviors, such as shoplifting and taking "little worthless things" from other people. The client states she has had a previous mental health diagnosis at age 21 and was prescribed medication, but it made her gain weight so she stopped taking it. She could not remember the name of the diagnosis or medication. When discussing drug use history, the client denies any use of marijuana or methamphetamine in over a week, and she denies using any alcohol in over five years. She reportedly does not like alcohol because her father was an alcoholic, and on several occasions when he was drinking, he had sexually abused her as a child. She states she started smoking marijuana at age 12, tried pain pills a few times as a teenager, and illicitly used antianxiety medication like Xanax from age 20 until she went to prison at age 31. The client indicates that she notices a desire to smoke marijuana and take antianxiety medication when she is "going through these times of craziness." She denies a desire to use methamphetamine again; she just "wanted to try it and did it without thinking." However, she reports difficulty in staying clean from marijuana and antianxiety medication because she tends to "feel more normal" when she uses those drugs. She understands that she has to stay clean as part of her parole requirement and is motivated to do so at this time, although the client reported a lower confidence in her ability to stay sober after parole is over. When discussing her needs, the client states she is financially strained, has never been able to "hold down a job because of [her] mind" and has never had independent living. The client has never received substance abuse counseling before and has only seen a psychiatrist in the past for a very short period of time.

Questions

1. As her therapist, what are the primary concerns at this time?
2. What potential mental health issues may be presenting? Were they preexisting or substance-induced? Why do you think so?
3. What could be the reasons for the client's behavior at the intake today?
4. What treatment goals, recommendations, and referrals would you make?

REFERENCES

Aase, D. M., Jason, L. A., & Robinson, W. L. (2008). 12-step participation among dually diagnosed individuals: A review of individual and contextual factors. *Clinical Psychology Review, 28*, 1235–1248.

Alegría, A., Hasin, D. S., Nunes, E. V., Liu, S-M., Davies, C., Grant, B. F., & Blanco, C. (2010). Comorbidity of generalized anxiety disorder and substance use disorders: Results from the national epidemiologic survey on alcohol and related conditions. *Journal of Clinical Psychiatry, 71*(9), 1187–1195.

Axelrod, A. R., Perepletchikova, F., Holtzman, K., & Sinha, R. (2011). Emotion regulation and substance use frequency in women with substance dependence and borderline personality disorder receiving dialectical behavior therapy. *American Journal of Drug and Alcohol Abuse, 37*, 37–42.

Berking, M., Margraf, M., Ebert, D., Wupperman, P., Hofmann, S. G., & Junghanns, K. (2011). Deficits in emotion-regulation skills predict alcohol use during and after cognitive-behavioral therapy for alcohol dependence. *Journal of Consulting and Clinical Psychology, 79*(3), 307–318.

Bizzarri, J. V., Sbrana, A., Rucci, P., Ravani, L., Massei, G. J., Gonnelli, C., ... Cassano, G. B. (2007). The spectrum of substance abuse in bipolar disorder: Reasons for use, sensation seeking and substance sensitivity. *Bipolar Disorder, 9*(3), 213–220.

Blume, A. W., Schmaling, K. B., & Marlatt, G. A. (2000). Revisiting the self-medication hypothesis from a behavioral perspective. *Cognitive and Behavioral Practice, 7*(4), 379–384.

Bolton, J. M., Robinson, J., & Sareen, J. (2009). Self-medication of mood disorders with alcohol and drugs in the National Epidemiologic Survey on Alcohol and Related Conditions. *Journal of Affective Disorders, 115*, 367–375.

Boschloo, L., van den Brink, W., Penninx, B. W. J. H., Wall, M. M., & Hassin, D. S. (2012). Alcohol-use disorder severity predicts first-incidence of depressive disorders. *Psychological Medicine, 42*, 695–703.

Brady, K. T., Back, S. E., Coffey, S. F. (2004). Substance abuse and posttraumatic stress disorder. *Current Directions in Psychological Science, 13*(5), 206–209.

Brown, S., Jun, M. K., Min, M. O., & Tracy, E. M. (2013). Impact of dual disorders, trauma, and social support on quality of life among women in treatment for substance dependence. *Journal of Dual Diagnosis, 9*(1), 61–71.

Cerullo, M. A., & Strakowski, S. M. (2007). The prevalence and significance of substance use disorders in bipolar type I and II disorder. *Substance Abuse Treatment, Prevention, and Policy, 2*, 1–9.

Center for Substance Abuse Treatment (2009). *Substance abuse treatment: Addressing the specific needs of women.* Treatment Improvement Protocol (TIP) Series 51. HHS Publication No. (SMA) 09-4426. Rockville, MD: Substance Abuse and Mental Health Services Administration.

Chen, K. W., Banducci, A. N., Guller, L., Macatee, R. J., Lavelle, A., Daughters, S., & Lejuez, C. W. (2011). An examination of psychiatric comorbidities as a function of gender and substance type within an inpatient substance use treatment program. *Drug and Alcohol Dependence, 118*, 92–99.

Coffey, S. F., Saladin, M. E., Drobes, D. J., Brady, K. T., Dansky, B. S., & Kilpatrick, D. G. (2002). Trauma and substance cue reactivity in individuals with comorbid posttraumatic stress disorder and cocaine or alcohol dependence. *Drugs and Alcohol Dependence, 65*, 115–127.

Conway, K. P., Compton, W., Stinson, F. S., & Grant, B. F. (2006). Lifetime comorbidity of DSM-IV mood and anxiety disorders: Results from the national epidemiologic survey on alcohol and related conditions. *Journal of Clinical Psychiatry, 67*(2), 247–257.

Dausey, D., & Desai, R. (2003). Psychiatric comorbidity and the prevalence of HIV infection in a sample of patients in treatment for substance abuse. *Journal of Nervous and Mental Disease, 191*(1), 10–17.

Davis, L. L., Frazier, E., Husain, M. M., Warden, D., Trivedi, M., Fava, M., ... Rush, A. J. (2006). Substance use disorder comorbidity in major depressive disorder: A confirmatory analysis of the STAR*D cohort. *American Journal on Addictions, 15*, 278–285.

Dennis, M. L., Chan, Y-F., & Funk, R. R. (2006). Development and validation of the GAIN short screener (GSS) for internalizing, externalizing, substance use disorders, and crime/violence patterns among adolescents and adults. *American Journal on Addictions, 15*(s1), s80–s91.

Dimeff, L. A., & Linehan, M. M. (2008). Dialectical Behavior Therapy for substance abusers. *Addiction Sciences and Clinical Practice, 4*(2), 39–47.

Dixon, L. (1999). Dual diagnosis of substance abuse in schizophrenia: Prevalence and impact on outcomes. *Schizophrenia Research, 35*(1), 93–100.

Eisen, S. V., Normand, S. L. T., & Belanger, A. J. (2004). The revised behavior and symptom identification scale: Reliability and validity. *Medical Care, 42*, 1230–1241.

Fazel, S., Khosla, V., Doll, H., & Geddes, J. (2008). The prevalence of mental disorders among the homeless in Western countries: Systematic review and meta-regression analysis. *PLOS Medicine, 5*(12). doi:10.1371/journal.pmed.0050225

Grant, B. F., Goldstein, R. B., Chou, S. B., Huang, B., Stinson, F. S., Dawson, D. A., ... Compton, W. M. (2009). Sociodemographic and psychopathologic predictors of first incidence of DSM-IV substance use, mood, and anxiety disorders: Results from wave 2 of national epidemiologic survey on alcohol and related conditions. *Molecular Psychiatry, 14*, 1051–1066.

Grant, B. F., Stinson, F. S., Dawson, D. A., Chou, P., Dufour, M. C., Compton, W., ... Kaplan, K. (2004). Prevalence and co-occurrence of substance use disorders and independent mood and anxiety disorders: Results from the national epidemiologic survey on alcohol and related conditions. *Archives of General Psychiatry, 61*(8), 807–816.

Gratz, K. L., & Roemer, L. (2004). Multidimensional assessment of emotion regulation and dysregulation: Development, factor structure, and initial validation of the difficulties in emotion regulation scale. *Journal of Psychopathology and Behavioral Assessment, 26*, 41–54.

Gross, J. J., & Thompson, R. A. (2007). Emotion regulation: Conceptual foundations. In J. J. Gross (Ed.), *Handbook of emotion regulation*. New York: Guilford Press.

Hayes, S. C., Wilson, K. G., Gifford, E. V., Bissett, R., Piasecki, M., Batten, S. V., ... Gregg, J. (2004). A preliminary trial of twelve-step facilitation and acceptance and commitment therapy with polysubstance-abusing methadone maintained opiate addicts. *Behavior Therapy, 35*(4), 667–688.

Hettema, J., Steele, J., & Miller, W. R. (2005). Motivational interviewing. *Annual Review of Clinical Psychology, 1*, 91–111.

Hudson, J. L., Hiripi, E., Pope, H. G., Kessler, R. C. (2007). The prevalence and correlates of eating disorders in the national comorbidity survey replication. *Biological Psychiatry, 61*, 348–358.

Kenneson, A., Funderburk, J. S., & Maisto, S. A. (2013). Substance use disorders increase the odds of subsequent mood disorders. *Drug and Alcohol Dependence*, in press.

Kessler, R. C., Berglund, P., Demler, O., Jin, R., Koretz, D., Merikangas, K. R., … Wang, P. S. (2003). The epidemiology of major depressive disorder: Results from the national comorbidity study replication (NCS-R). *JAMA, 289*(23), 3095–3105.

Kessler, R. C., Sonnega, A., Bromet, E., & Hughes, M. (1995). Posttraumatic stress disorder in the national comorbidity study. *Archives of General Psychiatry, 52*, 1048–1060.

Ledgerwood, D. M., Alessi, S. M., Hanson, T., Godley, M. D., & Petry, N. M. (2008). Contingency management for attendance to group substance abuse treatment administered by clinicians in community clinics. *Journal of Applied Behavior Analysis, 41*(4), 517–526.

Lezenweger, M. F., Lane, M. C., Loranger, A. W., & Kessler, R. C. (2007). DSM-IV personality disorders in the national comorbidity survey replication. *Biological Psychiatry, 62*(6), 553–564.

Linehan, M. M., Bohus, M., & Lynch, T. R. (2007). Dialectical behavior therapy for pervasive emotion dysregulation: Theoretical and practical underpinnings. In J. Gross (Ed.), *Handbook of Emotion Regulation* (pp. 581–605). New York: Guilford Press.

Linehan, M. M., Schmidt, H., Dimeff, L. A., Craft, J. C., Kanter, J., & Comtois, K. A. (1999). Dialectical behavior therapy for patients with borderline personality disorder. *American Journal of Addiction, 8*(4), 279–292.

Luoma, J. B., Kohlenberg, B. S., Hayes, S. C., & Fletcher, L. (2012). Slow and steady wins the race: A randomized clinical trial of acceptance and commitment therapy targeting shame in substance use disorders. *Journal of Consulting and Clinical Psychology, 80*(1), 43–53.

Mancebo, M. C., Grant J. E., Pinto, A., Eisen, J. L., & Rasmussen, S. A. (2009). Substance use disorders in an obsessive compulsive disorder sample. *Journal of Anxiety Disorders, 23*(4), 429–435.

Marmorstein, N. R. (2012). Substance use disorders: Different associations by anxiety disorder. *Journal of Anxiety Disorders, 26*, 88–94.

Martino, S., Carroll, K. M., O'Malley, S. S., & Rounsaville, B. J. (2000). Motivational interviewing with psychiatrically ill substance abusing patients. *American Journal of Addictions, 9*, 88–91.

McCambridge, J., & Strang, J. (2004). The efficacy of single session motivational interviewing in reducing drug consumption and perceptions of drug-related risk and harm among young people: Results from a multi-site cluster randomized trial. *Addiction, 99*, 39–52.

McCauley, J. L., Killeen, T., Gros, D. F., Brady, K. T., Back, S. E., & Johnson, R. H. (2012). Posttraumatic stress disorder and co-occurring substance use disorders: Advances in assessment and treatment. *Clinical Psychology Science and Practice, 19*(3), 283–304.

Miller, W. R., & Rollnick, S. (2004). Talking oneself into change: Motivational interviewing, stages of change, and therapeutic process. *Journal of Cognitive Psychotherapy: An International Quarterly, 18*(4), A1–A10.

Parakh, P., & Basu, D. (2013). Cannabis & psychosis: Have we found the missing links? *Asian Journal of Psychiatry, 6*(4), 281–287.

Pearlstein, T. (2002). Eating disorders and co-morbidity. *Archives of Women's Mental Health, 4*, 67–78.

Pietrzak, R. H., Goldstein, R. B., Southwick, S. M., & Grant, B. F. (2011). Medical comorbidity of full and partial posttraumatic stress disorder in US adults: Results from wave 2 of the national epidemiological survey on alcohol and related conditions. *Psychosomatic Medicine, 73*, 697–707.

Ritter, A., & Cameron, J. (2006). A review of the efficacy and effectiveness of harm reduction strategies for alcohol, tobacco, and illicit drugs. *Drug and Alcohol Review, 25*, 611–624.

Ruscio, A. M., Stein, D. J., Chiu, W. T., & Kessler, R. C. (2010). The epidemiology of obsessive compulsive disorder in the national comorbidity study replication. *Molecular Psychiatry, 15*, 53–63.

Santiago, P. N., Wilk, J. E., Miliken, C. S., Castro, C. A., Engel, C. C., & Hoge, C. W. (2010). Screening for alcohol misuse and alcohol-related behaviors among combat veterans. *Psychiatric Services, 61*(6), 575–581.

Sheehan, D. V., Lecrubier, Y., Sheehan, K. H., Amorim, P., Janavs, J., Weiller, E., … Dunbar, G. C. (1998). The Mini-International Neuropsychiatric Interview (M.I.N.I): The development and validation of a structured diagnostic interview for the DSM-IV and ICD-10. *Journal of Clinical Psychiatry, 59*(20), 22–33.

Spitzer, R. L., Kroenke, K., & Williams, J. B. W. (1999). Validation and utility of a self-report version of PRIME-MD: The PHQ primary care study. *Journal of the American Medical Association, 282*(18), 1737–1744.

Stinson, F. S., Dawson, D. A., Goldstein, R. B., Chou, S. P., Huang, B., Smith, S. M., … Grant, B. F. (2008). Prevalence, correlates, disability, and comorbidity of DSM-IV narcissistic personality disorder: Results from the wave 2 national epidemiologic survey of alcohol and related conditions. *Journal of Clinical Psychiatry, 69*(7), 1033–1045.

Substance Abuse and Mental Health Services Administration (2013). Results from the 2012 national survey on drug use and health: Summary of national findings, NSDUH Series H-46, HHS Publication No. (SMA) 13-4795. Rockville, MD: Substance Abuse and Mental Health Services Administration.

Substance Abuse and Mental Health Services Administration (2005). *Substance abuse treatment for persons with co-occurring disorders*. Treatment Improvement Protocol (TIP) Series, No. 42. HHS Publication No. (SMA) 133992. Rockville, MD: Substance Abuse and Mental Health Services Administration.

Trull, T. J., Jahng, S., Tomko, R. L., Wood, P. K., & Sher, K. J. (2010). Revised NESARC personality disorder diagnoses: Gender, prevalence, and comorbidity with substance dependence disorders. *Journal of Personality Disorders, 24*(4), 412–426.

Van den Bosch, L. M., Koeter, M. W., Stijnen, T., Verheul, R., & van den Brink, W. (2005). Sustained efficacy of dialectical behavior therapy for borderline personality disorder. *Behavior Research and Therapy, 43*(9), 1231–1241.

Watkins, K. E., Hunter, S. B., Wenzel, S. L., Tu, W., Paddock, S. M., Griffin, A., & Ebener, P. (2004). Prevalence and characteristics of clients with co-occurring disorders in outpatient substance abuse treatment. *American Journal of Alcohol and Drug Abuse, 30*(4), 749–764.

Weiss, N. H., Tull, M. T., Viana, A. G., Anestis, M. D., & Gratz, K. L. (2012). Impulsive behaviors as an emotion regulation strategy: Examining associations between PTSD, emotion dysregulation, and impulsive behaviors among substance dependent inpatients. *Journal of Anxiety Disorders, 26*, 453–458.

Wilson, K. G., Hayes, S. C., & Byrd, M. R. (2000). Exploring compatibilities between acceptance and commitment therapy and 12-step treatment for substance abuse. *Journal of Rational-Emotive & Cognitive Behavior Therapy, 18*(4), 209–234.

Zimmerman, M., & Mattia, J. I. (1999). The reliability and validity of a screening questionnaire for 13 DSM-IV Axis I disorders (the psychiatric diagnostic screening questionnaire) in psychiatric outpatients. *Journal of Clinical Psychiatry, 60*(10), 677–683.

APPENDIX A

Steps of Assessment of Co-Occurring Disorders

1. **Engage the client** through empathic listening, cultural sensitivity, validation of the client's learning history, and assessing the client's own motivation for treatment.
2. **Collect data from the client's environment.** Past providers, family members, and friends may be contacted to gather information, provided that the client consents to all communications.
3. **Screen for comorbid disorders.** All individuals presenting for SUD treatment should be routinely screened for concurrent mental health conditions. Within the screening process, the domains of imminent safety (e.g., suicidal behaviors, homicidal behaviors, risky sexual or drug-using behaviors), past and present disorders and problematic behaviors, learning and cognitive difficulties, and trauma history should be evaluated. Screening in these domains occurs regularly throughout the treatment process, as frequently as every session.
4. **Determine the severity of the mental health condition and the severity of substance abuse.** The four-quadrant grid (see Figure 4) can be used to determine the appropriate quadrant and level of treatment focus.
5. **Decide the appropriate level of care and context for that care.** Factors such as risk of harm, treatment history, environmental support, and ability to care for oneself are domains that may be considered in determining the best-fitting treatment environment.
6. **Assign a formal diagnosis.**
7. **Determine disability and functional impairment.** The individual's living environment, financial stability, social relationships, and cognitive abilities are all considered in this portion of the assessment.
8. **Identify the client's strengths and supports.** Focusing on strengths and supports can be a valuable area to emphasize in the treatment of SUDs and comorbid psychopathology, rather than exclusively emphasizing the individual's deficits.
9. **Assess potential cultural and linguistic service barriers.** Identifying any cultural or language difficulties that may arise throughout the course of recommended treatment is the function of this component of the assessment.
10. **Identify problem domains that may affect treatment success.** Potential medical, legal, financial, social, family, and occupational stressors may impact a client's success in treatment. Therefore, these areas are addressed and targeted in the assessment process.
11. **Determine the client's stage of change.** Understanding if the client has no interest in changing (precontemplation), might consider change (contemplation), is getting ready to change (preparation), is actively working to change target behaviors (action), and is attempting to maintain desired changes (maintenance) is necessary to separately assess in all SUDs and comorbid mental health conditions. Understanding motivation to change behavior(s) is an important component of treatment planning and recommendation.
12. **Develop the client's treatment plan.** Identifying the client's target behaviors, the goals for change, and the empirically supported interventions needed is the last step of the assessment process.

TIP 42; Source: SAMHSA, 2013

APPENDIX B

List of Additional Screeners, Assessments, and Measures

Diagnostic Tools for SUDs and/or Potential Co-Occurring Psychopathology
Anxiety Disorders Interview Schedule-IV (ADIS-IV; Silverman & Albano, 2004)
Global Appraisal of Individual Needs (GAIN; Dennis, White, Titus, & Unsicker, 2008)
Structured Clinical Interview for DSM-IV (SCID-I; Spitzer, Gibbon, & Williams, 2002)

Diagnostic Tools for Personality Psychopathology (including SUD subscales)
Minnesota Multiphasic Personality Inventory-2-RF (MMPI-2-RF; Ben-Porath, 2012)
Personality Assessment Inventory (PAI; Morey, 2007)
Schedule for Nonadaptive and Adaptive Personality-2 (SNAP-2; Clark, 2003)

Measures of Psychopathology That Commonly Co-Occur with SUDs
General Psychopathology
> Brief Symptom Inventory (BSI; Derogatis, 1982)
> Symptom Checklist-90 Revised (SCL-90R; Derogatis, 1994)

Depression
> Beck Depression Inventory-II (BDI-II; Beck, 1996)

Anxiety
> Anxiety Sensitivity Index-III (ASI-III; Taylor et al., 2007)
> Posttraumatic Stress Disorder Checklist (PCL; Weathers, Litz, Herman, Huska, & Keane, 1993)

Eating Disorders
> Eating Disorder Examination-Questionnaire (EDE-Q; Fairburn & Beglin, 2008)

Measures of Substance Use
Addiction Severity Index (ASI; McLellan et al., 1992)
Alcohol Use Disorder Identification Test (AUDIT; Bush, Kivlahan, McDonnell, Fihn, & Bradley, 1998)
Brief Addiction Inventory (BAM; Cacciola et al., 2013)

Measures of Emotion Regulation and Related Constructs
Acceptance and Action Questionnaire-II (AAQ-II; Bond et al., 2011)
Difficulties in Emotion Regulation Scale (DERS; Gratz & Roemer, 2004)
Emotion Regulation Questionnaire (ERQ; Gross & John, 2003)
Five Facet Mindfulness Questionnaire (FFMQ; Baer et al., 2008)
Toronto Alexithymia Inventory-20 (TAS-20; Parker, Taylor, & Bagby, 2003)

CHAPTER 13

PERSONS WITHIN THE CRIMINAL JUSTICE SYSTEM

The correctional system is comprised of many different types of facilities, hosting a variety of employee functions. Inmates are housed in jails, state and federal prisons, boot camps, work farms, transitional housing, etc. *Jails* are mainly designed to hold people during the adjudication process (i.e., presentencing). Usually, those in custody are referred to as detainees. Jails also confine those who have a sentence of one year or less. Often, jails are used for those who have violated probation, parole, or bond conditions, or who are waiting to be transferred to other facilities. *Prisons*, on the other hand, are usually for inmates who are serving longer periods of time (one year or longer) and have committed serious or repeated crimes. There are different categories of prisons based on levels of security (e.g., minimum or maximum security).

The United States incarcerates people at a rate almost five times higher than other countries. Approximately one in every 31 adults in America is subject to correctional supervision (Sheldon, 2010). According to the Bureau of Justice Statistics (2013), the U.S. prison system housed 1,571,013 individuals in 2012. This number has declined for the third consecutive year, from a high of 1,615,487 inmates in 2009. Of the total prison population in 2012, 1,353,198 were state inmates, and 217,815 were federal inmates. However, one year later, as of August 2013, there were almost 219,000 federally incarcerated individuals, which was an increase of almost 1,200 people (Federal Bureau of Prisons, 2013). Keep in mind that the average cost of one person in prison is $24,000 each year (Sheldon, 2010).

Many Americans in the criminal justice system are not incarcerated, but are under some form of community supervision, another form of correctional control that includes probation and parole. *Probation* is a court-ordered period of correctional supervision in the community and is generally an alternative to incarceration. In some cases, probation may be a combined sentence of incarceration, followed by a period of community supervision. While on probation, offenders are typically required to fulfill certain conditions of their probation such as: payment of fines; fees or court costs; urinalysis; participation in treatment programs; and adherence to specific rules of conduct while in the community. Failure to comply with conditions may result in incarceration. *Parole* differs from probation, in that it is a period of conditional supervised release in the community following a prison term. Parolees may also have specific conditions and report to a parole officer. Failure to comply with set conditions and reporting results in a return back to prison.

In the United States, at the end of 2011:

- approximately 4,814,200 adults were under community supervision (including probation and parole)
- the probation population fell below four million for the first time since 2002
- nearly 853,900 adults were on parole

CRIMINAL JUSTICE AND SUBSTANCE USE

There is a clear link between criminal activity and substance use. Sixty to 80 percent of those involved in the criminal justice system: (a) were under the influence of alcohol or other drugs at the time of their offense; (b) committed the offense to support their addiction; (c) were charged with a crime related to alcohol or other drugs; or (d) are regular substance users (Marlowe, 2011). The Office of National Drug Control Policy (ONDCP) has collected data for over a decade on arrestees to determine if drugs were used around the time of the offense. In 2012, ONDCP found 62 to 87 percent of males tested positive for a drug at the time of arrest (depending on booking site). In addition to illicit drug use, alcohol has also been known to be the cause of police contact. Thirty-five percent of jail inmates were under the influence of alcohol at the time of their offence (James, 2004). In 2012, alcohol-related arrests (i.e., driving under the influence, liquor law violations, drunkenness, disorderly conduct, and vagrancy) accounted for over 20 percent of all arrests (Sourcebook of Criminal Justice Statistics [SCJS], 2013).

Using alcohol and other drugs at the time of offense may be linked to criminal activity such as disorderly conduct, burglary, and homicide. However, when analyzing data regarding the most common offense of the federally incarcerated, drug offenses are listed as the most prevalent. By August 2013, drug offenses accounted for almost 47 percent of the federal crimes in that year, with the second most common crimes

Types of Offenses by Those Incarcerated in Federal Correctional Facilities

Drug Offenses:	89,506	(46.8 %)
Weapons, Explosives, Arson:	31,380	(16.4 %)
Immigration:	22,402	(11.7 %)
Robbery:	7,892	(4.1 %)
Burglary, Larceny, Property Offenses:	7,844	(4.1 %)
Extortion, Fraud, Bribery:	11,116	(5.8 %)
Homicide, Aggravated Assault, and Kidnapping Offenses:	5,733	(3.0 %)
Miscellaneous:	1,612	(0.8 %)
Sex Offenses:	11,800	(6.2 %)
Banking and Insurance, Counterfeit, Embezzlement:	822	(0.4 %)
Courts or Corrections:	654	(0.3 %)
Continuing Criminal Enterprise:	485	(0.3 %)
National Security:	83	(0.0 %)

Source: Federal Bureau of Prisons (2013). *Quick facts about the bureau of prisons.*

related to weapons, explosives, and arson at 16 percent (see above for a list of all offenses). This number has decreased over the past few years. More specifically, in 2010, the percentage of drug offenses was at 51.4 percent (Federal Bureau of Prisons, 2011).

AN INCREASE IN RATES OF INCARCERATION

In 2011, the number of people in federal prisons (i.e., 197,050) was almost nine times what it was in 1980 (i.e., 22,037). While this number is staggering, the number of people in prison for drug offenses in 2011 (94,472) is 20 times what it was 30 years ago (i.e., 4,749). Refer to Figure 13.1 below for a breakdown of total offenses and drug offenses by decade.

Several politicians have toted the ideology of being "hard on crime" and putting "dangerous criminals" away. This philosophy has resulted in laws causing an increase in the prison population. For example, approximately half of the states in America have harsh penalties for habitual offenders of serious or violent crimes, requiring minimum sentencing of 20 years or more for three convictions. In California, however, the "three strikes" law caused many nonviolent offenders (such as those convicted of drug crimes) to be given these harsh penalties, until changes were made in 2012 with the passing of Proposition 36.

The "War on Drugs" was a phrase that first came about after President Richard M. Nixon used it at a press conference in 1971. He described illicit drug use as "public enemy number one." The majority of

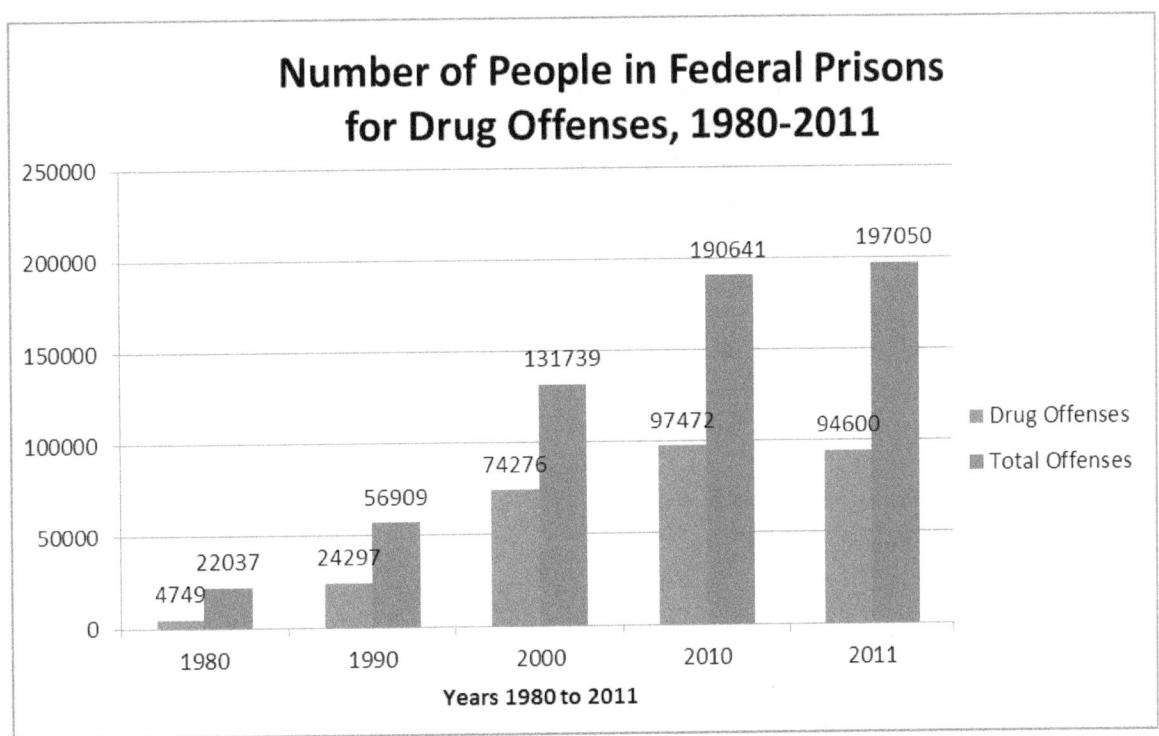

Figure 13.1: Number of Drug Offenses Compared to Total Offenses, from 1980–2011.

Source: The Sentencing Project (2012). *Trends in U.S. Corrections.* Federal Bureau of Prisons / Public Domain.

Americans think the war on drugs has been ineffective and has also led to the incarceration of nonviolent offenders such as those convicted of drug possession. Violent offenses only account for less than one-quarter (or 24.4 percent) of the crimes committed by jail inmates. Property offenses (e.g., burglary, larceny, and fraud) are just as common, at 24.4 percent; public order offenses (e.g., drinking while intoxicated, obstruction of justice, and traffic) constitute 24.9 percent; and drug offenses come in at 24.7 percent (Center for Substance Abuse Treatment [CSAT], 2005; James, 2004). Of the total drug offenses, trafficking was the most common (12.1 percent) and possession was second (10.8 percent).

As far as race and ethnicity, there are disparities among those incarcerated for drug offenses in the U.S. criminal justice system. More specifically, 44 percent are black/African American, and 20 percent are Hispanic/Latino (Sheldon, 2010). In California, racial disparities are clearly shown among those labeled as habitual offenders. Black/African American men, who constitute only about 3 percent of the state's population, represent approximately 33 percent of "second-strikers" and 44 percent of "third-strikers" (Chen, 2008). Later in this chapter, the author will discuss the reasons for the racial and class disparities in the criminal justice system.

SUBSTANCE ABUSE ISSUES

The potential for an individual to develop a substance use disorder and/or be involved in the court system can increase drastically, depending on various factors. For instance, researchers suggest issues related to education, employment, mental health status, and trauma influence the likelihood of criminal activity, including substance use. Approximately 44 percent of jail inmates have not graduated from high school or do not have a GED, and 29 percent were not working at the time of their arrest. Moreover, the average income for 59 percent of detainees was less than $1,000 (James, 2004). Regarding mental health, one in seven prisoners has a psychiatric illness or major depression, and of the inmates entering substance abuse treatment, 80 percent had a mental health disorder. In addition, over half of women in jail note they had been previously physically or sexually abused, compared to 10 percent of men.

In addition to education, employment, mental health status, and trauma, research has shown that experiences in childhood, adolescence, and young adulthood can influence substance use and criminal activity such as growing up in a single-parent household or with a guardian. Over half (56 percent) of jail inmates reportedly grew up in such a residence. Moreover, about one in nine had a history of living in a foster home or institution (James, 2004). Many inmates also report growing up with a parent or guardian who abused alcohol and other drugs (31 percent), and almost half (46 percent) had a family member who had been incarcerated in the past.

Below is a list of risk factors for substance use and criminal activity:

- No high school diploma or GED
- Unemployment
- Underemployment
- Housing issues
- Parent/guardian/family members using substances
- Family members with criminal involvement
- Gang affiliation

- Peers involved with substances and/or criminal activity
- Physical, emotional, sexual abuse history
- Mental health concerns
- Impulsivity
- Antisocial attitudes
- Limited recovery capital
- Quality-of-life issues

Barriers to Treatment

Abstinence from substance use has been shown to reduce crime by 40 to 75 percent; thus, treatment is recommended for those involved in the criminal justice system. However, there are many factors influencing accessing, obtaining, and successfully completing treatment for this specific population. Sometimes, the length of incarceration—such as a brief jail stay—is too short for substance abuse interventions. Some live in small, rural areas without local access to treatment or self-help meetings. Due to an arrest and/or pending charge(s), most people are under a substantial amount of stress. Increased anxiety and stress levels result from circumstances, including the uncertainty of legal outcomes, potentially getting fired from their job, and the possibility of losing custody of children. Obtaining treatment during the pretrial phase may not be a priority for many individuals.

Barriers to treatment for those convicted for crimes can be substantial, especially for inmates being released from prison. Transportation and housing issues, not having a driver's license, underemployment, and unemployment are a few examples of barriers. Research indicates after release, only 25 percent have a home to return to, and 37 percent of men have photo identification. Without a stable living environment or identification, employment is difficult to obtain, and most probationers and parolees are in debt. In fact, those released from prison owe approximately $650 on average, increasing to $900 after eight to ten months. These fees include debts associated with child support, court fines, supervision fees, and restitution.

TREATMENT RECOMMENDATIONS

For every dollar invested in treatment, California saves approximately $7 in future costs, including incarceration (Gerstein et al., 1994). Addressing substance use issues has been shown to reduce criminal activity and is cost effective; consequently, treatment is preferred versus placing someone into jail or prison (Peters & Matthews, 2002). Recidivism rates are less for inmates who have completed treatment (5 percent), than for those who have not (25 percent). Often, involvement in the criminal justice system is the first opportunity for those who need substance abuse treatment to obtain it. Of the 62 to 87 percent of arrestees testing positive in the previously mentioned ONDCP 2012 study, less than a third of those arrestees had ever been to a treatment program (ONDCP, 2013). Specific programs are put in place for people to link with substance abuse treatment and ancillary services. These programs may be available to people: (a) after arrest while their case is pending; (b) when placed on probation in lieu of jail or prison; (c) while incarcerated; and (d) after prison, many times as a condition of their parole.

In several states, pretrial diversion programs exist for nonviolent offenders with substance use disorders. These programs, such as Treatment Accountability for Safer Communities (TASC), have case managers that communicate with the courts while client cases are pending. An in-depth assessment is completed (usually within 72 hours of release from jail) and comprises: criminal justice history, the nature and extent of addiction, readiness for treatment, and likelihood of treatment success. TASC case managers develop individualized service plans that consist of linkages to community-based substance abuse treatment, medical/mental health services, vocational/educational programs, and other needed social services. Case managers monitor clients' substance use through toxicology screening and by continuously reevaluating client needs and providing reports to judges and court personnel. TASC programs can be strictly pretrial diversion programs, but some also serve as monitors for individuals placed on probation or parole.

TASC programs supervise people in the court system and serve as an adjunct to district and circuit courts. Many states have courts specific to the supervision of people with substance use disorders and have an alcohol- or illicit drug–related crime. Drug courts and sobriety courts (for driving offenses) have requirements for participants (e.g., urine analysis/Breathalyzer, 90 meetings in 90 days, obtaining a sponsor, weekly attendance at court) and provide sanctions (e.g., a weekend in jail) for noncompliance. If participants complete the requirements of drug court or sobriety court (usually for 12–18 months), then the offense is expunged off their record. Researchers have suggested that the most beneficial drug courts are those who use a multidisciplinary approach and have ongoing attendance by defense counsel, prosecutors, treatment providers, and law enforcement offers at staff meeting and status hearings. As of June 2012, there were 2,734 drug courts in the United States. In addition to drug courts, there are prebooking diversion programs, mental health courts, family drug treatment courts, and veterans' courts also available nationwide. Table 13.1 below is a listing of the various courts.

For those who are not placed in diversion programs or placed on probation but sentenced to prison, substance abuse treatment may be presented as an option to inmates. During 2010, 47,885 federal inmates participated in a drug abuse education course; 14,507 inmates received nonresidential treatment; 18,868 inmates participated in a residential drug abuse program (RDAP); and 16,912 participated in Transitional Drug Abuse Treatment (TDAT) at a residential reentry center. Of those offenders participating in

Table 13.1: * 2,734 Drug Courts in Operation in the United States and Its Territories as of June 30, 2012

COURT TYPE	NUMBER
Adult (*of which 401 are Hybrid DWI/Drug Courts)	1,438
Juvenile	458
Family Treatment	334
Driving Offenses	208
Veterans Treatment	104
Tribal Healing to Wellness	89
Mental Health	37
Federal Drug	31
Reentry Drug	30
Campus	5

Source: *National Drug Court Resource Center*. Retrieved on October 22, 2013, from http://www.ndcrc.org/content/how-many-drug-courts-are-there

nonresidential treatment, 13,634 successfully completed the program, and 16,038 successfully completed RDAP (Federal Bureau of Prisons, 2011).

Screening and Assessment

Regarding this population, the terms "screening" and "assessment" are equated with "eligibility" and "suitability," respectively. Does the offender meet the system's criteria for receiving treatment services (i.e., eligibility)? Eligibility is a quick screen (typically applicable in prisons and community corrections settings), which determines whether a person warrants an assessment to determine substance use problems. Suitability is determined by an assessment and establishes whether the offender is capable of benefiting from treatment or responding to a particular intervention. *The question of suitability arises once it has been determined that offenders meet the eligibility criteria for receiving services* (CSAT, 2005).

At this time, there are no comprehensive screening and assessment approaches in the criminal justice system on a national level. However, there are recommendations which are strongly endorsed. First, CSAT (2005) suggests specific information should be acquired by those working with offenders, including substance use, criminal involvement, and physical and mental health, etc. Refer to the box below in Table 13.2 for a listing of important details to obtain during the screening and assessment processes.

Counselors should take into consideration that individuals involved in the criminal justice system (especially during pretrial and presentencing) may not be honest during screening/assessment/treatment due to the potential consequences of doing so. Those who work with these clients must attend to confidentiality and ethical concerns related to not only suicidal and homicidal ideations, but also to substance use and criminal behavior. The client and counselor discuss these concerns in detail and if/when/how/to whom information will be communicated. This discussion with the client is completed during intake and is also reviewed continuously throughout treatment and therapy. Screening and assessment processes must be revisited as self-disclosure issues, and changes in motivation for treatment may change over time.

Programming Needs

Substance abuse treatment planning should focus on criminal thinking and criminal identities, as well as chemical use. This type of thinking should not be considered as a permanent fixture in a client's personality, but as an outcome of maladaptive coping skills. *Thinking for a Change* is an example of a curriculum that attends to criminal thinking and cognitive thinking errors (available online at http://nicic.gov/t4c). In addition to criminal thinking, other areas to target during treatment should also include: communication skills; anger management; domestic violence; problem-solving; trauma; prevention for diseases (e.g., HIV, hepatitis, etc.); social skills training; and conflict management. Other areas of consideration include clients who may have hidden deficits in basic life skills (e.g., balancing a checkbook) or instrumental skills (e.g., creating a résumé), and these should also be incorporated into treatment. As far as treatment strategies, the use of medications, motivational strategies, and contingency management is recommended for this population. Moreover, modalities that incorporate positive and supportive peers and family members are greatly encouraged.

Counselors must provide services on a continuum of care, and, as such, conceptualize clients in the criminal justice system as individuals with many needs (e.g., obtaining employment, housing, driver's license, etc.). If inpatient treatment is necessary, it should be followed by a recommendation for outpatient

Table 13.2: Suggested Information to Obtain During Screening and Assessment

Substance Use	• Substance use history • Motivation and desire for treatment • Severity and frequency of use • Detoxification needs, acute intoxication • Treatment history (e.g., number and type of episodes, outcomes)
Criminal Involvement	• Criminal thinking • Current offense(s) • Prior charges • Prior convictions • Age at first offense • Type of offense(s) • Number of incarcerations • Prior successful completion of probation or parole drug use offenses • Prior involvement in diversionary programs • History of diagnosis of any personality disorder
Physical Health	• Intoxication, infectious disease (e.g., tuberculosis, hepatitis, sexually transmitted diseases, HIV status) • Pregnancy • General health • Acute conditions
Mental Health	• Suicidality • History of treatment and prior diagnosis • Past diagnoses • Treatment outcome • Current and past medications • Acute symptoms • Psychopathy
Special Considerations	• Educational level • Reading level/literacy • Language/cultural barriers • Physical disability • Developmental disability • Learning disability • Health and biomedical record • Housing • Dependents/family issues • History of abuse (victim and/or perpetrator), including trauma experienced as a result of physical and sexual abuse

treatment. Research indicates offenders who have substance use disorders have better outcomes if they complete treatment that extends over nine to 12 months. More specifically, those involved in drug courts have been shown to have better outcomes if they saw a therapist or clinical case manager once a week during the first phase of the program.

SYSTEMIC FACTORS INFLUENCING PRISON POPULATION AND THE SOCIETAL IMPLICATIONS

The oppression of people of color exists at a systemic level within our many institutions, including the health care system, educational system, and the criminal justice system. This section will discuss some examples of how racism, classism, and oppression are—and have been—commonplace in the United States. Many of the current drug laws are based on racist ideologies, and our criminal justice system has been set up in a way that (a) targets people of color; (b) continues to perpetuate prejudices; and (c) maintains the power in our society for white people and for those of higher economic status.

Drug use rates among whites are not shown to be different from the drug use rates among black/African Americans; however, arrest rates for drug charges are higher among black/African Americans. There are reasons for this disparity. People of color are more likely to be profiled, searched, arrested, prosecuted, and sentenced (with harsher penalties). The result is a higher number of people of color under correctional supervision, thereby perpetuating the stereotypes that people of color are "dangerous," "drug addicts," and "criminals" (Sheldon, 2010).

Consider the following statistics:

- More than 6 in 10 persons in local jails were people of color; 40 percent were black/African American; 19 percent were Hispanic/Latino
- Black/African American males are 6 times more likely to be incarcerated than white males
- Black/African American males are 2.5 times more likely to be incarcerated than Hispanic/Latino males
- One of every 3 black/African American males born today can expect to go to prison in his lifetime
- One of every 6 Hispanic/Latino males born today can expect to go to prison
- One of every 17 white males born today can expect to go to prison (James, 2004; Sheldon, 2010; The Sentencing Project, 2013a)

Many of the drug laws in the United States have caused the racial disparity in our criminal justice system. Legislations such as the Harrison Act of 1914 and the Marijuana Tax Act of 1937 were passed due to racist fears perpetuated by unsubstantiated claims regarding people of color (Hart & Ksir, 2013). For instance, the *New York Times* published an article titled, "Negro Cocaine 'Fiends' are a New Southern Menace." The author warned of a cocaine epidemic in the South and professed black/African Americans were homicidal, "better marksmen," and resistant to bullets (Williams, 1914). Other laws have impacted the incarceration rates among people of color due to inequities in sentencing guidelines. Most notably, the Anti-Drug Abuse Act of 1986 imposed a mandatory five-year minimum federal sentence for possessing 500 grams of powder cocaine. That same five-year minimum sentence was also imposed for possessing *only five grams* of crack cocaine. Therefore, small-level crack cocaine street dealers were getting the same federal sentence mandates as those who are high-level powder cocaine dealers. In essence, this law appeared to be targeting people of color, who were more likely to sell small amounts of crack cocaine (Sheldon, 2010). After the law was enacted, there was a sharp increase in the number of imposed sentences for black/African Americans. Not only were they being incarcerated at high rates, but they also were receiving longer sentences than whites. In 1992, 91 percent of the sentences to federal prison for crack cocaine were for black/African Americans, and only 3 percent were for whites. Twenty years later, the disparity is still evident; 82 percent of those sentenced were black/African American, while only 9 percent were white (Hart & Ksir, 2013; U.S. Sentencing Commission, 2007). Otherwise known as the 100:1 law, this piece of legislature has been established as unfair. In 2010, President Barack Obama signed the Fair Sentencing Act into law, which reduced the ratio to 18:1. While this modification is considered a great step in the efforts to reduce inequities, many are still advocating for a 1:1 ratio.

In addition to profiling and targeting certain populations, a conviction of a crime subsequently comes with consequences that disproportionately impact people of color. As stated earlier, 1 in 3 black/African American males can expect to go to prison in his lifetime versus 1 in 6 Hispanic/Latino males and 1 in 17 white males. If people of color are more likely to be arrested, convicted, and sentenced (for longer periods of time), then the negative consequences of these events impact them more often and more severely, thus perpetuating racist fears and the systemic racism that exists in the United States. For example, in many states, those who are incarcerated are not allowed to vote in elections. Further, those who are not incarcerated, but have a prior felony conviction, can also be restricted from voting. Over the past 30 years, the number of Americans with voting restrictions has increased by 500 percent. In 1980, 1.17 million adults had some type of voting restriction, and by 2010 that number had increased to 5.85 million people. In the general population, 1 in 41 adults has lost the right to vote; however, 1 in 13 black/African Americans does not have this right (The Sentencing Project, 2013b). Not only are their votes not counted, but there are broader implications of losing this civil right. The implications of people of color losing the right to vote can be linked back to a courtroom and sentencing. Without the right to vote, one cannot serve on a jury, and thus it may be harder for a person of color to have a jury of one's own peers. (For more information on the restrictions by state, visit www.aclu.org; the American Civil Liberties Union website.)

In addition to voting restrictions, housing, educational, and employment opportunities become very limited for those with a criminal record. For instance, some institutions of higher education specifically ask about criminal records on their applications, and government financial aid is unavailable to a person after a drug-related conviction. Moreover, one's criminal background is taken into consideration for those who wish to obtain licensure or certifications in certain fields of employment (e.g., counseling, social work, health care). Due to the systemic racism and inequities in our society, people of color are socially excluded, disenfranchised, and controlled by taking away opportunities such as economic and educational advances (Sentencing Project, 2013).

Classism and the Criminal Justice System

The statement "The rich get richer and the poor get prison" represents how economic, employment, and educational status (i.e., class) not only impact opportunities for advancement in our society, but also how these aspects can influence who gets arrested, prosecuted, and sentenced (Reiman & Leighton, 2010). In *Our Punitive Society: Race, Class, Gender and Punishment in America*, Sheldon (2010) discusses the ideology that "those without capital, get punishment" and asserts that jails are temporary housing for the poor. Many people cannot afford to even bond out of jail, let alone pay for a private attorney. Subsequently, individuals who have less education, are underemployed or unemployed, and have a public defender can be perceived differently in court. This perception can influence sentencing.

Imagine the following:

A person is led to the jury box by an officer, wearing jail clothes and handcuffs. The person is waiting for the judge to attend to their case. Now, imagine someone whose name is called by the judge, who approaches the front of the courtroom wearing a suit, and who emerges from the benches of the public with a personal criminal defense attorney. Assumptions can be made about both of these individuals based on these scenarios. Reread the previous two descriptions. Describe the person led by the officer. Describe the person approaching from the public benches. Any differences in your assumptions?

CONCLUSION

Our criminal justice system is flawed. The war on drugs has not been successful, and many nonviolent offenders are behind bars. Substance use is linked to criminal activity, and research supports the correlation between providing treatment services and a reduction in crime. For many people in need of substance abuse treatment, contact with the criminal justice system is their first opportunity for treatment. For the first time, a substance use disorder may be recognized and diagnosed. Providing legal incentives to enter substance abuse treatment may motivate people to begin sobriety and recovery. For others, arrest and incarceration are part of a recurring cycle of drug use and criminal activity. Often, there are ingrained patterns of maladaptive coping skills, criminal values, and criminal identities that require a more intensive treatment approach. Resources must continue to be allocated for reentry programs, TASC programs, drug courts, and substance abuse treatment in correctional facilities. In addition, cross-training activities must occur. Judges, lawyers, police officers, correctional officers, probation/parole officers, and substance use professionals must learn from each other. These trainings can encourage the willingness to work with each other more and can help professionals manage the wide variety of services this population needs.

There must be transformation at a systemic level as well as an individual level. Ultimately, the scope of systemic reform can be measured only by our ability to level the playing field with regard to how we address substance use. Laws must be changed in order to address the racial and class inequities that exist in our court system and prison system; civil rights such as voting must be given to all Americans; and opportunities regarding housing, employment, and education must be available for anyone, regardless of their past criminal involvement. In certain communities, substance abuse is treated as a public health problem best addressed by prevention and treatment. In other communities, it is considered a criminal justice problem best addressed by more police, prosecutors, and prisons. A better model is available. Impeding the implementation of such a model, however, is the thinking of many Americans related to those who use substances and engage in criminal behavior.

Exercise

A client has been seeing you for group and individual therapy for the past six months due to her primary addiction to methamphetamines; she has reported no drug use since her arrest 16 months ago. Currently, she is in the final phase of drug court. At intake, she signed a release of information for her drug court case manager, and she is aware of the monthly reports you send in to the court about her progress. She is scheduled to graduate the drug court program next month. In two weeks, she will be completing the required treatment at your agency. She has been working with a sponsor for the past five months and has been attending NA meetings at least two times a week. Since you have known her, she has obtained employment, stable housing, and reports no criminal activity. During group today, she discloses that she smoked marijuana once last week. She told group members she took two "hits" and hated it and has no desire to ever smoke again. She said she told her sponsor about it immediately and has a prevention plan in place (e.g., changing her phone number, no longer associating with the person she got high with, etc.). The client asks during group that you not tell her case manager, and that she just wanted to "vent to the group and share." You are supposed to complete her monthly report by the end of this week, and you do not have an individual session scheduled until her discharge in two weeks. She has court on Friday for review, and they will be looking for your report.

Questions

1. How do you proceed in group? What do you say?
2. What would you write in the report?
3. What would be your next step with regard to treatment?
4. What ethical and confidentiality concerns are present?
5. What are your thoughts and feelings related to this case?

REFERENCES

Bureau of Justice Statistics (2013). *Prisoners in 2012–Advance courts.* United States Department of Justice. NCJ 242467. Retrieved on October 26, 2013, from http://www.bjs.gov/content/pub/pdf/p12ac.pdf

Center for Substance Abuse Treatment (2005). *Substance abuse treatment for adults in the criminal justice system.* Treatment Improvement Protocol (TIP) Series 44. HHS Publication No. (SMA) 13-4056. Rockville, MD: Substance Abuse and Mental Health Services Administration.

Chen, E. Y. (2008). Impacts of "three strikes and you're out" on crime trends in California and throughout the United States. *Journal of Contemporary Criminal Justice, 24*(4), 345–370.

Federal Bureau of Prisons (2013). *Quick facts about the bureau of prisons.* Retrieved on October 3, 2013, from http://www.bop.gov/news/quick.jsp#4

Federal Bureau of Prisons (2011). *State of the bureau, 2010.* Retrieved on October 3, 2013, from http://www.bop.gov/news/PDFs/sob10

Gerstein, D. R., Johnson, R. A., Harwood, H., Fountain, D., Suter, N., & Malloy, K. (1994). *Evaluating recovery series: The California drug and alcohol treatment assessment (CALDATA).* Sacramento, CA: Department of Alcohol and Drug Programs.

Hart, C. L., & Ksir, C. (2013). *Drugs, Society and Human Behavior* (15th ed.). New York: McGraw Hill.

James, D. J. (2004). *Profile of jail inmates, 2002.* Bureau of Justice Statistics.

Marlowe, D. B. (2011). Adult and juvenile drug courts. In C. Leukefeld, T. P. Gullotta, & J. Gregrich (Eds.), *Handbook of evidence-based substance abuse treatment in criminal justice settings* (pp. 123–141). New York: Springer Science.

Office of National Drug Control Policy (2013). *Arrestee drug abuse monitoring program II (ADAM II), 2012 annual report.* Executive Office of the President: Washington, DC. Retrieved on October 10, 2013, from http://www.whitehouse.gov/sites/default/files/ondcp/policy-and-research/adam_ii_2012_annual_rpt_final_final.pdf

Peters, R. H., & Matthews, C. O. (2002). Jail treatment for drug abusers. In C. G. Leukefeld, F. M. Tims, & D. F. Farabee (Eds.). *Treatment of drug offenders: Policies and issues* (pp. 186–203). New York: Springer Publishing.

Reinman, J., & Leighton, P. (2010). *The rich get richer and the poor get prison* (9th ed.). Boston: Pearson Higher Education.

The Sentencing Project (2013a). *Report of the sentencing project to the United Nations human rights committee: Regarding racial disparities in the United States criminal justice system.* Retrieved on October 11, 2013, from http://sentencingproject.org/doc/publications/rd_ICCPR%20Race%20and%20Justice%20Shadow%20Report.pdf

The Sentencing Project (2013b). *Felony disenfranchisement.* Retrieved on October 16, 2013, from http://www.sentencingproject.org/template/page.cfm?id=133

The Sentencing Project (2012). *Trends in U.S. Corrections.* Retrieved on October 16, 2013, from http://sentencingproject.org/doc/publications/inc_Trends_in_Corrections_Fact_sheet.pdf

Sheldon, R. G. (2010). *Our punitive society: Race, class, gender and punishment.* Long Grove, IL: Waveland Press, Inc.

Sourcebook of Criminal Justice Statistics (2013). *Arrests for alcohol-related offenses, by offense and State 2012.* Retrieved on October 11, 2013, from http://www.albany.edu/sourcebook/tost_4.html#4_c

Taxman, F. S. (2011). Parole: "What works" is still under construction. In C. Leukefeld, T. P. Gullotta, & J. Gregrich (Eds.), *Handbook of evidence-based substance abuse treatment in criminal justice settings* (pp. 205–227). New York: Springer Science.

U.S. Sentencing Commission (2007). *Cocaine and federal sentencing policy.* Washington, DC.

Williams, E. H. (1914, February 8). Negro cocaine "fiends" are a new southern menace. *New York Times*.

CHAPTER 14

PERSONS WITH DISABILITIES

*People with disabilities constitute our nation's largest minority group,
which is simultaneously the most inclusive and the most diverse.
Everyone is represented: of all genders, all ages, all religions,
all socioeconomic levels and all ethnic backgrounds.
The disability community is the only minority group that anyone can join at any time.*

—The Arc, 2014, para. 2

OVERVIEW

An estimated one in six Americans has a disability. Often, when people imagine a person with a disability, they envision a person in a wheelchair. One reason for this could be because the symbol that depicts such impairment (i.e., a figure in a wheelchair) is seen quite frequently in our society. However, there are various types of disabilities that impact functioning, and most are not problems with mobility. The Americans with Disabilities Act (ADA) defines a *person with a disability* as one who: (a) has a physical or mental impairment that substantially limits one or more major life activities; or (b) has a record of such impairment; or (c) is regarded as having such impairment. The ADA protects those who have a disability, including people who are blind, deaf, paraplegic, and those who are living with arthritis, HIV or AIDS, or mental illness.

In an effort to be clear and comprehensive about this topic, the author wishes to differentiate between the types of disabilities and provide some examples of each. Below is a list of terms and definitions. These are categorized as being physical, sensory, or cognitive. This text has a chapter devoted to affective disabilities (i.e., co-occurring disorders), and therefore, the author does not discuss mental illness as a disability in this chapter.

Types of Disabilities

Physical

> *Mobility Impairment:* Conditions that affect movement, which can range from chronic pain to quadriplegia. Impairment may be caused by accidents or other traumatic events, chronic events such as disease, or a condition that progresses slowly from birth. Examples include arthritis, cerebral palsy, multiple sclerosis, amputation, muscular dystrophy, spinal cord injury, or stroke.

Sensory

> *Visual Impairment:* Conditions including many degrees of vision loss (e.g., low vision, legally defined blindness, and total blindness).

> *Hearing Impairment:* Conditions that vary greatly from mild hearing loss to profound deafness. The term "hard of hearing" describes those who have mild to moderate hearing loss. Mild hearing loss is when a person can hear everything except very high-pitched sounds. Moderate hearing loss is when a person is unable to hear a conversation without amplification. "Deaf" is when a person has severe to profound hearing loss.

Cognitive

> *Learning Disability:* Conditions that can interfere with a person's ability to store, process, or produce information. These conditions affect one's ability to read, write, speak, or compute math, and can impede social skills. Examples include dyslexia, hyperactivity, hypoactivity, memory disorder, over-attention, and perceptual difficulties. Sometimes referred to as a "hidden" disability.

Physical and/or Cognitive

> *Developmental Disability:* Conditions that affect, or appear to affect, the mental and/or physical development of individuals, resulting in a severe impairment in the individual's ability to function in daily life. Life activities that may be affected are communication, learning, mobility, self-care, self-direction, economic self-sufficiency, and the capacity for independent living. Examples include traumatic brain injury (TBI), autism, cerebral palsy, and Down syndrome.

The purpose of this chapter is to focus only on the types of disabilities listed above. The term disability will refer to all physical, sensory, and cognitive disabilities unless otherwise specified. Although it will not be included as a disability in this chapter, the author wishes to note *a substance use disorder that substantially impairs major life activities, such as alcoholism, is a covered disability by the ADA.* Consequently, reasonable accommodations must be made for the individual (e.g., modified work schedule to attend AA meetings). Providing accommodation does not mean giving special preferences to the individual, but it refers to the act of reducing barriers to allow for equal opportunity and participation in employment, treatment programs, etc. Now that definitions, examples, and clarifications have been given, the next section presents the reader with statistics about people living with disabilities.

STATISTICS

According to the United States Census Bureau in 2010, there were 57 million people with a disability living in America, representing 19 percent of the civilian, noninstitutionalized population (Brault, 2012). Breaking the data down by age, the lowest prevalence of disabilities is among children under 15 years old (8 percent). For those who are 15 and older, 21 percent have a disability. Older adults have the highest rates of disability. When specifically looking at adults 65 and older, 50 percent have disabilities.

As stated in the previous section of this chapter, there is a variety of categories for disabilities. In 2010, eight million people (15 and older) had a hearing impairment; half of which were 65 and older. Eight million people (15 and older) had a visual impairment, and four million people used a wheelchair to assist with mobility.

The U.S. Census also gathered data regarding employment rates, income, government benefits, and health care coverage among those with disabilities. Less than half of those aged 21 to 64 were employed. In fact, 41 percent had employment. This undoubtedly impacts income disparities. The median monthly earnings for 21-to-64-year-olds with a disability was $1,961, compared with $2,724 for those with no disability. Indeed, almost a third of those with a severe disability (29 percent) lived in poverty, while 18 percent with non–severe disabilities were in poverty. As far as government benefits, 59 percent of people with severe disabilities received public assistance, and 33 percent received Social Security benefits. Twenty-eight percent of adults with severe disabilities received food stamp benefits, compared with 8 percent for those with no disability. Forty-eight percent of those with severe disabilities had government health coverage, while 40 percent had private health insurance coverage. Twenty-three percent had Medicare coverage and 35 percent received Medicaid, while 9 percent had dual coverage, receiving Medicare and Medicaid benefits. Last, despite the higher rates of health-related issues for this population, one in five of those aged 15 to 64 with a disability was uninsured (Brault, 2012).

Substance Use

Persons with disabilities experience substance abuse rates two to four times that of the general population. More specifically, 4.7 million American adults have a co-occurring disability and substance abuse problem, and an estimated 1.5 million people with disabilities may be in need of substance abuse treatment. People who have a particular disability appear to be more at risk for developing an issue with substance use than people with other disabilities. For instance, people with deafness, arthritis, or multiple sclerosis have higher substance abuse rates; these numbers are at least double the general population. Moreover, people with spinal cord injuries, orthopedic disabilities, visual impairment, and amputations have been classified as heavy drinkers in approximately 40–50 percent of cases. One study found 68 percent of people with spinal cord injuries resume drinking alcohol while undergoing rehabilitation for the injury, and 53 percent of clients with physical disabilities reported substance use problems as "substantial" or a "great" concern. In contrast to physical disabilities, those with developmental disabilities are shown to have the lowest rates of substance use, even compared to the general population.

One study compared alcohol and other drug use among those with disabilities to those without disabilities from 2002–2010 (Glazier & Kling, 2013). The data was taken from the National Survey on Drug Use and Health, which gathers information from in-person, household interviews of 70,000 randomly selected persons aged 12 and older. This research only examined data from persons aged 18 to 64. For all nine years, with the exception of alcohol, persons with disabilities used other drugs (e.g., cigarettes, heroin, and crack cocaine) more frequently than those without disabilities. For instance, the prevalence of smoking six or more cigarettes a day for those without disabilities was around 14 percent over the nine years; however, it was about 20 percent for those with disabilities. This study focused on odds-ratio differences, and revealed that in 2010, the odds ratio for overall substance abuse in the past month was 1.28. The following table (Table 14.1 below) is a comparison of odds ratios for past-month drug use between the two populations in 2010, as cited by Glazier and Kling (2013).

In essence, persons with disabilities were found to be almost five times more likely to have used heroin in the past month, three times more likely to have used sedatives and oxycodone, and a little over two and a half times more likely to have used methamphetamine and crack cocaine. They were almost one and a half times more likely to have smoked marijuana. Why do researchers find higher rates of use among those with disabilities?

The etiologies of substance abuse among this population are many. One theory is the desire for self-medication. As a result of issues surrounding a disability, some may use substances to avoid, numb out, and escape the negative emotions connected to these issues. Researchers have shown those with disabilities are more likely to experience social isolation and a lack of recreational activities. In addition, victimization (e.g., physical and sexual abuse), homelessness, and unemployment and underemployment are more common than in the general population. In fact, 30 percent of people with disabilities live below the poverty line. For the reasons stated above, substance use may become a coping mechanism for a person with a disability. The prevalence of use among those in vocational rehabilitation programs substantiates this assumption. Approximately 25 percent of persons with disabilities in such a program experience a significant problem with alcohol and other drugs. *On the other hand, alcohol and other drugs can be the cause of one's disability.* In the young adult population particularly, alcohol has been found to be a major cause of disabilities for those aged 20–21. Also, with people who have spinal cord injuries and TBIs (regardless of age), often intoxication was the cause of the disability.

Traumatic brain injuries (TBIs) often result in cognitive problems, excessive fatigue, and personality changes. As a result, the substance use rates among those with a TBI may increase due to the desire to self-medicate. Interestingly, researchers have shown that before injury, people who sustain a TBI were twice as likely as others in the community to be an abuser of substances (35 percent to 17 percent, respectively).

Table 14.1:

ODDS RATIO FOR DIFFERENCES BETWEEN PERSONS WITH AND WITHOUT DISABILITIES, 2010	
Heroin	4.72
Sedatives	3.02
Oxycodone	3.01
Methamphetamine	2.63
Crack Cocaine	2.60
Marijuana	1.43

Alcohol and other drug use can cause such impairment due to injury while intoxicated (e.g., car accident). In fact, 40–80 percent of TBIs occur while intoxicated. The use of substances after acquiring a TBI can be very harmful. Researchers have suggested continued substance use can result in slower recovery from the brain injury, further damage to an already injured brain, an increase in aggressive and/or antisocial behaviors, and interference with thinking processes.

SUBSTANCE ABUSE ISSUES

Historically, data on substance abuse and disabilities has been scarce (Ebener & Smedema, 2011). In fact, even among the substance abuse literature, only 12 percent of research references disability issues (West, 2007). Despite this dearth of information, there are specific substance abuse issues identified among scholars and practitioners that should be considered. This section will discuss the (a) functional capacities that may be impaired due to having a disability; (b) risk factors correlated with substance use among those with disabilities; (c) barriers impacting successful treatment outcomes; and (d) discrimination and oppression experienced by this population.

Functional Capacities

Disabilities and impairments can cause limitations in functional capacities, and these vary by person. Two people having the same disability can have different degrees of impairment in functionality. Clinicians should be familiar with the numerous functions of impairment in order to accurately create the most effective treatment plans with their clients. The following is a list of these functional capacities. An assessment of these areas is recommended not only at intake, but also throughout the course of therapy.

1. Self-care
   - Eating
   - Grooming
   - Bathing
   - Dressing
   - Bowel and bladder management
   - Medication usage

2. Mobility
   - Positioning
   - Walking, with or without assistive devices
   - Use of a wheelchair or other mobility aid
   - Use of stairs
   - Ability to operate motor vehicle
   - Use of public transportation (or other access to transportation)

3. Communication
   - Reading
   - Writing
   - Speaking
   - Listening

4. Learning
   - Attention
   - Comprehension
   - Retention
   - Application

5. Problem Solving
   - Awareness and recognition of problems
   - Identification of alternatives
   - Anticipation of possible consequences of various alternatives
   - Deciding on optimal alternatives

6. Social Skills
   - Understanding of social mores and values
   - Impulse control
   - Intimacy
   - Conversational skills
   - Empathy

7. Executive Functions
   - Planning and organization
   - Motivation and initiation
   - Monitoring and reviewing
   - Decision making (Center for Substance Abuse Treatment [CSAT], 2008, p.5)

Risk Factors

Persons with disabilities are at a disproportionately greater risk for substance abuse issues than those without disabilities. One factor increasing the risk of addiction is misidentification. Family members, friends, and professionals may focus on concerns related to the disability and miss the warning signs of substance abuse. Moreover, others tend to be more relaxed when persons with disabilities use alcohol and other drugs; at times, they can even rationalize use for one's disability (e.g., "He is an amputee, give him a break. If I had that disability, I would drink too"). This could lead to enabling behaviors and thus increase the risk for dependency. Another risk factor is the higher likelihood of prescription medication use among this population. Commonly, persons with disabilities have more medical and health problems than those without a disability. Therefore, this population usually takes medications and also has easy access to other drugs. While prescription medications may be helpful, the risk of abuse is present. Medications can be mixed with other drugs, including alcohol, and this can be deadly. One national telephone survey of 1,505 adults (aged 18–64) with permanent physical and/or mental disabilities reported 88 percent of their respondents took prescription medications (Kaiser Family Foundation, 2003). Some medications may be overprescribed and not needed. According to researchers, 41 percent of people with disabilities have stated they were given medications when they thought there was no necessity for the prescription. Other risk factors also include circumstances that create stress for those with disabilities. For instance, negative self-perceptions, adverse attitudes and a general lack of knowledge by others, and stigmatization all heighten the propensity for substance use, misuse, and dependency.

Barriers

According to CSAT (2008), there are four types of barriers for people with disabilities who are trying to access and complete substance abuse treatment. These four categories of barriers are: (1) attitudinal; (2) discriminatory policies, practices, and procedures; (3) communication; and (4) architectural. The following section offers some examples of these barriers, which continue to result in inadequate services for those with disabilities. Later in this chapter, treatment recommendations will be made to address these barriers.

Attitudinal

Substance abuse treatment outcomes may be affected by the way people without disabilities view and react to those with disabilities. Misperceptions are one such barrier. For instance, clinicians may think the same protocol should be used with everyone because people with disabilities do not want to be viewed or treated differently. Another misperception is the notion that people with disabilities will make other clients uncomfortable. Clinicians could also hold the belief that people with disabilities make too many demands and use their disability as an excuse for lack of participation in treatment. In addition, as stated before in the risk factors section of this chapter, professionals could also believe pity should be given to those with a disability and allow more latitude with regard to substance use.

Even further, stereotypes can impact the efficacy of servicing this population. For example, some people have inaccurate beliefs related to a specific type of disability. A counselor may hold the attitude that clients with a cognitive disability are not capable of learning about recovery and staying sober. In addition, counselors could have stereotypes about those with an addiction and view them as "resistant." One study of rehabilitation counselors substantiated this stereotype. The researchers asked these counselors (who work with people with visual impairments) about the prevalence of substance abuse among their clients and the extent of their education related to addiction. Over half of the clinicians had clients who struggle with addiction; however, 66 percent of the counselors reportedly did not have formal substance abuse education at a university, and 60 percent had no training on substance abuse case management or the use of 12-step programs (Davis, Koch, McKee, & Nelipovich, 2009). This lack of education may have impacted the counselors' attitudes toward their clients' participation in rehabilitation services. When asked about servicing these clients, 94 percent of the participants stated it was difficult to work with them because they were viewed as "uncooperative," "unreliable," and "unmotivated."

Discriminatory Policies, Practices, and Procedures

At a systemic level, addiction treatment programs can discriminate against those with disabilities. Administrators and staff must make a diligent effort in recognizing the macro-level barriers which impact their clients. Some programs have policies against providing services to clients on medication. Persons with disabilities may be prescribed pain medication, anxiety medication, or medication for attention-deficit disorders. Also, there may be discriminatory practices that must be considered, such as requiring all clients to read material in or out of the therapy room. Another practice that often occurs is discharging a client for missing their sessions. However, the client may have been absent or late due to issues with transportation (e.g., bus provided for the client broke down). Transportation is a barrier in and of itself, as some clients do not have a driver's license and/or have severe mobility problems, which may make it difficult to even leave the house.

Communication

Treatment programs must have a variety of auxiliary aids and services in order to communicate effectively with clients who have a disability. Physical, sensory, and cognitive disabilities can impact the ability for a person to communicate with their therapist and others in treatment. People may have speech impairments or respiratory problems, for example, and therapists must provide clients enough time to fully express their thoughts. Those with sensory disabilities, such as visual or hearing impairments, may require the use of an interpreter, Braille, large print, audiocassettes and/or transcription for communication. A treatment program should also have telecommunication devices for the deaf (TDDs) as well. This allows people to type and send messages over the telephone. Cognitive disabilities, like ones resulting from a TBI, may cause problems with comprehension and speaking. Often, people can have limited vocabularies or not have the ability for abstract thinking. For example, if a therapist talks about being powerless over substance use (as stated in Step One of the 12 Steps), clients with cognitive or developmental impairments may not understand this concept.

Architectural

Treatment programs may present barriers to people with disabilities because the architecture of some buildings makes accessibility difficult and impedes the ease of mobility for some clients. Several examples of architectural barriers include the absence of elevators or ramps, narrow hallways, loose rugs, and poor lighting.

To illustrate the barriers that exist in treatment facilities, the following data was collected by 159 substance abuse agencies and organizations nationwide in 2007:

- 20 percent did not have accessible parking spaces
- 20 percent did not have accessible restroom facilities
- 24 percent did not meet guidelines for accessible hallways or doors
- Of those with stairs leading to the entrance, 25 percent did not have a ramp, lifting device, etc.

- 24 percent did not have fire alarms with both auditory and visual alerts
- 84 percent did not have anyone on staff who knows sign language
- 95 percent did not have materials available in Braille (West, 2007)

As West (2007) states, "One would be hard-pressed to find another group so systematically excluded from health services today" (p. 4). Even with the passing of the ADA, substance abuse programs are still lagging behind in removing these barriers. Professionals must continue to advocate for change on behalf of their clients with disabilities.

Ableism

The barriers identified in the previous section indicate how people with disabilities can be oppressed and discriminated against, otherwise known as *ableism*. Unlike racism and sexism, ableism is a form of systemic oppression that any person may experience at any time in life. People without disabilities have certain unearned privileges related to their bodies. As Peggy McIntosh identifies privileges for whites, those without disabilities also have unearned benefits. Not having a disability is an asset that allows doors of opportunity to open and provides protection from harmful insensitivities (e.g., microaggressions), hostility, and violence; the things people with disabilities may not be privy to. The following five statements are privileges that people without disabilities can have:

- I can ignore the width of doors, the presence of steps, and other architectural features of buildings.
- I can use any bathroom stall I want without thought to accessibility, and I can do it without thinking of needing assistance.
- I am not expected to speak for all people who do not have a disability.
- I can be fairly sure that I am not viewed as subhuman, defective, or deviant due to the condition of my mind, body, or emotional self.
- I can assume that I will not be perceived as angry, incompetent, childlike, or helpless just because of the condition of my body. (May-Machunda, n.d.)

SCREENING AND ASSESSMENT

The process for screening and assessing for substance use disorders may take longer and can be very different with this population than the process for people without disabilities. In addition, clinicians should have the knowledge, skills and abilities, and self-awareness about this population in order to be competent screeners and assessors. This section addresses some problems and solutions with regard to these two processes.

As stated earlier, many disabilities are hidden and not as obvious as others (e.g., learning disabilities, seizure disorders, etc.). Therefore, counselors should be screening every client for potential disabilities. Allow the client to discuss any impairment, and identify what specific needs are warranted. A clinician should ask every client, "Do you need any accommodations in order to participate in our program?" Clinicians should also be aware of the fact that many clients will not disclose their disability, even when invited to do so. Some clients have spent their lives masking and hiding their disability and may not volunteer this information or admit to it when asked.

Besides hidden disabilities and nondisclosure of disabilities, clients may not even be aware of any impairment (e.g., hearing loss). Therefore, counselors should not only ask the appropriate questions outlined in intake paperwork, but they also need to assess for potential areas of impaired functioning that may appear during conversation and the interactions with clients. It should be noted that clients may appear to fully comprehend all the information presented during the intake; however, they may have problems with memory, decision making, planning, and learning comprehension. A counselor may realize these issues one session after the intake, or it could be months into the therapy process when the counselor understands the full extent of these impairments.

To address specific screening and assessment concerns for particular disabilities, the following recommendations are suggested. (1) For those who have visual impairments, the clinician should ask the client if they would like to have the intake paperwork in the medium of their choice (e.g., Braille, large print, audiocassette, or sighted assistance). (2) For persons who are deaf, paper-and-pencil methods should never be used. Sign language is the mode of communication to be employed. (3) For people with developmental and learning disabilities, clinicians should be very specific with their language. For instance, instead of asking clients if they "use alcohol," ask if they drink beer, wine, liquor, etc. Also, pictures of different sizes and types of alcohol can also be a means to gain the information needed for assessment purposes.

TREATMENT RECOMMENDATIONS AND CONSIDERATIONS

When working with persons with disabilities, helping professionals should consider several recommendations. For instance, discuss the apparent differences (i.e., use broaching behaviors in session), and explore the level of acculturation and phase of disability identity development. A person with a disability often goes through various phases of adjustment related to the disability. The client's current phase of adjustment is very important for clinicians to recognize in an effort to grasp a sense of the emotional state of their client. The phases of adjustment frequently displayed are:

- Shock
- Anxiety
- Denial
- Depression
- Internalized anger
- Externalized hostility
- Acknowledgment
- Adjustment and acceptance (Livneh & Antonak, 1997)

These are not linear in nature, and not all individuals experience them. For instance, a person born with a disability may not go through shock because it was not a loss, per se. It should be noted these phases can be reversed or revisited, and some of them can be omitted altogether.

Regardless of the phase of adjustment, counselors must have a competency-based view of clients and take on a strength-based perspective. They should view the person as one with a disability—not as a disabled person. Empowerment is very important in therapy. Counselors should encourage concepts of independence, choice, autonomy, and personal responsibility (i.e., self-determination) with their clients who have disabilities.

Moreover, accommodations must be made to decrease barriers for those attempting to access and complete substance abuse treatment. One accommodation is flexibility with counseling sessions; they can be shortened, lengthened, or more frequent, depending on the client's needs. Also, ask the client if breaks are needed throughout the session. In an effort to discuss the considerations needed for specific disabilities, the next section provides a list of recommendations by physical, sensory, and cognitive disability.

For Clients Who Have a Physical Disability

Make sure the table heights allow room for a wheelchair to fit beneath it

The counselor should not sit higher than the client is sitting

Do not touch the client's wheelchair or take control of the wheelchair without permission, as the wheelchair is regarded as an extension of the client; this can be considered offensive

For Clients with Visual Impairments

Keep pathways clear and raise low-hanging signs or lights

Use large-letter signs and add Braille labels to all signs and elevator buttons

Make oral announcements, and do not rely on visual announcements such as a bulletin board or dry-erase board

Give a guided tour of the facility on the first visit. Do so by having the client hold your arm and walk with the client, explaining where the doors, hallways, restrooms, and furniture are located

Put the client's hand on the back of the chair he or she will sit in

A service animal should not be distracted from its job; do not touch or pet the animal, and do not ask to do so

Be descriptive and detailed when communicating; avoid phrases like "over there" or "like this"

Ask if the lighting is appropriate and comfortable

Look directly at the person when communicating

For Clients Who Have Hearing Impairments

Look directly at the person when communicating. This will help the client read lips. If the person is using an interpreter, still look at your client when communicating

When appropriate, use an interpreter who uses sign language. Do not use the client's friend or family member as an interpreter

For Clients with Cognitive Disabilities

Ask simple questions, repeat questions, and ask the client to repeat in his or her own words what was discussed

Speak to the client's ability level; do not speak to the client as you would a child

Discussions should be concrete. Abstract concepts may be difficult to understand

Be aware that substance abuse materials may be written at too high a reading level for a person with an intellectual disability.

Use expressive therapy or role-playing

Use alternative media in place of writing

Use picture books, comic books, illustrated flashcards, art therapy techniques, and audio- and videotapes

Treatment Planning

Clinicians should focus on substance use issues when planning treatment, but all life areas must be taken into account. As stated earlier in this chapter, the various functional capacities (e.g., self-care, mobility, communication, learning, etc.) should be assessed throughout treatment. If limitations are identified, clinicians should employ efforts to address these deficiencies by removing barriers, providing education, and offering assistance to eliminating harmful circumstances that may exist. Some of these goals in treatment planning should include helping the client to:

- Leave, and also avoid, abusive situations
- Learn how to protect themselves from victimization
- Identify employment services available in area and assist with disability paperwork, if applicable
- Find volunteer work or other means of gaining a sense of productivity in lieu of paid employment
- Develop better self-care, mobility, and executive functioning (e.g., basic grooming, dressing appropriately, using public transportation, and cooking)
- Learn social skills that may be missing because of both substance use disorders and disability-related problems
- Learn to engage in healthy recreational activities
- Become educated about their legal rights to accessible environments and services, as well as employment
- Build new supportive, healthy peer networks
- Connect with case management services and partner with the various agencies in the area for a holistic approach to treating substance use issues (Adapted from CSAT, 2008).

The last goal listed above is an important part of advocacy, which clinicians should be engaged in when providing counseling to this population. Community partnerships are crucial with respect to the success of abstinence and harm-reduction strategies. The next section will address how linkages can assist with reducing substance use among those with disabilities.

Partnerships

Unlike some other culturally marginalized groups, persons with disabilities frequently do not have family members and other important people in their lives who have shared life experiences, can validate their sufferings, offer advice, or be role models. This is why it is important for treatment programs to link up with local agencies and groups which offer housing, vocational training, and other supports for those with disabilities. Counselors should be knowledgeable about the various resources available for this population. For example, there are Centers for Independent Living (CILs) that are run by and for people with disabilities. They offer support, advocacy, and information on attainment of independence from a peer viewpoint. Currently, there are over 400 Centers for Independent Living nationwide. (To search by state, visit http://www.ilru.org/html/publications/directory/index.html)

Some organizations assist those with specific disabilities who also struggle with addiction. In Ohio, a grant-funded program called Deaf off Drugs and Alcohol (DODA) was created to improve substance abuse treatment services for those with hearing impairments. All the counselors, case managers, and coordinators are fluent in American Sign Language and competent in the deaf culture. DODA does the following functions: (a) assists with finding and providing local treatment; (b) develops a communication plan based on the client's needs and preferences; (c) helps individuals in developing a sobriety plan; (d) provides additional counseling and case management services through videophone appointments; (e) consults with treatment providers about interpreting needs; (f) assists in finding interpreters for self-help meetings; and (g) advocates for additional services or accommodations when necessary. A treatment program similar to DODA is the Minnesota Chemical Dependency Program for Deaf and Hard of Hearing Individuals. If the reader is interested in learning more, the program's website offers materials and information that may assist counselors and administrators to more effectively treat those with hearing impairments.

Substance abuse treatment program staff must be proactive and have continuous contact with community agencies and organizations who serve those with disabilities. One reason is to provide cross-training to staff and personnel in both entities. Often, substance abuse counselors have expressed a lack of knowledge about how to work with those having disabilities, and those who serve persons with disabilities have reported they are unprepared to screen, assess, and treat those with addiction issues. Providing cross-training would (a) educate staff; (b) enhance sensitivity, empathy, and open-mindedness; (c) encourage mutual referrals; and (d) create a recovery-oriented system of care within the community. Moreover, programs that hire persons with disabilities have an advantage with regard to treating those with disabilities, as they can assist with removing barriers; they can also educate other staff about the needs of this specific population.

Language Considerations

The last treatment consideration to be addressed is related to language and what might be considered offensive to clients. Terms and phrases that are associated with disabilities which are commonly heard from others and through the media are ones like "special," "slow," "midget," "cripple," "the short bus," and "that's retarded." All of these are prejudicial and insulting. In addition to the overt insults, harmful language is also conveyed in more subtle and covert ways. For instance, the disability does not define a person, and therefore, people should not use language that labels a person. Use the phrase a "person with a disability" versus a "disabled person." Similarly, a "person with an addiction" should not be labeled as an "addicted person," "alcoholic," or "addict." Also, people should not state someone is "struggling with" or "afflicted with" a disability or an addiction. This implies the client is in constant misery without periods of pleasure or satisfaction. On the other hand, those without a disability should not be called "normal," or "able-bodied." By stating such, one implies that those with a disability are not normal, have bodies that do not function, and are lacking ability. Moreover, a client should not be referred to as a "patient," "case," "retarded," or "handicapped."

CONCLUSION

Throughout their careers, counselors will provide services to many people who have disabilities and co-occurring substance use issues. There are various types of disabilities that exist, and therapists must have the knowledge, skills, attitudes, and self-awareness to effectively help people who may have physical, sensory, and/or cognitive disabilities. This chapter addressed the specific substance abuse issues, risk factors, barriers, screening and assessment concerns, and treatment recommendations regarding this population. Take the time now to answer the questions below in an effort to explore your level of comfort and competency related to people with disabilities.

Exercises

1. Provide an example of each type of disability: physical, cognitive, and sensory. What thoughts, biases, attitudes, and beliefs could therapists have about each of these disabilities?
2. What biases do you hold about someone with a disability? Take the time to explore your thoughts about the various types of disabilities.
3. Describe two areas of competency related to this population that need to be strengthened. Are these competencies related to knowledge, ability/skills, and/or attitudes?
4. Identify three ways to increase these competencies.
5. If you work at an agency or organization currently, what types of barriers do you see (i.e., attitudinal; discriminatory policies, practices, and procedures; communication; or architectural)?

REFERENCES

The Arc. (2014). *What is people-first language?* Retrieved from http://www.thearc.org/page.aspx?pid=2523

Brault, M. W. (2012). Americans with disabilities; 2010. *Current Population Reports*, 70–131. U.S. Census Bureau: Washington, DC. Retrieved from http://www.census.gov/prod/2012pubs/p70-131.pdf

Center for Substance Abuse Treatment (2008). *Substance use disorder treatment for people with physical and cognitive disabilities.* Treatment Improvement Protocol (TIP) Series 29. Substance Abuse and Mental Health Services Administration: Rockville, MD.

Davis, S. J., Koch, D. S., McKee, M. F., & Nelipovich, M. (2009). AODA training experiences of blindness and visual impairment professionals. *Journal of Teaching in the Addictions, 8*, 42–50.

Ebener, D. J., & Smedema, S. M. (2011). Physical disability and substance use disorders: A convergence of adaptation and recovery. *Rehabilitation Counseling Bulletin, 54*, 131–141.

Grazier, R. E., & Kling, R. N. (2013). Recent trends in substance abuse among persons with disabilities compared to that of persons without disabilities. *Disability and Health Journal, 6*, 107–115.

Kaiser Family Foundation (2003). *Survey of People with Disabilities*. Retrieved from http://kaiserfamilyfoundation.files.wordpress.com/2013/01/survey-of-people-with-disabilities.pdf

Livneh, H., & Antonak, R. F. (1997). *Psychological adaptation to chronic illness and disability*. Gaithersburg, MD: Aspen.

May-Machunda, P. M. (n.d.). Exploring the invisible knapsack of able-bodied privilege. Retrieved from http://www.library.wisc.edu/EDVRC/docs/public/pdfs/LIReadings/ExploringInvisibleKnapsack.pdf

West, S. L. (2007). The accessibility of substance abuse treatment facilities in the United States for persons with disabilities. *Journal of Substance Abuse Treatment, 33*, 1–5.

CHAPTER 15

PERSONS WHO ARE ECONOMICALLY DISADVANTAGED

By Ashley J. Blount and Olivia Uwamahoro

Regardless of ethnicity, race, gender, culture, or age, individuals are expected to go through similar progressive stages of addiction (Van Wormer & Rae Davis, 2008). However, to avoid stereotyping and overgeneralization, a number of factors should be taken into account to ensure individuals are viewed holistically. Examples of such factors include acculturation, primary language, communication skills, family structure, religion, and socioeconomic status. It is essential that features such as these are evaluated so that treatment of addictions is tailored to the unique needs of every individual (Van Wormer & Rae Davis, 2008).

Socioeconomic status—often referred to as class—is of particular importance because it can be directly related to substance abuse (Van Wormer & Rae Davis, 2008). According to the Centers for Disease Control and Prevention (CDC), socioeconomic status is a composite measure that incorporates economic, social, and work status. Economic status is measured by income, social status determined by education, and work status established by occupation (CDC, 2013). Class is defined as any group sharing the same socioeconomic status or social status (Merriam-Webster, 2013). As such, class influences many aspects of an individual's life, and persons of lower socioeconomic status (i.e., economically disadvantaged populations) will be discussed in regard to substance use and abuse. For the purposes of this chapter, economically disadvantaged (ED) will refer to individuals who lack the financial resources necessary to function and achieve an equal position in society (Merriam-Webster, 2013). Reasons for substance use, risk and resiliency factors, treatment barriers, and assessment will be discussed and treatment methodology and interventions for working with ED populations will be highlighted.

A large portion of the United States population is comprised of ED and working-class populations. In 2012, the U.S. Census Bureau report on *Income, Poverty, and Health Insurance Coverage in the United States: 2011* demonstrated that 15 percent, or 46.2 million people, of the U.S. population were living in poverty. Poverty consists of individuals who fall under a recommended income amount and is based on how many people are in a family (Families USA, 2013). For example, the poverty line for a family of four in the United States is $23,550 (Families USA, 2013). According to the Trends in Substance Abuse Admissions (SAMSHA, 2010), individuals over the age of 18 admitted to alcohol and drug treatment facilities are more likely to be socioeconomically disadvantaged and showed higher rates of unemployment. Further, unemployed individuals showed double rates of admission into substance abuse treatment facilities, with around 40 percent of all admissions coming from unemployed individuals aged 16 years and older (SAMSHA, 2011). Additionally, the majority of individuals admitted had no primary source of income (SAMSHA, 2011), and according to the *Treatment Episode Data Set* (TEDS) admissions of individuals aged 16 and older, were less likely to be employed than the U.S. population within the same age range (National Admissions to Substance Abuse Treatment Services, 2011). Thus, there may be a correlation between socioeconomic status and substance use; consequently, individuals suffering from substance use disorders may also be economically disadvantaged.

Factors associated with socioeconomic status such as where people live and educational opportunities may also influence the propensity for addiction (Murphy & Rosenbaum, 1997). For instance, one may reside in a neighborhood with more liquor stores or in an area where drugs are commonly sold. Additionally, being economically disadvantaged can lead to increased levels of discrimination and financial hardship that are not experienced by more privileged individuals. As a result, ED individuals who also suffer from substance abuse are subject to even greater forms of discrimination and can be left feeling isolated in their problems. Before the authors discuss the treatment of ED individuals who present with substance misuse or abuse concerns, one must first explore why this population might use a particular substance in the first place.

ETIOLOGICAL THEORIES

The reasons or causes for abusing substances vary between individuals. However, people who are economically disadvantaged may experience substance use differently from those who are economically privileged. Literature on substance abuse contains many theories on why someone misuses a substance or becomes addicted, but the most popular theories are: (a) disease; (b) genetic; (c) behavioral; and (d) sociocultural theories (Stevens & Smith, 2009). When working with the ED population, it is important to gain an understanding of the distinct beliefs about addiction in order to tailor treatment on an individual basis. Furthermore, ED individuals who have substance-related issues are likely to fall into one of the aforementioned theoretical categories. The disease model of addiction centers on a belief that individuals are not responsible for having addictions, but rather are responsible for managing their disease and finding a Higher Power in order to fully recover from the disease (Fisher & Harrison, 2009; Stevens & Smith, 2009). An example of a recovery group that practices from the disease model ideology is Alcoholics Anonymous (AA). ED individuals who follow the disease etiology believe their substance abuse is a direct result of a disease. That is, they seek help in overcoming their substance abuse similar to someone who has a disease like cancer needs help in the treatment process.

The genetic model posits substance abuse or addiction as biologically inherited. Certain traits are passed down through generations, and essentially, a mother or father suffering from alcoholism would pass down the propensity for addiction to their children. For example, individuals may have a predisposition to alcohol abuse (e.g., high tolerance and personality characteristics) because their parent or relative was an alcoholic. Thus, a relative or parent with an addiction would increase the chances of ED individuals having an addiction or substance abuse problem themselves.

Behavioral theory, on the other hand, focuses on substance abuse as a learned behavior. From this perspective, ED individuals learned substance abuse behaviors from parents, peers, etc. For example, modeling of drug use and misuse could result in drug experimentation and use in later generations. In addition, behaviors that were positively or negatively reinforced would be increased. As a result, economically disadvantaged individuals may increase use of substances if they had a positive experience with it in the past. Thus, behavioral-based substance abuse revolves around learned actions that are taken in order to achieve a positive experience (e.g., obtaining a euphoric feeling) or avoid/escape a negative experience (e.g., coping with a depressive state).

Lastly, sociocultural theory postulates substance abuse is caused by environmental influences. Such influences that ED individuals might experience are peer pressure, living with an individual who abuses substances, stress, life events (e.g., death of family member or loss of job), increasing poverty, availability of drugs, and violence (Stevens & Smith, 2009). Environmental factors directly influence an individual's path toward substance use and could affect the amount used, as well as the specific substance used. For instance, in lower socioeconomic neighborhoods where alcohol is the cheapest and availability of illegal drugs is increased, people may use these substances out of convenience and accessibility.

Economically disadvantaged individuals face additional stressors than economically privileged individuals. Stressors are typically categorized into two categories: *psychosocial stressors* or *material stressors* (Droomers, Schrijvers, Stronks, Mheen, & Mackenback, 1999). Psychosocial stressors include negative life events such as divorce or loss of employment (Droomers et al., 1999). Material stressors include quality of housing, air pollution, other neighborhood aspects (e.g., level of crime and community resources), income, and material deprivation (Droomers et al., 1999). For example, individuals with a low socioeconomic status have a higher chance of: (a) living in poverty; (b) residing in unsafe neighborhoods; (c) being unemployed; (c) having limited income; and (d) limitations on affordable material goods. As a direct result of material stressors, ED individuals have an increased chance of experiencing psychosocial stressors throughout their lifetime. Additionally, ED persons are more likely to experience high levels of psychosocial and material stressors as a result of economic hardship.

Economically disadvantaged individuals with lower education levels are at greater risk for illicit substance abuse and excessive drinking than individuals with higher education (Droomers et al., 1999). Droomers and colleagues (1999) noted material stressors such as financial problems, deprivation, and lower income contributed to excessive drinking. Further, the identified material stressors were linked to educational level. Of all individuals admitted for substance abuse issues, roughly 60 percent of individuals admitted had received education levels of a high school degree or below (SAMSHA, 2011). Consequently, excessive alcohol use is associated with educational level and ultimately may be correlated with being economically disadvantaged. For example, individuals who never graduated from high school have more limitations regarding employment and face decreased benefits (e.g., health care, maternity leave, and job security). As individuals continue to work through different life situations that result from being socioeconomically disadvantaged, stress increases, and life satisfaction tends to decrease.

STIGMAS

As with most mental health concerns, the general public views substance use issues negatively. This negative perception hinders individuals from seeking treatment for substance use concerns. Picture individuals who present with alcohol abuse and are unemployed. What are the first thoughts that come to mind? What types of stereotypes come into play?

The spiritual and religious beliefs of ED individuals may also contribute to a stigmatized view of substance abuse. For example, some religious groups view drunkenness as a sin, while others such as the Mormon Church prohibit drinking and intake of other substances altogether (Fisher & Harrison, 2009). Consequently, ED individuals may not be able to afford treatment on their own, and at the same time, may feel uncomfortable seeking support from their religious/spiritual leaders.

Cultural values of ED individuals also contribute to stigmatized views of substance abuse. For instance, drinking is accepted among individuals of Jewish heritage, as evidenced by alcohol use during various social and ceremonial events by both young people and adults. However, though alcohol use is accepted, excessive use of alcohol is prohibited (Fisher & Harrison, 2009). Another illustration where culture plays a role in how substance use is viewed is that in some cultures, there is a feeling that issues and concerns should stay within a family, so as to save face for the family. An example includes someone suffering from substance abuse in a household where familial values are strong. In this case, family members might dislike or disapprove of the substance abuse, but no outside action or intervention would be taken in order to keep the abuse a secret within the family. As one can see, culture plays a large role in how substance abuse is viewed, how the abuse is handled by family members and peers, and what actions are taken.

RISK FACTORS

There are a number of risk factors for substance abuse for ED individuals. Some of these factors include: (a) increased mental health problems; (b) lower quality of life; (c) decreased well-being; (d) higher rates of addiction, morbidity, and mortality; (e) higher levels of stress; (f) increased discrimination; (g) decreased levels of education; (h) increased crime; (i) lack of opportunities and support; and (j) food insecurity (Caron, 2012; Kennedy, Kawachi, Glass, & Prothrow-Stith, 1998; Mackenbach, 1997; Williams & Collins, 1995). Risk factors could lead to increased levels of substance misuse and abuse in ED populations. For example, depression may result from economic status, and individuals may use substances to self-medicate and find relief from their depressive symptoms.

Another risk factor deserving of mention is that of access to treatment. ED individuals may not have access to treatment centers or outpatient services to address substance abuse issues. Therefore, ED individuals may have a more difficult time overcoming substance use disorders than privileged populations. When discussing access to treatment with ED individuals, it is essential to look at the physical accessibility of treatment centers, as well as the quality of treatment provided.

Finally, education is another risk factor which influences ED individuals presenting with substance abuse concerns. Casswell, Pledger, and Hooper (2003) looked at drinking patterns among young adults and found a relationship between the frequency and quantity of alcohol consumption and socioeconomic status and educational level. Participants who consumed significantly more quantities of alcohol were less educated. As stated previously, lower education correlates with lower socioeconomic status; as a result, there is a potential risk factor for ED individuals. Consequently, only 25 percent of individuals admitted for substance abuse issues had higher than a high school degree (SAMSHA, 2011). A lower level of education can be viewed as the highest risk factor because it is linked to employment, which is connected to income and socioeconomic status.

BARRIERS TO TREATMENT

Along with risk factors for the ED populations, researchers have identified specific barriers to treatment. Such barriers include: (a) being uninsured; (b) family instability; (c) limited time to seek treatment services; (d) competing priorities; (e) inconvenient clinic locations; (f) transportation; (g) loss of wages from missing work; (h) child care difficulties; and (i) communication issues (Armstrong, Ishike, Heiman, Mundt, & Womack, 1984; Maynard, Ehreth, Cox, Peterson, & McGann, 1997). For example, ED individuals seeking treatment for substance abuse problems may have a high desire to get help; however, due to low socioeconomic status, they lack transportation and health insurance, which automatically influences access to treatment. An evaluation of these barriers will lead to a better understanding of what the ED person is experiencing in his or her own environment and point the way to a better appreciation of how best to help the client.

Lastly, when treating ED individuals, it is important to consider violence as a potential barrier to treatment. The prevalence of intimate partner violence (IPV) is higher among the urban poor population than in the general population (Oshiro, Poudyal, Poudel, Jimba, & Hokama, 2010). Oshiro et al. (2010) found that approximately 33 percent of ED individuals showed the prevalence of IPV in their relationships, compared to around 20 percent for the general population. Given this, ED individuals are at a higher risk for physical violence than privileged populations; consequently, those ED individuals who are in violent relationships might use substances as a way to cope with experienced violence. As a result, violence is a risk factor that could influence substance use and abuse of ED individuals and affect the treatment outcomes of ED populations who seek treatment.

RESILIENCY AND PREVENTIVE FACTORS

Now that some of the risk factors, barriers to treatment, and stigmas associated with ED individuals have been discussed, the authors now address the potential resiliency and preventive factors (also referred to as *protective factors*). Newcomb and Felix-Ortiz (1993) define protective factors as "influences that prevent, limit, or reduce" the use of alcohol and other drugs (p. 281). Level of education has been identified as a resiliency and preventive factor to the misuse and abuse of alcohol. Casswell, Pledger, and Hooper (2003) looked at the relationship between socioeconomic status and the consumption of alcohol. Socioeconomic status was measured on three levels: educational achievement, income, and occupational activity. The authors found no significant relationship between the frequency of drinking and socioeconomic status. However, participants who were more educated consumed lower quantities of alcohol across age and gender (Casswell, Pledge, & Hooper, 2003). Here, one can see a link between a person's educational level and how much alcohol he or she consumes.

An additional preventive factor is that of support. Individuals coming from families who provide sources of support are more likely to seek treatment for their substance abuse issues. Further, having external support and resources available may increase the probability of individuals seeking help for substance abuse concerns.

SCREENING AND ASSESSMENT

When working with ED individuals, it is important to have a thorough understanding of the quality of life of the population. It is essential to determine if the basic needs of the individual are being met (e.g., proper nutrition, shelter, etc.) before treatment begins. The Schalock and Keith (1993) *Quality of Life Questionnaire* (QOL-Q) is an assessment that can be used with ED individuals seeking substance abuse treatment. The QOL-Q is a 40-item instrument that assesses an individual's quality of life. The questionnaire consists of four domains: (a) personal life satisfaction; (b) individual competence and productivity at work; (c) feelings of empowerment and independence in the living environment; and (d) feelings of belonging and community integration (Schalock & Keith, 1993).

Additionally, it is imperative to assess for mental health disorders such as depression and anxiety. The Beck Depression Inventory (BDI) is a screening measure that identifies current depressive symptomology via a 21-item self-report assessment (Beck, Steer, & Garbin, 1988). The Beck Anxiety Inventory (BAI) is a similar measure that is used to assess anxiety-related symptomology that could be beneficial when working with ED individuals (Beck, Epstein, Brown, & Steer, 1988). Thus, BDI and BAI could be effective assessments for use with ED individuals to screen for anxiety or depression symptomology.

The Global Assessment of Individual Needs (GAIN) is another assessment instrument that may benefit individuals with substance abuse concerns (Dennis, Titus, White, Unsicker, & Hodkgins, 2002). The GAIN assesses substance use and abuse, treatment, health, and risk behaviors of individuals. It also looks at mental health, self-efficacy, and anxiety symptoms (Dennis et al., 2002), which may be advantageous when treating ED populations.

Cultural-specific interventions may be particularly impactful when working with ED populations and substance abuse issues. For example, treatments can be tailored to the specific cultural group one is working with by: (a) discovering individual cultural beliefs and values regarding the use of substances; (b) determining individual definitions of substance use problems; (c) finding out what *help* looks like within the particular culture; (d) defining the meaning and consequences of relapse; and (e) searching for resources and available support (Van Wormer & Rae Davis, 2008). Within cultural-specific interventions, it is important to determine the person's feelings regarding the substance abuse. For example, determining individual beliefs as to whether substance abuse is viewed as a disease, genetically or behaviorally based, or socially based is essential to treatment planning (Stevens & Smith, 2009). As a result, treatment differs, depending on the individual's feelings regarding the etiology of their substance abuse, available resources, and readiness for change. For additional screening and assessment tools for substance abuse, see Juhnke's (2002) *Substance Abuse Assessment and Diagnosis: A Comprehensive Guide for Counselors and Helping Professionals*.

TREATMENT RECOMMENDATIONS AND THERAPEUTIC CONSIDERATIONS

Multicultural Systemic Approach

The authors of this chapter recommend that counselors complete necessary assessment(s) in order to gather adequate information on the individual and the presenting concern(s). Counselors also need to develop a rapport with clients in order to facilitate a therapeutic alliance. Research findings across the mental health field hold that a strong therapeutic alliance contributes to positive client outcomes (Norcross, 2011). In addition, the authors recommend a culturally tailored treatment for ED persons with substance abuse concerns. Dass-Brailsford (2012) states that, "as psychotherapists we have an ethical responsibility to offer clients the best possible treatment that is inclusive of their values and cultural context" (p. 38). A culturally sensitive treatment plan allows for treatment to be individualized based on culture, environment, and personal wants and needs. Further, culturally sensitive treatment promotes resiliency by using the individual's strengths and resources to help them overcome their substance abuse issues.

Hays (2008) suggests working from the ADDRESSING model in order to take into account an individual's culture. The ADDRESSING model accounts for: (a) **A**ge and generational influences; (b) **D**evelopmental disabilities; (c) **D**isabilities acquired later in life; (d) **R**eligion and spiritual orientation; (e) **E**thnic and racial identity; (f) **S**ocioeconomic status; (g) **S**exual orientation; (h) **I**ndigenous heritage; (i) **N**ational origin; and (j) **G**ender (Hays, 2008). The ADDRESSING model can be implemented as a tool for exploration of culture and could result in the facilitation of a culturally based discussion with ED individuals.

Dass-Brailsford (2012) emphasizes the following interventions when working with individuals of low socioeconomic status: (a) empathic understanding and respect; (b) using an ecological framework; and (c) empowerment. By using empathic understanding and respect, counselors and/or individuals in other helping professions decrease the likelihood of psychologically distancing themselves from ED individuals due to an inability to make meaningful connections. Furthermore, empathic understanding allows counselors to broaden their worldviews, which promotes learning and understanding of ED individuals and their cultures (Dass-Brailsford, 2012). Empathic understanding fosters respect, which, in turn, helps develop and maintain the therapeutic alliance.

Working from an ecological framework allows counselors to presume that an ED individual's presenting concern(s) are influenced by multiple factors (i.e., individual characteristics, family, community, etc.) (Dass-Brailsford, 2012). As the counselor gains a greater understanding of the ED individual's ecological system, engagement in treatment is likely to increase. Additionally, with increased understanding, counselors are better able to assist ED individuals in assessing and identifying resources already present in their ecological system.

Empowerment has been found to have a positive influence on individual change (Liden, Wayne, & Sparrowe, 2000). Counselors can empower ED individuals by "helping them gain mastery and control of challenging and destabilizing issues and increasing an awareness of prevalent societal injustices" (Dass-Brailsford, 2012, p. 40). Further, counselors assess how an ED individual's present concern(s) has been influenced by external factors. Finally, the counselor is to ensure that the ED individual's involvement is a central aspect of treatment and encourage participation in the decision-making progress of their treatment.

Another intervention that can be used to gain a better understanding of an ED person's history, family of origin, current lifestyle, and culture is the genogram (Lim & Nakamoto, 2008; Young, 2013). For example, ED individuals can see the lines of substance abuse existing in their backgrounds. Further, the genogram aids in understanding the influences of the past that may be affecting present addiction, substance abuse and misuse, and lifestyle choices. The genogram is a tool that counselors and helping professionals can use to gain an understanding of an ED person's world and establish empathy early on in the therapeutic process.

The sandtray and family art draw can also be used as interventions when working with ED individuals. In the sandtray activity, ED clients construct their world using miniatures (i.e., an array of figurines including people, nature, animals, etc.). Through this construction, an understanding of their culture, background, and current lifestyle is construed. The family art draw activity is similar, in that ED individuals develop a picture of their family. As with the genogram and the sandtray interventions, the art draw allows for gaining a better understanding of a person's culture and allows for discussions about past and present substance use or addiction(s).

Two Case Studies

CASE 1 Paul

Paul is a 43-year-old man who currently lives in public housing with his wife and two small children. Paul has a 10th grade education and has worked on getting his GED in the past. For the past six months, he has been employed as a restaurant cook part-time, but states he is searching for "better work." Paul reports that he consumes up to a "case of beer" a day and that he "occasionally smokes marijuana" to calm himself down. Due to a domestic violence conviction, he is presenting for an assessment as part of his probation requirements.

At this time, Paul has concerns about his relationship with his wife and children. He feels that his wife is "always on his case about drinking" and that his children require a lot time and attention from him. Additionally, Paul feels he would like to live in a better neighborhood so that the children could go outside and play and that his "wife would be happier in a house." Paul also states that he believes he works hard, but has nothing to show for it because his money goes to bills.

Paul does not feel he has a problem with alcohol or marijuana and states that he functions very well, even when he works morning shifts at the restaurant. Paul's wife disagrees and says that Paul "is often hung over and needs to drink in the morning to get going." Paul's mother and father were both alcoholics, but he feels that he is different because he has a job and supports his family.

Paul has no car. He takes the bus to work or wherever he needs to go. He also says that it is often difficult to see extended family because the public transportation only goes so far. Paul states that "money is tight right now," and that he needs to get a better job so that his family can have better health insurance in the near future.

CASE 2 Jova

Jova is a 35-year-old female who currently works full time at a hospital as a registered nurse (RN). Jova lives in a gated apartment complex in the suburb of a city with her boyfriend. She appears well dressed, with good hygiene. Jova admits to being a social drinker and states she started drinking when she was in high school.

Jova was referred for treatment through the hospital's Employee Assistance Program (EAP) after her supervisor noted that she was "a little out of it" during a few of her shifts. Jova has worked at this hospital for ten years, and this was the first disciplinary action taken against her.

Jova reports consuming four to five liquor drinks within a three hour period when she goes out with her coworkers, friends, or family. She does this a few times a month. Jova also states she "enjoys" two to three glasses of wine at home after a long work day. When asked about the frequency of use at home, she says she drinks wine about three times a week and it is often alone. Jova's boyfriend has previously expressed concern about her drinking; however, Jova discounted it because according to her, "He is just jealous because I make more money than him."

Jova confirmed that the majority of the adults in her family drink; however, no one (to her knowledge) has a history of alcoholism or any other type of substance misuse or abuse. Jova visits with her family and her boyfriend's family regularly. Jova expresses a desire to be engaged and married and have her first child within the next three years.

CASE QUESTIONS

1. How would you define the socioeconomic status or class of Paul and Jova? Identify three indicators for each case.
2. After evaluating both cases, discuss why Paul or Jova has a better chance at working through substance abuse issues.
3. Develop a plan of action as to what might be the best treatment for Paul and Jova. What recommendations would you make?

REFERENCES

Armstrong, H., Ishike, D., Heiman, J., Mundt, J., & Womack, W. (1984). Service utilization by black and white clientele in an urban community mental health center: Revised assessment of an old problem. *Community Mental Health Journal, 20*, 269–281.

Beck, A. T., Epstein, N., Brown, G., & Steer, Robert A. An inventory for measuring clinical anxiety: Psychometric properties. *Journal of Consulting and Clinical Psychology, 56*(6), 893–897. doi:10.1037/0022-006X.56.6.893

Beck, A. T., Steer, R. A., & Garbin, M. G. (1988). Psychometric properties of the Beck Depression Inventory. *Clinical Psychology Review, 8*, 77–100.

Casswell, S., Pledger, M., & Hooper, R. (2003). Socioeconomic status and drinking patterns in young adults. *Addiction, 98*, 601–610.

Caron, J. (2012). Predictors of quality of life in economically disadvantaged populations in Montreal. *Social Indicators Research, 107*, 411–427. doi:10.1007/s11205-011-9855-0

Centers for Disease Control and Prevention (2013). Social Determinants of Health. Retrieved from http://www.cdc.gov/socialdeterminants/Definitions.html

Dass-Brailsford, P. (2012). Culturally sensitive therapy with low-income ethnic minority clients: An empowering intervention. *Journal of Contemporary Psychotherapy, 42*, 37–44.

Dennis, M., Titus, J., White, M., Unsicker, J., & Hodkgins, D. (2002). Global Appraisal of Individual Needs (GAIN): Administration guide for the GAIN and related measures. Bloomington, IL: Chestnut Health Systems. Retrieved from www.chestnut.org/li/gain/gadm1299.pdf

Droomers, M., Schrijvers, C. T. M., Stronks, K. M., Mheen, D. V. D., & Mackenback, J. P. (1999). Educational differences in excessive alcohol consumption: The role of psychosocial and material stressors. *Preventive Medicine, 29*, 1–10.

Families USA. (2013). 2013 Federal Poverty Guidelines. Retrieved from http://www.familiesusa.org/

Fisher, G. L., & Harrison, T. C. (2009) *Substance abuse: Information for school counselors, social workers, therapists, and counselors* (4th ed.). Boston: Pearson Education, Inc.

Hays, P. A. (2008). *Addressing cultural complexities in practice: Assessment, diagnosis, and therapy*. Washington, DC: American Psychological Association.

Kennedy, B., Kawachi, I., Glass, R., & Prothrow-Stith, D. (1998). Income distribution, socioeconomic status, and self-rated health in the United States: Multilevel analysis. *British Medical Journal, 317*, 917–921.

Liden, R. C., Wayne, S. J., & Sparrowe, R. T. (2000). An examination of the mediating role of psychological empowerment on the relation between the job, interpersonal relationships, and work outcomes. *Journal of Applied Psychology, 85*, 407–416.

Lim, S., & Nakamoto, T. (2008). Genograms: Use in therapy with Asian families with diverse cultural heritages. *Contemporary Family Therapy: An International Journal, 30*(4), 199–219. doi:10.1007/s10591-008-9070-6

Mackenbach, J. (1997). Socioeconomic inequalities in morbidity and mortality in Western Europe. *Lancet, 349*, 1655–1659.

Maynard, C., Ehreth, J., Cox, G., Peterson. P., & McGann, M. (1997). Racial differences in the utilization of public mental health services in Washington state. *Administration and Policy in Mental Health, 24*, 411–424.

Merriam-Webster. (2013). In *Merriam-Webster online dictionary*. Retrieved from http://www.merriam-webster.com/browse/dictionary/a.htm?&t=1366032939

Murphy, S., & Rosenbaum, M. (1997). Two women who used cocaine too much: Class, race, gender, crack, and coke. In C. Reinarman & H. Levine (Eds.), *Crack in America: Demon drugs and social justice* (pp. 98–112). Berkeley: University of California Press.

National Admissions to Substance Abuse Treatment Services. *Treatment Episode Data Set (TEDS): 2001–2011*. Retrieved from: http://www.samhsa.gov/data/2k13/TEDS2011/TEDS2011NTOC.htm

Newcomb, M., & Felix-Ortiz, M. (1993). Multiple protective and risk factors for drug use and abuse: Cross-sectional and prospective findings. *Journal of Personality and Social Psychology, 63*, 280–296.

Norcross, J. C. (2011). *Psychotherapy relationships that work: Evidence-based responsiveness* (2nd ed.). New York: Oxford University Press, Inc.

Oshiro, A., Poudyal, A. K., Poudel, K. C., Jimba, M., & Hokama, T. (2010). Intimate partner violence among general and urban poor populations in Kathmandu, Nepal. *Journal of Interpersonal Violence, 26*(10), 2073–2092. doi:10.1177/0886260510372944

Schalock, R. L., & Keith, K. D. (1993). *Quality of life questionnaire*. Worthington, OH: IDS Publishers.

Stevens, P., & Smith, R. L. (2009). *Substance abuse counseling: Theory and practice* (4th ed.). Upper Saddle River, NJ: Pearson Education, Inc.

Substance Abuse and Mental Health Services Administration (SAMHSA). (2011). *Results from the 2010 National Survey on Drug Use and Health: Summary of National Findings*. Retrieved from http://www.samhsa.gov/data/NSDUH/2k10NSDUH/2k10Results.htm#7.1.5

U.S. Bureau of the Census. (2010). *2010 census data.* Retrieved from http://www.census.gov/2010census/data/

U.S. Bureau of the Census. (2012). *Income, poverty, and health insurance coverage in the United States: 2011.* Retrieved from http://www.census.gov/prod/2012pubs/p60-243.pdf

Van Wormer, K., & Rae Davis, D. (2008). *Addiction treatment: A strengths perspective* (2nd ed.). Belmont, CA: Brooks/Cole.

Williams, D. R., & Collins, C. (1995). U.S. socioeconomic and racial differences in health: Patterns and explanations. *Annual Review of Sociology, 21,* 349–386.

Young, M. E. (2013). *Learning the art of helping* (5th ed.). Upper Saddle River, NJ: Pearson.

CHAPTER 16

PERSONS WHO IDENTIFY AS LESBIAN, GAY, BISEXUAL, TRANSGENDER, AND QUESTIONING

By Cher N. Edwards and Christy Bauman

This chapter will address the unique strengths and needs of lesbian, gay, bisexual, transgender, and questioning (LGBTQ) populations when providing substance abuse treatment. The literature reviewed for this chapter includes articles specific to LGB, LGBT, transgender, and LGBTQ populations; therefore, these varying terms will be used throughout to describe the appropriate population. The following pages hope to serve the reader with an overview of the LGBTQ community, an awareness of treatment-specific needs, and recommendations for best practice. The chapter concludes with reflective questions for the treatment provider, as well as resources that may be helpful to LGBTQ populations and the support systems in their lives.

OVERVIEW OF POPULATION

In our society, there has been a steady, continuing progression toward acceptance of sexual minority populations. Even within the LGB community, acceptance and advocacy for alternative sexuality, such as transgender and questioning, have been demonstrated. In areas of research among same-sex and both-sex attraction, there is cooperative growth around issues of health and psychology. Where psychologists once classified same-sex attraction as a mental health disorder, these relationships are now recognized with civil unions and same-sex marriages. In fact, in 2004, Massachusetts was the first state to issue marriage licenses to same-sex couples, and ten years later, in 2014, 17 states now recognize same-sex marriages (Ring, 2014).

Despite the progress made toward acceptance and interest in health concerns experienced by this population, there still appears to be challenges influencing substance use rates. Compared to the general population, the LGBTQ population is more likely to use and abuse alcohol and other drugs (Anderson, 2009; Brewster & Tillman, 2012; Marshal et al., 2008; Russell, Driscoll, & Truong, 2002). In fact, current research contends alcohol abuse is more prevalent among lesbians than the general population. Also, transgender and gay men are estimated to abuse substances around 20–30 percent, in comparison to about 9 percent of the general population (Hunt, 2013). Hunt (2013) reports men who have sex with other men are over 9.5 times more likely to use heroin and 12.2 times more likely to use amphetamines than heterosexual men.

It should be noted, however, that researchers are not in agreement about the prevalence and trends noted in substance use among the LGBT community. Green and Feinstein (2012) indicate there are trends seen in this population such as a decreased likelihood of alcohol abstention, an increased risk for alcohol-related problems, and a lack of typical protective factors. However, methodological flaws exist in the research, which makes one question these findings. Some of these flaws include the specific recruitment strategies used and a lack of comparison groups. These flaws may impact the validity of the research completed with the LGBT populations

Although there has been a growth in exposure, research, advocacy, and treatment for substance abuse, issues continue to exist that impact the health of LGBTQ individuals. For instance, a lack of awareness by others and the microaggressions experienced around homosexuality contribute to the stress of those in the LGBTQ community. Consequently, using alcohol and other drugs is a way to relate and cope with this stress. Moreover, correlations between substance use and shame have been identified, which insinuates addiction for LGBTQ individuals is often perpetuated by embarrassment and guilt from societal pressures and judgments (DiClemente, 2003). Sexual minorities tend to experience high levels of stress associated with social prejudice and discriminatory laws in the areas of employment, relationship recognition, and health care (Center for Substance Abuse Treatment [CSAT], 2001; Hunt, 2013; Jordan, 2000). In order to help combat the misuse of substances in this population, a societal commitment must be made to increase awareness and education related to the particular substance abuse issues faced by the LGBTQ community. The next section addresses several of these substance abuse concerns that may explain the higher rates of chemical use among some people in this population.

SUBSTANCE ABUSE ISSUES

The etiological theories of substance use and abuse for the general population have a long history of research, and these should be considered for specific populations as well. For instance, biological predisposition and environmental stressors are causes that no doubt apply to the LGBTQ population; however, unique issues for this population should also be taken into account (Jordan, 2000). With research indicating the vulnerability of LGBTQ individuals using or abusing substances, the application of social learning theory (Bandura, 1977) may help to provide an understanding related to reasons for use. Current scholarly literature identifies a correlation between individual substance use and peer and partner substance use (Homish & Leonard, 2008). This is based on the notion that behavior is learned through observation and imitation (Bandura, 1977), and individuals are most likely to mirror behaviors of those with whom they spend a significant amount of time.

In addition to social learning theory, several sociocultural factors are also often cited in the literature as influencing substance use in the LGBT populations. Age, gender, bisexuality, affiliation with gay culture, sexual minority stress, "outness," human immunodeficiency virus (HIV) status, and body image are some of these identified factors (Green & Feinstein, 2012). Age is typically a significant protective factor among the general population; however, this is less robust within the LGBT community. In other words, as a person gets older, the frequency and amount of alcohol and other drug use usually decreases. This is not the case in LGBTQ populations. Another sociocultural factor cited to influence rates of use is gender differences. More specifically, female gender status has been identified as a protective factor in the general population, but this is not seen within LGBT populations. One reason for this could be the possibility that LGBT populations may be less conforming to typical gender roles. In addition to age and gender, bisexuality also appears to be a significant risk factor associated with substance abuse. Those who are bisexual indicate a higher likelihood to use and abuse substances to a greater extent than both the heterosexual and gay and lesbian populations. This may be attributed to a lack of social support or potential bias from both communities (Balsam & Mohr, 2007).

Affiliation with gay culture may impact substance use and should be viewed as a critical risk factor for abuse and dependency. As stated earlier, the social learning theory posits behavior may be learned by one's association with peers, partners, and family members. Therefore, the typical social outlets for LGBT populations may impact behaviors, including substance use. Green and Feinstein (2012) note "although LGB communities are not as confined to bars and clubs as in the past, gay bars remain one of the main social outlets in LGB communities" (p. 272). With these places as common settings for socializing, the stigma associated with LGBT populations and substance abuse is perpetuated.

Sexual minority stress is also a contributor to use and abuse, pointing to the social pressure of being part of a marginalized group. An additional consideration related to this issue is that of support systems. Compared to other marginalized groups (e.g., people of color), LGBTQ individuals may not have the typical support systems such as family of origin, who understand or share their experiences as a member of a minority group. Often, LGBTQ individuals face discrimination and rejection by family and other typical supportive networks (Brewster & Tillman, 2012).

"Outness" is described as the degree to which an individual has made others aware of his or her sexual orientation or affection (Green & Feinstein, 2012). The literature (e.g., Green & Feinstein) purports that the more "out" an individual is, the greater propensity for potential discrimination or harassment. This is likely due to the potential for family, friends, and acquaintances to respond negatively to the individual coming out or being out.

Yet another factor to address regarding substance abuse issues in the LGBTQ population is HIV status. Researchers indicate HIV status is positively correlated with substance use and abuse, perhaps due to the anxiety and stress associated with the diagnosis. Alternatively, substance abuse may place an individual at increased risk for HIV infection due to intravenous (IV) drug use and decreased inhibitions, leading to high-risk sexual behavior. In particular, LGB youth may engage in behaviors that put them at higher risk for HIV infection to cope with the stigma associated with sexual orientation/affection and sexual violence (Saewyc et al., 2006).

Substance use is also attributed to body-image issues within the gay community. Researchers noted participants indicated that some members of the gay community use drugs (crystal meth was specifically identified) as an appetite suppressant. These individuals report stress associated with maintaining a certain body image and use to achieve fitness goals (Mutchler, McKay, McDavitt, & Gordon, 2013).

Of the sociocultural factors previously discussed, the most prevalent factor in the literature is related to the stress of being a part of this marginalized population. The application of a minority stress model to the LGBTQ population is one that conceptualizes substance use as a stress reliever (Meyer, 2003). There is a large amount of stress created by the "hostility, discrimination, and violence due to a largely homophobic culture" (Marshal et al., 2008, p. 553). This issue is particularly significant for LGBTQ youth, as substance use may be an attempt to fit into the subculture and rationalize same-sex attraction (Jordan, 2000). The next section outlines the various difficulties the LGBTQ population faces related to substance abuse services.

BARRIERS TO TREATMENT

Substance abuse treatment providers will benefit from being mindful of potential barriers to treatment when working with LGBTQ populations. The social stigma associated with being a sexual minority is compounded when group members are also identified as an alcohol or addict. This phenomenon is referred to as *double stigmatization* and is cited as an obstacle to individuals seeking treatment (Green & Feinstein, 2012).

Implicit and explicit attitudes of treatment providers toward LGBTQ populations, as well as an individual's own internalized heterosexism, may also present as barriers to substance abuse treatment. Even though the attitudes of counselors working with this population are likely to impact treatment retention and outcome, there is a dearth of research focused on the potential bias among mental health providers. Despite the lack of research, ethical codes mandate professional counselors to be culturally competent, and they must provide a safe environment for LGBT clients (Cochran, Peavy, & Cauce, 2007; Cochran, Peavy, & Robohm, 2007). Among this particular population, transgender clients are noted as the group often discriminated against by health care providers, as well as our health care system (Bockting, Robinson, Benner, & Scheltema, 2004).

Additional barriers include the lack of resources available to the person seeking services. For example, homelessness is identified as a major hindrance to treatment among the LGBT population, particularly among sexual minority adolescents (Corliss, Goodenow, Nichols, & Austin, 2011). Without stable housing or a permanent residence, continuity of care and ongoing treatment may be difficult. Another concern that causes problems with treatment is related to health care coverage. LGBTQ minors who need parental consent may avoid treatment because of confidentiality concerns regarding billing and coverage. Moreover, due to the obstacles regarding insurance benefits between people who are gay and lesbian, insurance coverage may be limited. Therefore, the accessibility and attractiveness of treatment, as well as the retention in treatment, may be negatively impacted.

A final barrier significantly represented in the research is the co-occurrence of substance abuse and other mental health issues. LGBT youth tend to experience more bullying, harassment, and physical victimization than their heterosexual peers, and this may contribute to higher rates of depression, anxiety, self-harm behaviors, and suicide attempts (Almeida, Johnson, Corliss, Molnar, & Azrael, 2009; Suicide Prevention Resource Center, 2008). Researchers indicate there is a rise in suicidal ideation, as well as suicidal attempts, around the time of coming out. In fact, LGB youth who had disclosed to their families were more than four times as likely to have attempted suicide as LGB youth who had not disclosed (Suicide Prevention Resource Center, 2008). The severity and prevalence of mental health conditions among this population do not lessen as a person ages. As stated earlier, the stress encountered due to (a) the prejudice, discrimination, and marginalization of being LGBT; (b) internalized homophobia; and (c) the coming-out process can all lead to an increase in depression and anxiety as an adult (Meyer, 2003). In a study focusing on LGBT individuals in a substance abuse treatment program, approximately 94 percent were diagnosed with at least one personality disorder. The most common diagnoses (listed in order of prevalence) were borderline, obsessive-compulsive, and avoidant (Grant, Flynn, Odlaug, & Schreiber, 2011). In summary, a mental health condition may facilitate substance use and can become a barrier for treatment. Given the likelihood that LGBT individuals experience high levels of stress—as well as depression, anxiety, or even a personality disorder—counselors must consider the implications for treatment access, retention, and outcomes.

SCREENING AND ASSESSMENT

Culturally competent and sensitive screening is imperative when working with LGBTQ populations. In essence, the most important screening and assessment consideration is the clinician. Substance abuse treatment clinicians must seek out appropriate training and assess their own biases and stereotypes prior to attempting to serve as advocates and providers for this population. Recognizing the contributing factors and barriers to substance abuse treatment is useful when identifying treatment options. Through formal (instruments) or informal (interview) assessments, counselors should be mindful of how the client's internalized oppression, cultural identity, and co-occurring challenges (e.g., homelessness, mental health diagnosis, HIV status, discrimination) impact current use and potential outcomes. Cochran, Peavy, and Cauce (2007) provide an example of an instrument (the *Measure of Attitudes Toward Gay, Lesbian, Bisexual, and Transgender Clients*) that may be useful for clinicians to assess their competency related to serving clients who are LGBTQ.

Specific assessment foci are recommended when interviewing a client who identifies as LGBTQ. Counselors are to be intentional in their understanding about the client's (a) self-identity and the coming-out process; (b) available social supports; (c) relationship with family of origin; (d) romantic and sexual history; (e) present attraction and relationships; and (f) spirituality and religious beliefs (Ratner, 1993). Exercise caution when attending to the aforementioned recommendations, as some topics may be better broached once rapport is further established. A premature discussion of sexual history, for example, could evoke shame or perceived judgment and may inadvertently impact treatment negatively.

This chapter has predominantly focused on treatment for individuals who self-report as LGBTQ. However, given the importance of culturally relevant treatment that includes sexual identity, it is relevant to consider how to best serve LGBTQ clients who do not readily identify as such. In an effort to address this concern, Barbara, Chaim, and Doctor (2002) developed an assessment titled, "Asking the right questions: Talking about sexual orientation and gender identity during assessment for drug and alcohol concerns." Refer to Appendix A for sample questions. Whether or not an assessment specifically designed for reaching a non–self-reporting audience is utilized or not, it is important that practitioners consider factors related to affection, sexual orientation, and relationship history and attraction when assessing for substance abuse issues. To clarify, the purpose of this inclusion is not to identify an individual as lesbian, gay, bisexual, or transgender. More importantly, counselors should consider how factors associated with affection and attraction may impact substance use and treatment and acknowledge that the individual has the right not to self-disclose and is on a journey of identity development.

RESILIENCY FACTORS

Fostering resiliency in clients is extremely important in the work of a substance abuse treatment provider. Some clients may present with a fierce strength from within, while others appear broken and weak. A counselor must take on a strengths-based perspective that encourages clients to become aware of the support systems and personal attributes that will serve them well in their recovery. Thus, being knowledgeable regarding typical resiliency factors among LGBTQ clients is useful in treatment planning.

Identifying, utilizing, and creating support networks, recognizing role models, visualizing self as a potential role model for others, and being able to self-advocate are identified as resiliency factors (Holmes & Cahill, 2013). Counselors may support clients by assisting them in identifying existing and available support systems in their lives and helping clients find their voices to advocate for themselves and others. Clients may be unaware of organized resources in their schools and communities that are well positioned to serve as a means of support and an opportunity for them to help others. Although internalized heterosexism is often referred to as a source of pain, being able to resolve it through faith and spirituality can be a source of resiliency as well (Kubicek et al., 2009). Counselors may serve clients effectively by: (a) considering the role of spirituality in the lives of their clients; (b) acknowledging the pain that may be associated with faith or religion; and (c) assisting clients in attending to themselves as spiritual beings.

RECOMMENDATIONS FOR TREATMENT AND THERAPEUTIC CONSIDERATIONS

There are therapeutic considerations that counselors must take into account regarding those within the LGBTQ population. First, the authors will address and define terminology that is particular to this population. Next, the therapeutic relationship and issues of sponsorship will be explored. Last, concerns about the coming-out process, families of origin and families of choice, and clinical issues pertaining to lesbians, gay males, bisexual, transgender, and questioning clients will be presented.

Terminology for LGBTQ

Counselors would benefit to use and understand appropriate language when working with LGBTQ clients. For instance, sexual identity, sexual orientation, gender role, gender identity, heterosexism, and homophobia are basic terminology one needs to understand to offer constructive therapeutic work. *Sexual identity* is the awareness a person has toward his or her own sexual desires. Exploring and distinguishing the client's sexual identity in a safe environment is an imperative part of therapy. Once there has been foundational work around sexual identity, the client moves on to exploring sexual orientation. *Sexual orientation* is considered to be the romantic attraction to the opposite sex, the same sex, or both sexes (McCabe, Hughes, Bostwick, Morales, & Boyd, 2012). Sexual behavior does not equal sexual orientation; one's sexual orientation refers to self-concepts and feelings. Only more recently have lawmakers and activists fought to make sexual orientation treated with equality, nondiscrimination, and dignity. Because of the negativity and prejudices in the past tied to sexual behaviors of the LGBTQ community, it is mandatory to differentiate sexual behavior from orientation (Human Rights Education Associates, 2011).

Indicators of one's *biological sex* include sex chromosomes, gonads, internal reproductive organs, and external genitalia. *Transgender* refers to persons whose gender identity, expression, or behavior does not correspond to that typically correlated with the sex to which they were ascribed at birth, whereas a *transsexual* shifts from one gender to another and may involve transitioning to a gender that is neither traditionally male nor female. A *transvestite*, who is more often a male, is a person who adopts the dress and sometimes the behavior emblematic of the opposite sex, especially for purposes of emotional or sexual gratification. *Questioning* or *queer* is often referred as the "Q" in LGBTQ and encompasses any exploration or uncertainty of one's sexual orientation, gender, or identity (American Psychological Association, 2014).

Gender role is customary to a particular culture's view of behaviors, which are either perceived as masculine or feminine. Gender roles and sexual orientation are not to be confused with *gender identity*, which is one's sense of self as either male or female. Within the therapeutic process, each individual will choose how to relate these definitions to oneself within culture, family, religion/spirituality, and society. This type of dialogue will occur after clients have established how to admit, accept, and engage their own sexual identity and orientation (Substance Abuse and Mental Health Services Administration [SAMHSA], 2012).

In correlation with understanding the terminology and psychological complexities of gay, lesbian, bisexual, and transgender issues, a counselor must also recognize the transference and countertransference of heterosexism and homophobia. *Heterosexism* is a bias for opposite-sex relationships and can mirror racism or sexism toward nonheterosexual relationships. Examples of heterosexism are acts such as internal beliefs, ideologies, and societal patterns that support superiority over same-sex couples. *Homophobia* is defined as an irrational fear or aversion toward LGBT sexuality or persons. Acts of homophobia might include interpersonal incidents such as conversations or jokes misrepresenting or putting down LGBT individuals. Counselors must not only define, but also understand, these perceptions as an imperative part of doing effective therapeutic work with LGBTQ clients (CSAT, 2001).

The Therapeutic Relationship

Countertransference issues are important concerns to address because they can impact the therapeutic relationship. Therapists with the same sexual minority identity as their client might minimize the client's substance abuse more easily and might also anticipate idealization of the client (Greene & Faltz, 1992). Alternatively, a heterosexual therapist's inaccurate beliefs about homosexuality might complicate therapy. Moreover, a therapist may assume that the client's sexual orientation is the cause of substance abuse problems and might lean toward inappropriately making a therapeutic goal of changing the client's sexual orientation. It is imperative for therapists to have done their own work and identify their personal story, prejudices, and beliefs around sexuality.

Sponsorship

Another consideration for substance abuse counselors is sponsorship in recovery. Alcoholics Anonymous, Narcotics Anonymous, or other self-help groups encourage clients to obtain a sponsor. Although there is little research discussing sexual orientation and sponsorship, consideration must be given when choosing whether a sponsor has the same gender and sexual orientation (Ratner, 1993). In addition to self-help group considerations, substance abuse treatment programs and counselors should make efforts to provide competent services to this population. A counselor's spoken awareness and willingness to understand these issues can allow clients to speak openly and lessen their fears about their sexual orientation.

The Coming-Out Process

Counselors must be familiar with the "coming-out" process and the implications it has for clients. This process refers to the course of changing a negative self-identity to a positive self-identity with regard to sexual orientation. This process is particularly important to many gay and lesbian people who are recovering from substance abuse, as recovery from addiction requires an affirming and positive feeling about oneself. Cass (1979) proposes six stages within the framework of interpersonal congruency theory, in which individuals form their own identity and self-concept with homosexuality. The six stages of sexual identity development are: (1) identity confusion; (2) identity comparison; (3) identity tolerance; (4) identity acceptance; (5) identity pride; and (6) identity synthesis. It is understood these stages play only a framework to the conversation of "coming out." See Appendix B for more detailed information regarding the six stages of the Cass (1979) model.

Using these stages to conceptualize the client's self-identification as lesbian or gay would benefit a clinician to cultivate work facilitating client movement toward an affirming identity. Often, degradation and shame are leading issues interfering with the attainment of a healthy and constructive sexual identity (Bradshaw, 1988). Addressing and combating the shame in context of coming out is a positive step in the abstention or moderation of substance use. After sexual identity has been established, the counselor will move toward working with the client's family systems within his or her family of origin.

There are other issues that can arise in therapeutic work, as some individuals do not wish to come out or openly identify themselves as lesbian, bisexual, gay, transgender, or questioning. Clients may identify and "own" their sexuality in the therapy office, while choosing to not make their sexual identity known elsewhere. The therapist must continue to offer a safe place for clients to continue to explore their sexuality and way of life.

Further, the category of Questioning includes people who are still uncertain about their sexual identity, gender, and sexual orientation and who may be still exploring these areas of their lives. Many times, Questioning individuals are reluctant to put a name on their sexuality due to societal stigmas and labels. Although therapeutic work around naming sexual identity is helpful to those in confusion identity stage, it does not alleviate the pressure of social and familial judgments. Therapy with clients who are questioning should incorporate discussions around gender identification and whom they have crushes on and/or fantasize about being with sexually (i.e., sexual identity).

To assist clinicians with clients who may be coming out, SAMHSA (2012) provides the following recommendations. The counselor can:

- encourage a discussion of how the client hid his or her LGBT feelings from others
- explore the emotional costs of hiding and denying one's sexuality
- discuss attempts the client has made to change in an effort to fit in
- examine negative feelings of self-blame, feeling "bad" or "sick," and the impact of shaming messages on the client
- foster the client's courage to accept and speak up about who he or she is (SAMHSA, 2012, p. 117).

Family of Origin and Family of Choice

One of the most noteworthy elements of treating issues of substance abuse is exploring the family dynamics a client has encountered. A comprehensive biopsychosocial assessment includes exploration of family systems and origin. Thoughtfulness should be used when addressing family-of-origin matters, as unresolved issues with family members are common in regard to disclosure of sexual identity. To assist with these issues, the support group Parents, Families and Friends of Lesbians and Gays (PFLAG) works with families of origin. The LGBTQ community may have also built close relationships with what is called *family of choice*. Family of choice is usually comprised of people who are most noted for helping and caring for someone who has been rejected from his or her family due to sexual orientation. These usually include friends who have been accepting and understanding through the process of coming out.

Clinical Issues to Consider with LGBTQ Clients

This section of the chapter has mostly discussed treatment considerations for the LGBTQ population as a whole. It is also imperative to look at the specific concerns that arise for those who identify as lesbian, gay, bisexual, transgender, or questioning. The following is a summary of the particular clinical issues among the sexual minority populations, as identified in the literature:

Clinical Issues with Lesbian Clients (Hughes & Wilsnack, 1997)
- Patterns of substance abuse vary
- Alcohol problems are higher for lesbians than for heterosexual women
- Stressors to coming out or "passing" as heterosexual
- Effects of trauma from violence or abuse

Clinical Issues with Gay Male Clients (CSAT, 2001)
- "Gay ghetto," which refers to the area in each city where gay men tend to congregate and often is associated with alcohol and drug use
- HIV/AIDS continues to be a major factor
- Substance use allows men to act on suppressed feelings, but harder to integrate sex and intimacy
- Males who do not fit the stereotypical male role
- Being effeminate in the gay community is sometimes condemned and increases shame

Clinical Issues with Bisexual Clients (CSAT, 2001)
- Bisexuals may feel alienated, not just from the heterosexual majority, but also the lesbian and gay community
- Internalized biphobia may result in self-abasement
- Bias counselors who might see bisexuality as borderline personality disorder with fluctuating sexual behavior as a symptom of acting out or poor impulse control

Clinical Issues with Transgender Clients (Lewis, Dana, & Blevins, 1994)
- Transsexualism has historically been viewed as psychopathological and classified as gender identity disorder
- Extremely high rates of substance abuse in the transgender community
- Treatment must be multimodal to address multiple problems and patterns of abuse
- Societal, internalized transphobia, violence, discrimination, family problems, isolation, low self-esteem, lack of educational and job opportunities

- Often distrustful of health care providers because of many negative experiences
- Hormone treatment and therapy must be monitored closely through treatment for substance abuse
- In-patient treatment faces multiple issues with housing, rest rooms, and sleeping arrangement logistics
- Open-ended questions should be asked regarding sexual and gender orientation

Clinical Issues with Questioning clients (APA, 2014)
- Often, adolescents are in a period of experimentation, and many youths may question their sexual feelings
- Affirmation that awareness of sexual feelings is a normal developmental task that is beneficial to explore
- Exploring and talking through same-sex feelings or experiences that cause confusion about their sexual orientation
- This confusion appears to decline over time, with different outcomes for different individuals
- Open-ended questions should always be used when working with Questioning clients
- Inquiring about stereotypes and prejudices that might obstruct the client's desire to explore further

CONCLUSION

This chapter serves as an introduction to the distinctive needs of many individuals within the LGBTQ community. It is important to note that many factors impact culture. Therefore, the information presented is based on social norms and should not be considered as an absolute for individuals within this specific population. Cultural competency and sensitivity are imperative when serving all populations, but particularly those who are often marginalized and underserved. Counselors providing substance abuse treatment to LGBTQ populations will benefit from ongoing self-reflection, professional development and training, and consultation/supervision. This chapter ends with questions for reflection, as the reader begins or continues the journey of advocating for the health and wellness of LGBTQ clients. References and resources are also found in the appendices that may be of further support.

Reflection Questions

1. How prepared are you to work with LGBTQ clients? Why?
2. Identify at least two areas of additional training that would help you be a more effective advocate and supporter of LGBTQ clients.
3. What bias or stereotypes about lesbians, gays, bisexuals, and transgenders do you hold?
4. When is the last time you participated in an LGBT event or have been socially engaged with people who are lesbian, gay, bisexual, or transgender?
5. What plans do you have to continue to grow professionally (e.g., professional development), personally (e.g., your own work), and socially that will best support you to serve the LGBT population?

REFERENCES

Almeida, J., Johnson, R. M., Corliss, H. L., Molnar, B. E., & Azrael, D. (2009). Emotional distress among LGBT youth: The influence of perceived discrimination based on sexual orientation. *Journal of Youth and Adolescence, 38,* 1001–1014.

American Psychological Association. (2014). Lesbian, Gay, Bisexual, and Transgender concerns. Retrieved at http://www.apa.org/pi/lgbt/index.aspx

Anderson, S. C. (2009). *Substance use disorders in lesbian, gay, bisexual, and transgender clients: Assessment and treatment.* New York: Columbia University.

Balsam, K. F., & Mohr, J. J. (2007). Adaptation to sexual orientation stigma: A comparison of bisexual and lesbian/gay adults. *Journal of Counseling Psychology, 54*(3), 306–319. doi:10.1037/0022-0167.54.3.306

Bandura, A. (1977). *Social learning theory.* Englewood Cliffs, NJ: Prentice Hall.

Barbara, A. M., Chaim, G., & Doctor, F. (2002). *Asking the right questions: Talking about sexual orientation and gender identity during assessment for drug and alcohol concerns.* Toronto: Centre for Addiction and Mental Health.

Bockting, W., Robinson, B., Benner, A., & Scheltema, K. (2004). Patient satisfaction with transgender health services. *Journal of Sex & Marital Therapy, 30*(4), 277–294. doi:10.1080/00926230490422467

Bradshaw, J. (1988). *Healing the shame that binds you.* Deerfield Beach, FL: Health Communications.

Brewster, K. L., & Tillman, K. H. (2012). Sexual orientation and substance use among adolescents and young adults. *American Journal of Public Health, 102*(6), 1168–1176.

Cass, V. C. (1979). Homosexuality identity formation: A theoretical model. *Journal of Homosexuality, 4*(3), 219–235. doi:10.1300/j082v04n03_01

Center for Substance Abuse Treatment (2001). *A provider's introduction to substance abuse treatment for lesbian, gay, bisexual and transgender individuals.* Rockville, MD: The Center.

Cochran, B. N., Peavy, K., & Cauce, A. (2007). Substance abuse treatment providers' explicit and implicit attitudes regarding sexual minorities. *Journal of Homosexuality, 53*(3), 181–207. doi:10.1300/J082v53n03_10

Cochran, B. N., Peavy, K. M., & Robohm, J. S. (2007). Do specialized services exist for LGBT individuals seeking treatment for substance misuse? A study of available treatment programs. *Substance Use & Misuse, 42*(1), 161–176. doi:10.1080/10826080601094207

Corliss, H. L., Goodenow, C. S., Nichols, L., & Austin, S. B. (2011). High burden of homelessness among sexual-minority adolescents: Findings from a representative Massachusetts high school sample. *American Journal of Public Health, 101*(9), 1683–1689. doi:10.2105/AJPH.2011.3000155

DiClemente, C. C. (2003). *Addiction and change: How addictions develop and addicted people recover.* New York: Guilford Press.

Grant, J. E., Flynn, M., Odlaug, B. L., & Schreiber, L. R. (2011). Personality disorders in gay, lesbian, bisexual, and transgender chemically dependent patients. *American Journal on Addictions, 20*(5), 405–411. doi:10.111/j.1521-0391.2011.00155.x

Green, K. E., & Feinstein, B. A. (2012). Substance use in lesbian, gay, and bisexual populations: An update on empirical research and implications for treatment. *Psychology of Addictive Behaviors, 26*(2), 265–278. doi:10.1037/a0025424

Greene, D., & Faltz, B. (1992). Chemical dependency and relapse in gay men with HIV infection: Issues and treatment. *Journal of Chemical Dependency Treatment, 4*(2), 79–90. doi:10.1300/J034v04n02_08

Holmes, S., & Cahill, S. (2003). School experiences of gay, lesbian, bisexual and transgender youth. *Journal of Gay & Lesbian Issues in Education, 1*(3), 53–66. doi:10.1300/J367v01n03_06

Homish, G. G., & Leonard, K. E. (2008). The social network and alcohol use. *Journal of Studies on Alcohol and Drugs, 69*(6), 906–914.

Hughes, T. L., & Wilsnack, S. C. (1997). Use of alcohol among lesbians: Research and clinical implications. *American Journal of Orthopsychiatry, 67*(1), 20–36. doi: 10.1037/h0080208

Human Rights Education Associates (2011). Sexual Orientation and Human Rights. Retrieved from http://www.hrea.org/index.php?base_id=161

Hunt, J. (2013). *Why the gay and transgender population experiences higher rates of substance use.* Center for American Progress. Retrieved from http://www.americanprogress.org/issues/lgbt/report/2012/03/09/11228/why-the-gay-and-transgender-population-experiences-higher-rates-of-substance-use/

Jordan, K. M. (2000). Substance abuse among gay, lesbian, bisexual, transgender, and questioning adolescents. *School Psychology Review, 29*(2), 201–206.

Kubicek, K., McDavitt, B., Carpineto, J., Weiss, G., Iverson, E. F., & Kipke, M. D. (2009). "God made me gay for a reason": Young men who have sex with men's resiliency in resolving internalized homophobia from religious sources. *Journal of Adolescent Research, 24*(5), 601–633. doi:10.1177/0743558409341078

Lewis, J. A., Dana, R. Q., & Blevins, G. A. (1994). *Substance abuse counseling* (2nd ed). Belmont, CA: Brooks/Cole Publishing.

Marshal, M. P., et al. (2008). REVIEW: Sexual orientation and adolescent substance use: A meta-analysis and methodological review. *Addiction, 103*(4), 546–556. doi:10.1111/j.1360-0443.2008.02149.x

McCabe, S. E., Hughes, T. L., Bostwick, W., Morales, M., & Boyd, C. J. (2012). Measurement of sexual identity in surveys: Implications for substance abuse research. *Archives of Sexual Behavior, 41*(3), 649–657. doi:10.1007/S10508-011-9768-7

Meyer, I. H. (2003). Prejudice, social stress, and mental health in lesbian, gay, and bisexual populations: Conceptual issues and research evidence. *Psychological Bulletin, 129*(5), 674–697. doi:10.1037/0033-2909.129.5.674

Mutchler, M. G., McKay, T., McDavitt, B., & Gordon, K. K. (2013). Using peer ethnography to address health disparities among young urban Black and Latino men who have sex with men. *American Journal of Public Health, 103*(5), 849–852. doi:10.2105/AJPH.2012.3000988

Ratner, E. F. (1993) Treatment issues for chemically dependent lesbians and gay men. In L. D. Garnets & D. C. Kimmel (Eds.), *Psychological perspectives on lesbian and gay male experiences* (567–578). New York: Columbia University.

Ring, T. (2014, January). Judge says OK to marriage equality in Oklahoma. *Advocate*. Retrieved from http://www.advocate.com/politics/marriage-equality/2014/01/14/breaking-judge-says-ok-marriage-equality-oklahoma

Russell, S. T., Driscoll, A. K., & Truong, N. (2002). Adolescent same-sex romantic attractions and relationships: Implications for substance use and abuse. *American Journal of Public Health, 92*(2), 198–202. doi:10.2105/AJPH.92.2.198

Saewyc, E., Skay, C., Richens, K., Reis, E., Poon, C., & Murphy, A. (2006) Sexual orientation, sexual abuse, and HIV-risk behaviors in the Pacific Northwest. *American Journal of Public Health*, 1104–1110. doi:10.2105%2FAJPH.2005.065870

Substance Abuse and Mental Health Services Administration (2012). *A provider's introduction to substance abuse treatment for Lesbian, Gay, Bisexual, and Transgender individuals.* Rockville, MD: Substance Abuse and Mental Health Services Administration.

Suicide Prevention Resource Center (2008). Suicide risk and prevention for lesbian, gay, bisexual, and transgender youth. Newton, MA: Education Development Center, Inc.

APPENDIX A

"Asking the Right Questions"

Part A

Are you currently dating, sexually active or in a relationship(s)? Yes_____ No_____

If yes... is (are) your partner(s) __ female __ male __ transgender __ transsexual __ other _____

How long have you been dating or in a relationship? _____

How important is this (are these) relationship(s) to you? __ not much __ somewhat __ very much

If you have had previous relationships, was (were) your partner(s) __ female __ male __ transgender __ transsexual __ other _____

In terms of your sexual orientation, do you identify with a particular group? gay_____, lesbian_____, straight/heterosexual_____, bisexual_____, unsure_____, or none of the above_____

Are there concerns or questions related to your sexual orientation/identity or do you ever feel uncomfortable about your sexuality? Yes_____ No_____

Part B

Can you tell me about any interactions you have encountered because of homophobia?

How open are you about your sexual orientation? How do you feel about the orientation with which you identify yourself?

Where are you at regarding your coming out process?

How has your sexual orientation affected your relationship with your family?

Is your family supportive of you?

Can you tell me about your involvement and acceptance in the gay, lesbian, bi, and trans community?

For gay/bisexual men only: Do you ever worry about HIV?

If yes... In what ways?

Have you ever used substances to cope with any of the issues we mentioned above? Yes_____ No_____

If yes... In what ways?

Adapted from Barbara, A. M., Chaim, G., & Doctor, F. (2002). *Asking the right questions: Talking about sexual orientation and gender identity during assessment for drug and alcohol concerns.* Toronto: Centre for Addiction and Mental Health.

APPENDIX B

Cass Model of Homosexual Identity Development

1. **Identity Confusion:**

   "Could I be gay?" Person is beginning to wonder if "homosexuality" is personally relevant. Denial and confusion is experienced.

   Task: Who am I? –Accept, Deny, Reject.

   Possible Responses: Will avoid information about lesbians and gays; inhibit behavior; deny homosexuality ("experimenting," "an accident," "just drunk"). Males: May keep emotional involvement separate from sexual contact. Females: May have deep relationships that are nonsexual, though strongly emotional.

   Possible Needs: May explore internal positive and negative judgments. Will be permitted to be uncertain regarding sexual identity. May find support in knowing that sexual behavior occurs along a spectrum. May receive permission and encouragement to explore sexual identity as a normal experience (like career identity and social identity).

2. **Identity Comparison:**

   "Maybe this does apply to me." Will accept the possibility that she or he may be gay. Self-alienation becomes isolation.

   Task: Deal with social alienation.

   Possible Responses: May begin to grieve for losses and the things she or he will give up by embracing their sexual orientation. May compartmentalize their own sexuality. Accepts lesbian, gay definition of behavior but maintains "heterosexual" identity of self. Tells oneself, "It's only temporary"; "I'm just in love with this particular woman/man," etc.

   Possible Needs: Will be very important that the person develops own definitions. Will need information about sexual identity, lesbian, gay community resources, encouragement to talk about loss of heterosexual life expectations. May be permitted to keep some "heterosexual" identity (it is not an all or none issue).

3. **Identity Tolerance:**

   "I'm not the only one." Accepts the probability of being homosexual and recognizes sexual, social, emotional needs that go with being lesbian and gay. Increased commitment to being lesbian or gay.

   Task: Decrease social alienation by seeking out lesbians and gays.

   Possible Responses: Beginning to have language to talk and think about the issue. Recognition that being lesbian or gay does not preclude other options. Accentuates difference between self and heterosexuals. Seeks out lesbian and gay culture (positive contact leads to more positive sense of self, negative contact leads to devaluation of the culture, stops growth). May try out variety of stereotypical roles.

Possible Needs: Be supported in exploring own shame feelings derived from heterosexism, as well as external heterosexism. Receive support in finding positive lesbian, gay community connections. It is particularly important for the person to know community resources.

4. **Identity Acceptance:**
"I will be okay." Accepts, rather than tolerates, gay or lesbian self-image. There is continuing and increased contact with the gay and lesbian culture.

Task: Deal with inner tension of no longer subscribing to society's norm, attempt to bring congruence between private and public view of self.

Possible Responses: Accepts gay or lesbian self-identification. May compartmentalize "gay life." Maintains less and less contact with heterosexual community. Attempts to "fit in" and "not make waves" within the gay and lesbian community. Begins some selective disclosures of sexual identity. More social coming out; more comfortable being seen with groups of men or women that are identified as "gay." More realistic evaluation of situation.

Possible Needs: Continue exploring grief and loss of heterosexual life expectations. Continue exploring internalized "homophobia" (learned shame for heterosexist society). Find support in making decisions about where, when, and to whom he or she self-discloses.

5. **Identity Pride:**
"I've got to let people know who I am!" Immerses self in gay and lesbian culture. Less and less involvement with heterosexual community. Us-them quality to political/social viewpoint.

Task: Deal with incongruent views of heterosexuals.

Possible Responses: Splits world into "gay" (good) and "straight" (bad). Experiences disclosure crises with heterosexuals, as he or she is less willing to "blend in." Identifies gay culture as sole source of support; all gay friends, business connections, social connections.

Possible Needs: Receive support for exploring anger issues. Find support for exploring issues of heterosexism. Develop skills for coping with reactions and responses to disclosure of sexual identity. Resist being defensive!

6. **Identity Synthesis:**
Develops holistic view of self. Defines self in a more complete fashion, not just in terms of sexual orientation.

Task: Integrate gay and lesbian identity so that instead of being the identity, it is an aspect of self.

Possible Responses: Continues to be angry at heterosexism, but with decreased intensity. Allows trust of others to increase and build. Gay and lesbian identity is integrated with all aspects of "self." Feels all right to move out into the community and not simply define space according to sexual orientation.

Adapted from: Vivienne C. Cass, "Cass Model of Homosexual Identity Development," Journal of Homosexuality, vol. 4, no. 3.

CHAPTER 17

PERSONS WITHIN THE MILITARY

By Joan McDowell and Jessica Rodriguez

OVERVIEW OF SUBSTANCE ABUSE IN MILITARY POPULATIONS

Veterans and military personnel are a unique subset of the United States (U.S.) population related to their experiences serving in the Army, Navy, Air Force, Marine Corps, or Coast Guard. As of 2010, approximately nine percent of the population consisted of individuals who previously served in the U.S. Armed Forces (i.e., veterans; U.S. Census Bureau, 2012). Additionally, nearly one percent of the population maintains active involvement in the U.S. Armed Forces (i.e., active duty, Reserves, or National Guard; Office of the Deputy Under Secretary of Defense, 2010). Evans (2012) reports that "as of September 2011, there were 1,468,364 active duty military personnel and in 2010, there were 21.8 million veterans in the United States" (p. 470). The vast majority of veterans are male (93 percent), Caucasian (84 percent), and age 55 or older (67 percent; U.S. Census Bureau, 2012). Active duty personnel are, by comparison, somewhat more diverse: predominantly male (86 percent), Caucasian (63 percent), and an average age of 28.5 (Office of the Deputy Under Secretary of Defense, 2010).

Definitions and Prevalence of Substance Use

While definitions of substance use difficulties vary, *risky alcohol use* or *binge drinking* may be defined as consuming greater than three alcoholic drinks per occasion or greater than seven alcoholic drinks per week for women and greater than four drinks per occasion or greater than 14 drinks per week for men (Department of Veteran Affairs, Department of Defense, 2009). *Substance misuse* is defined as substance use that results in negative consequences for the individual, but remains under the threshold for diagnosis of a substance use disorder (SUD). *Substance abuse* and *substance dependence* are disorders defined by the fourth edition of the *Diagnostic and Statistical Manual of Mental Disorders* (DSM-IV-TR; American Psychiatric Association, 2000). Most recent research studies utilize these criteria to classify subjects. At the time of this text, the fifth edition of the DSM (DSM-V) was published, and with its publication, the diagnostic criteria for substance use disorders have changed. Substance use and substance dependence have been combined into one diagnostic category (substance use disorders), based on the substance and quantified by level of severity (i.e., mild, moderate, or severe). Certainly, as research on SUDs progresses, additional findings based on this newer classification will be forthcoming.

Alcohol use

A nationally representative study of veterans and civilians conducted in 2004 reveals less alcohol use (58.5 percent), binge drinking (13.3 percent), and heavy alcohol use (5.0 percent) among veterans than nonveterans (63.7 percent, 25.7 percent, and 6.3 percent, respectively) after controlling for sociodemographic factors (Bohnert et al., 2012). Exceptions to this finding include veterans aged 61 to 70, who reported higher rates of heavy drinking than nonveterans. Studies sampling military personnel and veterans from more recent conflicts such as Operation Enduring Freedom and Operation Iraqi Freedom (OEF/OIF), find that National Guard and Reserve personnel demonstrate a heightened risk of alcohol use difficulties over and above that of regular active-duty personnel (Bray et al., 2009; Jacobson et al., 2008). Rates of alcohol use disorders in female veterans (4.8 percent alcohol use disorder, 2.4 percent drug use disorder) tend to be lower than that of male veterans (10.5 percent and 4.8 percent, respectively; Seal et al., 2011). When comparisons are made by age group/war era, studies show that younger males (predominantly from OEF/OIF) have higher rates of alcohol misuse (21.8 percent) than older (non–OEF/OIF) males (10.5 percent; Hawkins, Lapham, Kivlahan, & Bradley, 2010). No differences in war eras were found for female veterans (Hawkins et al., 2010). Taken together, these results indicate individuals who are young, male, active duty, or have Reserve or National Guard status are the populations with the highest likelihood of alcohol use difficulties.

Use of other substances

Studies of illicit drug misuse, including prescription drug misuse, show rates of approximately 12 percent among active-duty military personnel (Bray et al., 2009). This percentage is a sharp increase from previous estimates, and the increase is primarily attributed to rising rates of prescription drug abuse (Bray et al., 2009; Jeffery, Babeu, Nelson, Kloc, & Klette, 2013). However, rates of illicit drug use among military personnel continue to be lower than civilians (14 percent; Bray et al., 2009). Excluding prescription drug abuse, rates of illicit drug abuse have remained relatively stable among military personnel: two percent in 2005 and 2008. Among OEF/OIF veterans receiving care through the Department of Veterans Affairs (VA), Seal et al. (2011) found rates of illicit drug abuse and dependence at 3.9 percent and 2.7 percent, respectively. Cannabis is the most commonly used illicit drug among veterans, with a rate of use of 3.5 percent in the previous month (Bray et al., 2009; National Survey on Drug Use and Health, 2005).

Cigarette use among active military members has been decreasing since 2002. Use of cigarettes during the previous month was reported at 31 percent in 2008, similar to civilian rates (30 percent, Bray et al., 2009). Rates of cigarette use for veterans have been reported at approximately 20 percent (Department of Veterans Affairs Veterans Health Administration, Office of the Assistant Deputy Under Secretary for Health for Policy and Planning, 2012); however, risk for use of cigarettes among veterans with mental health difficulties is reported as twofold that of individuals without mental health difficulties (e.g., Duffy et al., 2012). Tobacco use is an important health concern and is addressed within the VA and Department of Defense (DoD)

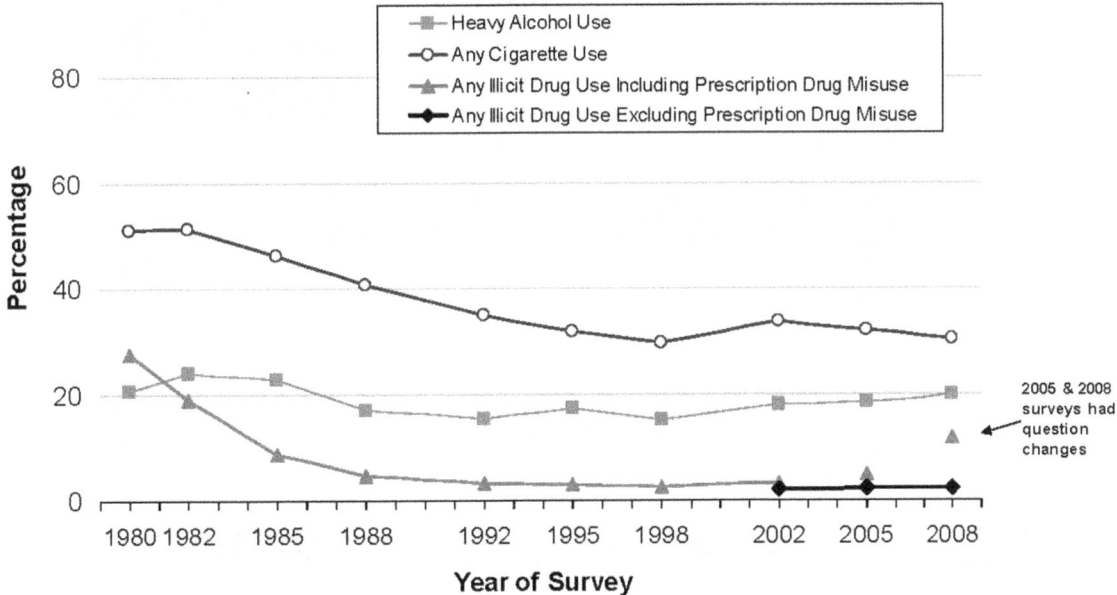

Heavy Alcohol Use = 5 or more drinks __n the same occasion at least once a week in past 30 days.
Any Illicit Drug Use Including Prescription = use of marijuana, cocaine (including crack). hallucinogens (PCP, MDA, MDMA, and other hallucinogens), heroin, methamphetamine, inhalants, GHB/GBL, or non-medical use of prescription-type amphetamines/stimulants, tranquilizers/muscle relaxers, barbiturates/sedatives, or pain relievers.
Any Illicit Drug Use Excluding Prescription Drug Misuse- use of marijuana, cocaine (including crack), hallucinogens (PCP, MDA. MDMA, and other hallucinogens), heroin, inhalants, or GHB/GBL.

Figure 17.1. Substance Use Trends for DoD Services, Past 30 Days, 1980–2008

Source: Karen H. Seal, et al., from "Substance Use Disorders in Iraq and Afghanistan Veterans in VA Healthcare, 2001-2010: Implications for Screening, Diagnosis and Treatment Drug and Alcohol Dependence, vol. 116, nos. 1-3. Copyright © 2011 by Elsevier Science and Technology. Reprinted with permission.

through regular screenings, education, and treatment. Due to space limitations, it will not be addressed in depth in this chapter. (Refer to Hamlett et al., 2009, for more information See Figure 17.1 for information on substance use trends from 1980 to 2008.)

Substance Abuse Etiology

Several studies have examined the etiology of substance use problems in current and previous military personnel. The two most common explanations for the onset of SUDs include the self-medication hypothesis and the high-risk hypothesis (e.g., Kessler, 2004; Kessler et al., 1996). Most risk factors associated with the likelihood of substance abuse (e.g., co-occurring mental disorders, low socioeconomic status) can be classified under these two theories. Protective factors, which are aspects of one's life that reduce the likelihood of developing a SUD, will also be discussed. Refer to Table 17.1 below for a list of both risk and protective factors.

Table 17.1: A Summary of Factors Increasing or Decreasing Risk of SUDs in the Military Population

FACTORS THAT INCREASE RISK
Self-medication hypothesis
Comorbid psychiatric condition (e.g., post-traumatic stress disorder, depression)
Co-occurring condition (e.g., chronic pain, traumatic brain injury)
High-risk hypothesis
Caucasian
Unmarried
Younger age
Low socioeconomic status
Lack of social support
Disruptive life events
Antisocial behavior
Personality factors (e.g., low level of agreeableness, disconstraint, low positive emotionality)
Military factors (e.g., combat deployment, traditions and rituals)
FACTORS THAT DECREASE RISK
Social support
Positive temperament
Resiliency
Spirituality
Adequate income
Self-help behaviors
Structured activities
Self-efficacy related to sobriety

The self-medication hypothesis

The self-medication hypothesis posits that mental health problems precede substance use difficulties, and substance use develops as a means of coping with and decreasing distress. One well-established relationship is the association of SUDs with mental health problems. For individuals diagnosed with a SUD, rates for a co-occurring mental disorder have been found to be as high as 50 percent (see Figure 17.2 below; Kessler et al., 1996; Seal et al., 2011).

Self-medication is often cited and supported in literature examining the relationship between post-traumatic stress disorder (PTSD) and SUDs among military personnel and veterans (e.g., Chilcoat & Breslau, 1998; Ouimette, Read, Wade, & Tirone, 2010; Seal et al., 2011). One study examines SUDs pre- and post-deployment among OIF National Guard soldiers (Kehle et al., 2012). Five percent of the soldiers without a diagnosis of a SUD pre-deployment were diagnosed with a disorder post-deployment. *For this group of combat personnel, the biggest predictor of a substance use diagnosis was the presence of symptoms of PTSD.* Individuals who have PTSD often have lower rates for successful treatment. For example, Bernhardt (2009) reports that those diagnosed with PTSD and an SUD who do seek treatment report significantly more drug use at admission, have poorer treatment adherence, and exhibit more substance use at their three-month follow-up.

However, PTSD is not the most common disorder associated with SUDs. Petrakis, Rosenheck, and Desai (2011) examined the occurrence of dual diagnosis (co-occurrence of mental illness and a SUD) in

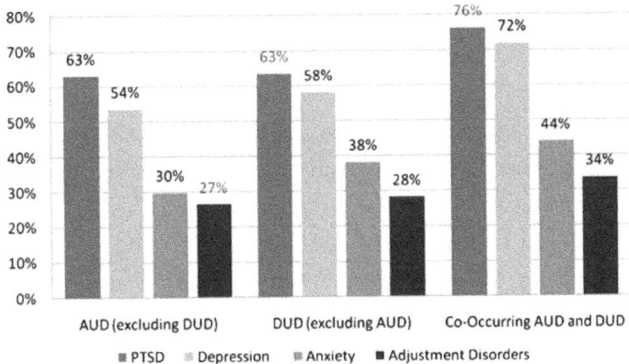

Figure 17.2. Unadjusted prevalence of comorbid military service-related mental health diagnoses (PTSD, depression, anxiety and adjustment disorders) associated with alcohol use disorders (AUD), drug use disorders (DUD), and both among active duty and National Guard and Reserve veterans of Iraq and Afghanistan.

Source: Seal, K. H., et. al. Substance use disorders in Iraq and Afghanistan veterans in VA healthcare, 2001–2010: Implications for screening, diagnosis and treatment. *Drug and Alcohol Dependence, 116*(1–3), 93–101. (2011).

over one million veterans receiving care through the VA during a one-year period, from 2007 to 2008. Results showed that 21 percent of veterans were assigned dual diagnoses. Veterans with affective disorders (e.g., major depression) and serious mental illness were most likely to be assigned a dual diagnosis. To put this information in perspective, compared to veterans with PTSD, veterans with bipolar disorder had a 1.92 greater likelihood of a dual diagnosis, and veterans with other affective disorders had a 1.66 greater likelihood of a dual diagnosis. Based on this information, clinicians should assess for the possibility of self-medication by veterans attempting to cope with various mental health concerns.

Also consistent with the self-medication hypothesis is the misuse of prescription medication. One possible reason the prevalence of prescription drug abuse has risen is the increased rate of survived physical injuries incurred while in the military (e.g., Anderson, Stewart, & Unger, 2007). Better body armor and advanced medical care have increased the rates of personnel who survive serious injuries, thereby increasing the number of pain issues. Combat veterans receiving a mental health diagnosis and a pain diagnosis have been shown to be more likely to receive opioids for pain, have high-risk opioid use, and adverse outcomes such as accidents or overdose (Seal et al., 2012).

Another possible reason for SUD that falls under the self-medication hypothesis is the presence of traumatic brain injury (TBI). TBIs have been called the signature injury of the recent conflicts due to the risk of improvised explosive devices. Nearly 50 percent of individuals post-TBI report an alcohol use disorder (West, 2011). For individuals with TBI, the presence of SUDs has been shown to negatively impact treatment outcomes.

The high-risk hypothesis

The high-risk hypothesis states genetic and environmental factors predispose individuals to use substances (Kessler, 2004). For example, being Caucasian, unmarried, and of a younger age have been shown to increase the likelihood of having a substance use disorder (Calhoun, Elter, Jones, Kudler, & Straits-Tröster,

2008; Seal et al., 2012). Furthermore, low socioeconomic status, lack of social relationships, disruptive life events, and a history of antisocial behavior (e.g., fighting, arrest, school sanctions, relationships with deviant peers) have been linked to enlistment in the military and are also risk factors for substance use difficulties (e.g., Elder, Wang, Spence, Adkins, & Brown, 2010; Fu et al., 2002).

Personality factors also help predict the risk for substance abuse. Individuals who join the military have lower levels of agreeableness compared to those who do not enter the military (Jackson, Thoemmes, Jonkmann, Lüdtke, & Trautwein, 2012), and low levels of agreeableness have been linked to substance use disorders (Kotov, Gamez, Schmidt, & Watson, 2010). Personality factors also helped differentiate soldiers who did and did not develop substance use disorders post-deployment (Kehle et al., 2012). Soldiers with a substance use disorder post-deployment had higher disconstraint (tendency toward impulsivity, risk taking, and noncompliance with societal standards) and lower positive emotionality (tendency toward decreased life engagement and negative affect), compared to soldiers without a diagnosis pre- and post-deployment.

While the Department of Defense has made significant efforts to decrease the incidence of SUDs in the military (Department of Defense, 1997), the very culture of the military is often implicated for increasing the risk of misuse. Traditions and rituals involving substance use, removal of alcohol use restrictions during relaxation and recreational activities, and inconsistently applied alcohol policies have all been cited as contributing to substance use difficulties in the military (Ames, Cunradi, Moore, & Stern, 2007). Furthermore, aspects of military-related work such as number of deployments, combat exposure, increased work-related stress, and lack of sleep have been linked to increased rates of substance use (Bray et al., 2009; Seal et al., 2012; Wilk et al., 2010).

Protective factors

While the factors noted above have been shown to increase the risk for SUDs, other factors have been shown to protect individuals from the likelihood of having such problems. Social support, a positive temperament, resiliency, and spirituality are known protective factors (Institute of Medicine, 2013; Hawkins, Catalano, & Miller, 1992). Adequate income; engagement in self-help behaviors (e.g., attending 12-step meetings); engagement in prosocial, structured activities (e.g., work, school); and self-efficacy related to maintaining sobriety have also been shown to protect against substance use difficulties (Cacciola et al., 2013). These factors can also qualify as recovery capital for military personnel who have a SUD, but are attempting to reduce use or abstain.

Barriers to Treatment

Among members of the National Guard who reported misuse of substances, only 31 percent received any form of treatment (Burnett-Zeigler et al., 2011). Even more surprising, only 2.5 percent of these individuals received treatment specifically for substance use difficulties, which is similar to rates of treatment found within the VA (Glass et al., 2010). Several factors serve as barriers to appropriate care and treatment among military personnel and veterans.

Even if treatment is offered or recommended to an individual, the client may decline treatment. One study conducted by Burnett-Zeigler et al. (2011) examines beliefs that interfere with treatment engagement among OEF/OIF National Guard members. Beliefs that substance use difficulties will be documented in their military record; seeking treatment is a sign of weakness; leaders will review those receiving treatment in a negative manner; and substance use will be viewed as shameful or embarrassing were among the top reasons for not seeking treatment. Another reason for not seeking care is many veterans and service members view their drinking as normal and believe everyone is engaging in similar behavior (Amos et al., 2007).

The fear of treatment and what treatment may entail also can impact the choice to receive care. For example, many veterans and military personnel with comorbid PTSD and substance use difficulties use substances to avoid painful trauma reminders (Kehle et al., 2012). A key component of many evidence-based treatments involves facing, rather than avoiding, painful memories and associated distress. The fear of having to face what one has avoided can prohibit individuals from initially engaging in treatment.

Finally, a lack of identification of substance use difficulties by staff in clinical settings may also limit access to appropriate care. Specifically, the lack of standardized screening for illicit drug use (Department of Veteran Affairs, Department of Defense, 2009) may be a significant barrier to treatment.

SCREENING AND ASSESSMENT

Screening for alcohol misuse is an important priority for service members and veterans due to the prevalence of high risk substance use, especially among newly returning combat personnel. Screening helps identify those who may benefit from interventions. Within the military, Health Reassessments (HRAs) are conducted annually, as well as pre- and post-deployment, to screen for physical and mental health problems, including substance abuse. However, the only branch to utilize a validated instrument is the Air Force. Furthermore, only a small proportion of service members who screen positive receive treatment. In one study of Army personnel, of 12 percent who screened positive, only .05 percent engaged in SUD treatment during the next 90 days (Institute of Medicine, 2013).

The VA has implemented an annual screening process for every patient receiving care at a medical center through the use of the Alcohol Use Disorders Identification Test-Consumption (AUDIT-C; Bush, Kivlahan, McDonell, Fihn, & Bradley, 1998). Although various measures may be utilized, the AUDIT-C is recommended because it allows the flexibility to identify those who may be at risk for alcohol misuse, rather than only those who may meet criteria for a SUD (Bradley et al., 2006). However, no comparable screening process for drug abuse is recommended within the VA at the time of this writing due to the lower prevalence of drug use disorders (Department of Veteran Affairs, Department of Defense, 2009). Alternatively, clinicians can order individual urine drug screens at any point during treatment for veterans who are suspected of misusing substances as a way to help identify patients who may be at risk for complications due to their medication regimen.

Outreach through the Internet is also available to help service members and veterans gain information about possible problems and treatment options through websites such as afterdeployment.org, which may be especially useful for those who have not accessed medical care. The DoD promotes several training programs that utilize websites and social media to enhance substance abuse prevention efforts, such as Military Pathways and the Real Warriors Campaign. In addition, Veteran Justice Outreach coordinators, assigned by the VA, visit jails to identify incarcerated veterans who may benefit from treatment.

If a veteran is referred to a specialty SUD clinic for treatment, assessment includes a full biopsychosocial interview to identify risk and protective factors, comorbid disorders that also may require intervention, and to gather other information that would be helpful in treatment (e.g., medical issues, strengths and weaknesses specific to the individual). Careful questioning during an interview may elicit answers that are underreported on self-report measures or checklists (Bradley, Kivlahan, & Williams, 2009). For example, it is not uncommon for a veteran to report "one or two" drinks; however, further questioning may reveal that one glass was filled with 12 ounces of liquor, or the equivalent of eight drinks.

Assessment instruments may also be employed to assist in the process. For instance, the Addiction Severity Index (ASI; McLellan, Luborsky, O'Brien, & Woody, 1980) serves as an all-inclusive structured assessment instrument to assess current and lifetime factors, including use, risk, and resilience factors, and other psychosocial factors important to treatment planning. More recently, the Brief Addiction Monitor (BAM; Cacciola et al., 2013) was developed for assessment of substance use, as well as ongoing assessment of progress in treatment. This measure also tracks risk and resilience factors as the veteran makes improvements in his or her psychosocial situation. The BAM can be administered repeatedly to track progress in treatment. As of the present writing, the VA recommends administering the BAM to assess levels of use and monitor progress at regular intervals throughout treatment.

Difficulties with assessment are typically related to barriers described in a previous section. Service members commonly report that they were not interested in discussing problems during a post-deployment HRA. They were eager to get back to their families and reluctant to admit possible issues in the presence of commanding officers. Even when enrolling for services at the VA, veterans may minimize issues. Sometimes this is due to beliefs about stigma, but it also can be due to inaccurate beliefs about what constitutes an alcoholic drink or about typical levels of use related to the military culture or developmental stage of the veteran. Careful questioning and psychoeducation may help individuals recognize misuse patterns and make changes or address the issues before significant negative consequences occur.

RECOMMENDATIONS FOR TREATMENT

Within the military, substance abuse treatment programs are available with a comprehensive range of services. The strongest programs were identified in the Air Force (the Alcohol and Drug Abuse Prevention and Treatment Program; ADAPT) and in the Navy (the Substance Abuse Rehabilitation Program; SARP) (Institute of Medicine, 2013). These programs were recognized for their focus on evidence-based practices, treatment monitoring, and follow-up care. The ADAPT program includes regular assessments for substance use and duty performance during the 12-month aftercare. A particular strength of this program is the availability of brief interventions integrated with primary care appointments that may help counter the stigma associated with seeking SUD treatment. The Navy's SARP program utilizes online support and a recovery coach available for 18 months after treatment.

The Army Substance Abuse Program utilizes several evidence-based practices, but requires command notification; there is no formal evaluation of effectiveness, and there is no treatment available for comorbid conditions. However, the Army has several promising pilot programs, including the Confidential Alcohol Treatment and Education Pilot and the Intensive Outpatient Program at Fort Hood, Texas. The former is based on self-referral and does not compromise one's career, while the latter provides intensive treatment that includes comorbid disorders.

The Marine Corps Substance Abuse Program does not use standardized screening instruments, and treatment modalities vary widely, with no standardized or required methods. However, the Battalion Alcohol Skills Intervention Curriculum (BASIC) is an evidence-based prevention program utilized within the Marine Corps. Unfortunately, outcome studies showed that it did not have a significant effect on drinking behavior among marines (Institute of Medicine, 2013).

Recommendations for substance abuse treatment include interventions based on stepped levels of care (Department of Veteran Affairs, 2012a), described in more detail below. If individuals do not respond to a particular level of care, the intensity of treatment can be increased. Stepped care approaches also provide a step-down approach for follow-up care after a successful intervention, creating opportunities for contacts with providers to develop relapse prevention strategies. Services can be based on each veteran's unique needs, creating a treatment plan with the least restrictive environment necessary for safety and recovery. Not all veterans require all levels of care.

Within the VA, initial interventions for SUDs typically begin in primary care after a positive AUDIT-C screening. Brief interventions are provided such as focusing on increasing insight and awareness about alcohol use and motivation for behavior change. This may include expressing concern about using at unhealthy levels, personalized feedback about alcohol use and health, and advice to abstain or drink below recommended limits. If individuals do not respond to interventions, or for certain groups of patients at high risk, referral to a specialty SUD clinic is indicated. Detoxification services, outpatient treatment, intensive outpatient programs, and residential treatment can be considered, based on assessment of each veteran's needs. Generally, the more co-occurring problems and severity of use, the more intensive care is indicated (Department of Veterans Affairs, Department of Defense, 2009).

The VA has implemented policies to enhance provision of care by ensuring that all veterans have access to evidence-based treatments. These recommended treatments cover a wide range, but have in common a convincing research base that demonstrates positive outcomes in controlled studies. Evidence-based protocols typically require 9–16 sessions delivered on a weekly basis. Recommended treatments include, but are not limited to, Motivational Enhancement Therapy, Behavioral Couples Therapy for Substance Use Disorders, Cognitive Behavioral Coping Skills Training, Community Reinforcement, and Contingency Management (Department of Veterans Affairs, 2012b).

In addition, pharmacotherapy is highly recommended and should be made available to all veterans who might benefit from this form of treatment. There is a strong evidence base for opioid agonists, partial agonists, and antagonists (e.g., methadone, buprenorphine, naltrexone) for opiate dependence. For treatment of alcohol dependence, naltrexone, acamprosate, and disulfiram are recommended (Department of Veterans Affairs, 2012a).

Finally, practitioners working with veterans who choose to engage in care outside the VA may find it helpful to complete the appropriate forms for release of information to obtain medical records from the VA/DoD. The computerized record systems allow for a wealth of information that may inform treatment, including lab tests, treatment notes, and assessments.

SPECIAL ISSUES

There are multiple complications to consider when working with a military population. As is common among any population treated for SUD, relapse rates are high, and substance use disorders are considered a chronic condition (Department of Veteran Affairs, Department of Defense, 2009). Multiple-treatment episodes are the rule, rather than the exception. In addition, many veterans treated for SUDs have complicating psychosocial factors such as homelessness, unemployment, or lack of a social support system (Department of Veterans Affairs, 2012a). Reducing risk factors, building resilience, and providing services through a recovery-oriented system of care enhance the likelihood of treatment success.

As noted previously, military factors such as deployments, availability of substances, and culture appear to promote drinking and prescription medication misuse, with the most problematic use among active duty and Reserve/National Guard military personnel. Some service members and veterans are unaware that their use exceeds recommended levels and may be problematic. Psychoeducation regarding these factors and assessing the negative consequences of use may help veterans decide to change. However, the military norms that promoted a high level of use may make change difficult. It is common to hear from clients, "I don't know anybody that doesn't drink." Treatment choices might focus on strengthening the veteran's ability to reduce/abstain through cognitive behavioral coping skills training in order to teach and model how to create new relationships or activities that do not revolve around drinking.

Within the VA, the consequences of reporting may encourage veterans to appear to comply with treatment requirements. For instance, veterans may underreport substance use because the computerized patient record is available to all providers involved in the veterans' care. The communication of substance use may result in changes from medication prescribers concerned about the consequences of combining certain medications with substances or of possible prescription medication misuse. Secondly, active-duty personnel are not provided the same limits of confidentiality as a typical patient, which may affect their careers. Faced with the possibility of such consequences, military personnel may be reticent to provide accurate reports.

The 85 percent prevalence rate for legal arrest among veterans engaged in VA SUD programming (Weaver, Trafton, Kimerling, Timko, & Moos, 2013) also suggests that involvement with the legal system may have a large impact on treatment. Justice-involved veterans frequently present for treatment under orders from the court. Special programs designated as "veterans' courts" are increasing, in which veterans are diverted from jail into treatment to receive follow-up for legal issues. Court orders typically require treatment prior to sentencing or as a condition of probation. These agreements include having judges and other legal personnel communicate with mental health providers to ensure the veteran is progressing in treatment. Based on reports, judges may adjust court orders accordingly. In addition, the VA has designated Veteran Justice Outreach (VJO) coordinators, who travel to jails and identify incarcerated veterans who may benefit from treatment. The VJO coordinators then advocate for the veterans and serve as liaisons for communication between the treatment providers and legal personnel.

Many veterans seeking treatment have chronic pain, which increases the likelihood for prescription medication misuse, as well as other substance abuse, in efforts to mitigate unresolved pain. Similarly, when comorbid mental health disorders such as PTSD or depression are included in the profile, veterans may be more likely to increase substance use in order to self-medicate psychiatric symptoms (Seal et al.,

2012). Addressing the relationships and interactions among these problems and substance use can create a challenging treatment environment.

Evidence suggests that comorbid conditions, including chronic pain, escalate the severity of symptoms and result in poorer treatment outcomes (Caldiero et al., 2008; Kessler et al., 1996; Ouimette, 1998; Watkins, Burnam, Kung, & Paddock, 2001). In such cases, integrated treatments that address several problems at the same time by the same provider are considered the treatments of choice, although convincing evidence for the superiority of integrated treatments is still lacking. Integrated treatments allow for efficient use of resources and eliminate the possibility that parallel treatments may provide conflicting strategies. One caveat is to recognize treatment for a comorbid condition may potentially intensify a veteran's distress, increasing the likelihood of substance abuse if careful monitoring and attention to addressing symptoms is neglected.

Due to the high rates of comorbid disorders, particularly depression and PTSD, familiarity with integrated treatments is indicated for professionals working with this population. Several treatments for comorbid depression and SUD have been studied, including Integrated Cognitive Behavioral Therapy (ICBT) and Building Recovery by Improving Goals, Habits, and Thoughts (BRIGHT; Substance Abuse and Mental Health Services Administration, 2012). ICBT was compared against Twelve-Step Facilitation Therapy and showed that the ICBT group had less substance use and depressive symptoms than the Twelve-Step group. BRIGHT, an adapted CBT group treatment, was compared against treatment as usual (TAU) in four residential SUD treatment programs. Results showed that the BRIGHT participants reported fewer depressive symptoms and fewer days of substance abuse than TAU participants at six-month follow-up.

For comorbid PTSD, there are reports on a large number of integrated treatments. A recent publication focuses on stringent criteria to select articles for review (van Dam, Vedel, Ehring, & Emmelkamp, 2012). Studies need to include outcomes for both PTSD and SUD, have formal diagnoses for both disorders, and be published in a peer-reviewed journal. The authors separated the studies into trauma-focused and non–trauma-focused treatments. Among non–trauma-focused therapies, outcomes for Seeking Safety, CBT for PTSD in SUD treatment, Substance Dependency-Posttraumatic Stress Disorder Therapy, and Transcend were reported. Overall, the studies support the effectiveness of these treatments for PTSD and SUD. However, the five randomized controlled studies identified in this category show that the integrated treatments did not result in outcomes superior to control treatments focused on SUD only. Among the trauma-focused treatments in this review, Concurrent Treatment of PTSD and Cocaine Dependence, Seeking Safety plus Exposure Therapy-Revised, and a parallel treatment with imaginal exposure provided along with CBT for SUD all demonstrated positive outcomes for PTSD and SUD. However, only one (parallel treatment with imaginal exposure) was a controlled study that demonstrated superior effectiveness, compared to an active control relaxation training group.

Another relatively common complication among the military population is the possibility of sequelae from a TBI sustained in combat. TBI increases the likelihood the client is unable to learn from previous experiences and continues to make the same choices, regardless of the consequences. Impulsivity associated with TBI is also likely to negatively influence substance abuse treatment outcomes by contributing to frequent relapses. These factors again suggest the importance of integrating treatments to address issues that are likely to affect treatment for either condition alone.

Finally, it is important to note there is a connection between substance abuse and the likelihood of suicide (Wilcox, Conner, & Caine, 2004). The common co-occurring conditions discussed above are also associated with suicide, compounding the risk (Mills, Teesson, Ross, & Peters, 2006; Simpson & Tate, 2005; Waller, Lyons, & Costantini-Ferrando, 1999). In addition to suicide, VA patients with an alcohol use disorder appear more likely to die from homicide than those without an alcohol use disorder (Chermack, Bohnert, Price, Austin, & Ilgen, 2012). Therefore, careful assessment and attention to suicidal ideation and risky lifestyle factors are crucial.

With all of these additional issues to consider, treatment for a SUD requires careful attention to prioritizing and addressing co-occurring biopsychosocial problems that may decrease the likelihood of a positive clinical outcome. Integrated or concurrent treatment and coordination of care with additional services should be based on a collaboratively established treatment plan.

SUMMARY

Veterans and military personnel make up a significant proportion of the population; consequently, addressing substance abuse among this population is a public health concern. Regular screenings using validated instruments will help with earlier identification of individuals who may benefit from interventions. Illicit drug use has declined, following efforts from the DoD to implement "zero tolerance" policies. However, the misuse of alcohol and prescription medication continues to rise. Stepped levels of care, based on individual needs, are highly recommended. In addition, prioritizing evidence-based treatments such as Motivational Enhancement Therapy, Behavioral Couples Therapy for Substance Use Disorders, Cognitive Behavioral Coping Skills Training, Community Reinforcement, and Contingency Management is likely to produce more positive outcomes. Pharmacotherapy may also be a useful adjunct for a select group of clients. Attention to special issues among this population is also important for positive treatment outcomes. Careful assessment of and attention to co-occurring conditions (e.g., depression, PTSD, TBI, chronic pain), legal issues, homelessness, unemployment, underreporting use, and risks for suicide and homicide are strongly indicated.

Chapter Review Questions

1. Identify 5 risk factors for substance abuse within the military population.
2. Describe three special issues salient to military populations with SUDs and why these issues are important to consider.
3. List three evidence-based treatments (EBTs) for substance use disorders (SUDs).
4. Name three recommended practices for SUD treatment in military populations.

REFERENCES

American Psychiatric Association (2000). *Diagnostic and statistical manual of mental disorders* (4th ed., text rev.). Washington, DC: Author.

Ames, G. M., Cunradi, C. B., Moore, R. S., & Stern, P. (2007). Military culture and drinking behavior among U.S. navy careerists. *Journal of Studies on Alcohol and Drugs, 68*(3), 336–344.

Anderson, C., Stewart, K., & Unger, D. (2007). Recent advances in lower-extremity amputations. *Current Opinion in Orthopedics, 18*, 137–144.

Bernhardt, A. (2009). Rising to the challenge of treating OEF/OIF veterans with co-occurring PTSD and substance abuse. *Smith College Studies in Social Work, 79*, 344–367.

Bohnert, A. S. B., Ilgen, M. A., Bossarte, R. M., Britton, P. C., Chermack, S. T., & Blow, F. C. (2012). Veteran status and alcohol use in men in the United States. *Military Medicine, 177*(2), 198–203.

Bradley, K. A., Kivlahan, D. R., & Williams, E. C. (2009). Brief approaches to alcohol screening: Practical alternatives for primary care. *Journal of General Internal Medicine, 24*(7), 881–883.

Bradley, K. A., Williams, E. C., Achtmeyer, C. A., Volpp, B., Collins, B. J., & Kivlahan, D. R. (2006). Implementation of evidence-based alcohol screening in the Veterans Health Administration. *American Journal of Managed Care, 12*, 597–606.

Bray, R. M., Pemberton, M. R., Hourani, L. L., Witt, M., Olmsted, K. L. E., Brown, J. M., … Bradshaw, M. (2009). *2008 Department of Defense survey of health related behaviors among active duty military personnel.* Research Triangle Park, NC: Research Triangle Institute.

Burnett-Zeigler, I., Ilgen, M., Valenstein, M., Zivin, K., Gorman, L., Blow, A., … Chermack, S. (2011). Prevalence and correlates of alcohol misuse among returning Afghanistan and Iraq veterans. *Addictive Behaviors, 36*(8), 801–806.

Bush, K., Kivlahan, D. R., McDonell, M. B., Fihn, S. D., & Bradley, K. A. (1998). The AUDIT alcohol consumption questions (AUDIT-C): An effective brief screening test for problem drinking: Ambulatory Care Quality Improvement Project (ACQUIP): Alcohol Use Disorders Identification Test. *Archives of Internal Medicine, 158*, 1789–1795.

Cacciola, J. S., Alterman, A. I., Dephilippis, D., Drapkin, M. L., Valadez, C. Jr., Fala, N. C., … McKay, J. R. (2013). Development and initial evaluation of the Brief Addiction Monitor (BAM). *Journal of Substance Abuse Treatment, 44*(3), 256–63.

Caldiero, R. M., Malte, C. A., Calsyn, D. A., Baer, J. S., Nichol, P., Kivlahan, D. R., & Saxon, A. J. (2008). The association of persistent pain with out-patient addiction treatment outcomes and service utilization. *Addiction, 103*(12), 1996–2005.

Calhoun, P. S., Elter, J. R., Jones, E. R., Kudler, H., & Straits-Tröster, K. (2008). Hazardous alcohol use and receipt of risk-reduction counseling among U.S. veterans of the wars in Iraq and Afghanistan. *Journal of Clinical Psychiatry, 69*(11), 1686–1693.

Chermack, S. T., Bohnert, A. S. B., Price, A. M., Austin, K., & Ilgen, M. A. (2012). Substance use disorders and homicide death in veterans. *Journal of the Study of Alcohol and Drugs, 73*, 10–14.

Chilcoat, H. D., & Breslau, N. (1998). Investigations of causal pathways between PTSD and drug use disorders. *Addictive Behaviors, 23*, 827–840.

Department of Defense (1997). *Drug and Alcohol Abuse by DoD Personnel* (Directive No. 1010.4). Washington, DC: Author.

Department of Veterans Affairs. (2012a). *VHA programs for veterans with substance use disorders* (VHA Handbook 1160.04). Washington DC: Veterans Health Administration.

Department of Veterans Affairs. (2012b). *Local implementation of evidenced based psychotherapies for mental and behavioral health conditions* (VHA Handbook 1160.05). Washington DC: Veterans Health Administration.

Department of Veterans Affairs, Department of Defense. (2009). *VA/DoD clinical practice guideline for management of substance use disorders (SUD).* Washington DC: Author.

Department of Veterans Affairs, Veterans Health Administration, Office of the Assistant Deputy Under Secretary for Health for Policy and Planning (2012). *2011 Survey of Veteran enrollees' health and reliance upon VA with selected comparison to the 1999–2010 surveys.* Washington, DC.

Elder, G. H., Wang, L., Spence, N. J., Adkins, D. E., & Brown, T. H. (2010). Pathways to the all-volunteer military. *Social Science Quarterly, 91*(2), 455–475.

Evans, K. (2012). Serving those who served us: Resources for active duty soldiers and veterans. *College & Research Libraries News, 73*(8), 470–480.

Fu, Q., Heath, A. C., Bucholz, K. K., Nelson, E., Goldberg, J., Lyons, M. J., … Eisen, S. A. (2002). Shared genetic risk of major depression, alcohol dependence, and marijuana dependence: Contribution of antisocial personality disorder in men. *Archives of General Psychiatry, 59*(12), 1125–1132.

Glass, J. E., Perron, B. E., Ilgen, M. A., Chermack, S. T., Ratliff, S., & Zivin, K. (2010). Prevalence and correlates of specialty substance use disorder treatment for Department of Veterans Affairs healthcare system patients with high alcohol consumption. *Drug and Alcohol Dependence, 112*(1–2), 150–155.

Hamlett-Berry, K., Davison, J., Kivlahan, D. R, Matthews, M. H., Hendrickson, J. E., & Almenoff, P. L. (2009). Evidence-based national initiatives to address tobacco use as a public health priority in the Veterans Health Administration. *Military Medicine, 174*(1), 29–34.

Hawkins, J. D., Catalano, R. F., & Miller, J. Y. (1992). Risk and protective factors for alcohol and other drug problems in adolescence and early adulthood: Implications for substance abuse prevention. *Psychological Bulletin, 112*(1), 64–105.

Hawkins, E. J., Lapham, G. T., Kivlahan, D. R., & Bradley, K. A. (2010). Recognition and management of alcohol misuse in OEF/OIF and other veterans in the VA: A cross-sectional study. *Drug and Alcohol Dependence, 109*(1–3), 147–153.

Institute of Medicine (2013). *Substance use disorders in the U.S. armed forces.* Washington, DC: National Academies Press. Retrieved from: http://www.nap.edu/openbook.php?record_id=13441

Jackson, J. J., Thoemmes, F., Jonkmann, K., Lüdtke, O., & Trautwein, U. (2012). Military training and personality trait development: Does the military make the man, or does the man make the military? *Psychological Science, 23*(3), 270–277.

Jacobson, I. G., Ryan, M. A. K., Hooper, T. I., Smith, T. C., Amoroso, P. J., Boyko, E. J., … Bell, N. S. (2008). Alcohol use and alcohol-related problems before and after military combat deployment. *Journal of the American Medical Association, 300*(6), 663–675.

Jeffery, D. D., Babeu, L. A., Nelson, L. E., Kloc, M., & Klette, K. (2013). Prescription drug misuse among U.S. active duty military personnel: A secondary analysis of the 2008 DoD survey of health related behaviors. *Military Medicine, 178*(2), 180–195.

Kehle, S. M., Ferrier-Auerbach, A., Meis, L. A., Arbisi, P. A., Erbes, C. R., & Polusny, M. A. (2012). Predictors of postdeployment alcohol use disorders in National Guard soldiers deployed to Operation Iraqi Freedom. *Psychology of Addictive Behaviors, 26*(1), 42–50.

Kessler, R. C. (2004). Impact of substance abuse on the diagnosis, course, and treatment of mood disorders: The epidemiology of dual diagnosis. *Biological Psychiatry, 56*(10), 730–737.

Kessler, R. C., Nelson, C. B., McGonagle, K. A., Edlund, M. J., Frank, R. G., & Leaf, P. J. (1996). The epidemiology of co-occurring addictive and mental disorders: Implications for prevention and service utilization. *American Journal of Orthopsychiatry, 66*(1), 17–31.

Kotov, R., Gamez, W., Schmidt, F., & Watson, D. (2010). Linking "big" personality traits to anxiety, depressive, and substance use disorders: A meta-analysis. *Psychological Bulletin, 136*(5), 768–821.

McLellan, A. T., Luborsky, L., O'Brien, C. P., & Woody, G. E. (1980). An improved diagnostic instrument for substance abuse patients: The Addiction Severity Index. *Journal of Nervous & Mental Diseases, 168*, 26–33.

Mills, K. L., Teesson, M., Ross, J., & Peters, L. (2006). Trauma, PTSD, and substance use disorders: Findings from the Australian National Survey of Mental Health and Well-Being. *American Journal of Psychiatry, 163*(4), 652–658.

National Survey on Drug Use and Health. (2005). *Substance use, dependence, and treatment among veterans.* Office of Applied Studies, Substance Abuse and Mental Health Services Administration (SAMHSA). Retrieved from: http://www.samhsa.gov/data//2k5 /vets/vets.htm

Office of the Deputy Under Secretary of Defense (Military Community and Family Policy). (2010). *Demographics 2010: Profile of the military community.* Washington, DC: Author.

Ouimette, P. C. (1998). Course and treatment of patients with both substance use and posttraumatic stress disorders. *Addictive Behaviors, 23*(6), 785–795.

Ouimette, P., Read, J. P., Wade, M., & Tirone, V. (2010). Modeling associations between posttraumatic stress symptoms and substance use. *Addictive Behaviors, 35*, 64–67.

Petrakis, I. L., Rosenheck, R., Desai, R. (2011). Substance use comorbidity among veterans with posttraumatic stress disorder and other psychiatric illness. *American Journal of Addictions, 20*(3), 185–189.

Seal, K. H., Cohen, G., Waldrop, A. E., Cohen, B. E., Maguen, S., & Ren, L. (2011). Substance use disorders in Iraq and Afghanistan veterans in VA healthcare, 2001–2010: Implications for screening, diagnosis and treatment. *Drug and Alcohol Dependence, 116*(1–3), 93–101.

Seal, K. H., Shi, Y., Cohen, G., Cohen, B. E., Maguen, S., Krebs, E. E., & Neylan, T. C. (2012). Association of mental health disorders with prescription opioids and high-risk opioid use in US veterans of Iraq and Afghanistan. *JAMA, 307*(9), 940–947.

Simpson, G., & Tate, R. (2005). Clinical features of suicide attempts after traumatic brain injury. *Journal of Nervous and Mental Disorders, 193*(10), 680–685.

Substance Abuse and Mental Health Services Administration. (2012). *Managing depressive symptoms in substance abuse clients during early recovery: A review of the literature—updates.* Treatment Improvement Protocol 48. (SMA12-4353). Rockville, MD: Substance Abuse and Mental Health Services Administration. Retrieved from: http://store.samhsa.gov/shin/content//SMA12-4353/TIP48_Lit_Review_Updates.pdf

U.S. Census Bureau (2012). *Statistical Abstract of the United States: 2012.* Washington, DC: Author. Retrieved from: http://www.census.gov/compendia/statab/2012edition.html

van Dam, D., Vedel, E., Ehring, T., & Emmelkamp, P. M. G. (2012). Psychological treatments for concurrent posttraumatic stress disorder and substance use disorder: A systematic review. *Clinical Psychology Review, 32*, 202–214.

Waller, S. J., Lyons, J. S., & Costantini-Ferrando, M. F. (1999). Impact of comorbid affective and alcohol use disorders on suicidal ideation and attempts. *Journal of Clinical Psychology, 55*(5), 585–595.

Watkins, K. E., Burnam, A., Kung, F-Y., & Paddock, S. (2001). A national survey of care for persons with co-occurring mental and substance use disorders. *Psychiatric Services, 52*, 1062–1068.

Weaver, C. M., Trafton, J. A., Kimerling, R., Timko, C., & Moos, R. (2013). Prevalence and nature of criminal offending in a national sample of veterans in VA substance use treatment prior to the Operation Enduring Freedom/Operation Iraqi Freedom conflicts. *Psychological Services, 10*(1), 54–65.

West, S. L. (2011). Substance use among persons with traumatic brain injury: A review. *Neuropsychological Rehabilitation, 29*(1), 1–8.

Wilcox, H. C., Conner, K. R., & Caine, E. D. (2004). Association of alcohol and drug use disorders and completed suicide: An empirical review of cohort studies. *Drug and Alcohol Dependence, 76 Supplement*, S11–19.

Wilk, J. E., Bliese, P. D., Kim, P. Y., Thomas, J. L., McGurk, D., & Hoge, C. W. (2010). Relationship of combat experiences to alcohol misuse among U.S. soldiers returning from the Iraq war. *Drug and Alcohol Dependence, 108*(1–2), 115–121.

CHAPTER 18

MULTICULTURAL AND ADDICTION-RELATED COUNSELING COMPETENCIES

We see the world, not as it is, but as we are ...
Or as we are conditioned to see it.

—Stephen Covey, author

Humans are conditioned and socialized to assess and interpret their surroundings and other humans in a certain manner. Consequently, we develop deeply ingrained thoughts, beliefs, attitudes, stigmas, prejudices, and behaviors toward others, often without self-awareness of how they are acquired, how they are maintained, and how harmful they can be. For those with privilege, these aspects may not be explored fully (or at all) and can impact their competency as therapists. By definition, the term competency describes an individual's knowledge and skill to complete a task. In the counseling profession, however, *cultural competency* encompasses more than knowledge and skill; it also includes an awareness of the thoughts, beliefs, biases, and attitudes about one's own culture and the culture of others. Cultural competency is an active, developmental, and continual process that is aspirational rather than accomplished. Counselors must strive for competency in matters of race and ethnicity, sexual orientation, gender, age, disabilities, social class, etc. This chapter will present information on (a) specific facets of cultural competency; (b) the importance of discussing cultural differences in session with clients (i.e., broaching); (c) social justice and advocacy; and (d) addiction-related counseling competencies.

This author wishes to note the term "cultural intelligence" has been recently used in the counselor education literature to refer to multicultural competency (e.g., Ang & Van Dyne, 2008; Peterson, 2013). Cited often in global business resources, this term refers to the extent to which an individual has cognitive, motivational, and behavioral capacities to understand and effectively respond to the beliefs, values, attitudes, and behaviors of diverse group members in order to achieve an intended goal. For the purposes of this book, the author will continue to use the term competency in lieu of any other designation.

FACETS OF CULTURAL COMPETENCY

At the beginning of the text, the author discussed a framework of personal identity that includes the universal, group, and individual levels (Sue, 2001). At the universal level, all *Homo sapiens* share (a) common life experiences; (b) biological and physical similarities; (c) the ability to have self-awareness; and (d) the ability to use symbols for communication. At a group level, people have similarities and differences regarding gender, age, race, marital status, abilities, socioeconomic status, etc. Humans also have distinctive qualities at an individual level, such as genetic endowment and experiences unique to self. In an effort to be a competent counselor, one must adopt a holistic approach and attempt to understand how a client's personal identity is influenced by all three levels.

Personal identity is not the only thing impacted by these levels. How a person thinks, makes decisions, defines experiences, and behaves results from one's lived experiences as an individual, as well as a part of a group. Culture can determine how one interprets reality, views others, conceptualizes the origins of disorders, and defines normality and abnormality. Therefore, counselors should be cognizant of their own three levels of personal identity and how their worldview can affect the analysis and understanding of client problems, behaviors, thoughts, attitudes, and motivations.

The following is a list of well-known identity models. Counselors are encouraged to review them in an effort to develop a better understanding of their clients' personal identities and cultures. Counselors should keep in mind that some of these models are linear in nature, and they may not apply to everyone. For example, Erikson's (1968) psychosocial developmental model primarily focuses on the development of white, American men who do not have disabilities; the model may not be applicable to a Latina born in Colombia who has a disability. Having the unique experiences due to one particular identity (e.g., a Latina, a woman, a person with a physical disability) has the potential to impact how a person interacts, socializes, and views self and others throughout the developmental stages.

Multicultural Identity Models

Racial
    Black Racial Identity (Cross, 1971, 1991)
    White Racial Identity (Helms, 1984)
    Biracial Identity Development (Poston, 1990)
    Multidimensional Identity (Reynolds & Pope, 1991)
    Minority Identity Development (Atkinson, Morten, & Sue, 1993)

Gender
    Feminist Identity Development (Downing & Roush, 1985)
    Womanist Identity Development (Ossana, Helms, & Leonard, 1992)

LGBT
    Sexual Identity (Cass, 1979)
    Sexual Identity Development (Coleman, 1982)
    Identity Development among People of Color Who Are Gay and Lesbian (Morales, 1989)
    Lesbian, Gay, and Bisexual Identity Development (D'Augelli, 1994)
    Lesbian Identity Development Model (McCarn & Fassinger, 1996)
    The Gay and Lesbian Affirmative Development (GLAD) (Marszalek & Cashwell, 1999)

Age
    Theory of Psychosocial Development (Erikson, 1968)

Ego Identity Development (Marcia, 1980)
Identity Development from Adolescence to Adulthood (Waterman, 1982)

Disability
Four Types of Integration in Disability Identity Development (Gill, 1997)
Disability Identity Development (Gibson, 2006)

Understanding the various developmental models and frameworks for personal identity assists with becoming a culturally skilled counselor; however, there is much more to this process. Over the past few decades, counselors have discussed and researched this topic in an effort to ascertain what defines competency. The Association of Multicultural Counseling and Development (AMCD), a division of the American Counseling Association (ACA), created 31 competencies. These are divided into three categories: (a) Counselor Awareness of Own Cultural Values and Biases; (b) Counselor Awareness of Client's Worldview; and (c) Culturally Appropriate Intervention Strategies. Table 18.1 below highlights nine of the 31 AMCD competencies (see Appendix A for the full list). Notice each category includes attitudes and beliefs, knowledge, and skills.

Table 18.1: AMCD Multicultural Competencies

	COUNSELOR AWARENESS OF OWN CULTURAL VALUES AND BIASES
Attitudes and Beliefs	Recognizes sources of discomfort with differences that exist between self and clients in terms of race, ethnicity, and culture
Knowledge	Knows and understands how oppression, racism, discrimination, and stereotyping affect self and work with clients
Skills	Constantly seeks to understand self as racial and cultural beings and actively seek a nonracist identity
	COUNSELOR AWARENESS OF CLIENT'S WORLDVIEW
Attitudes and Beliefs	Is aware of own stereotypes and preconceived notions held toward other groups
Knowledge	Understands how race, culture, ethnicity, and so forth may affect personality formation, vocational choices, manifestation of psychological disorders, help-seeking behavior, and the appropriateness or inappropriateness of counseling approaches
Skills	Is actively involved with marginalized individuals outside of the counseling setting (e.g., community events, social and political functions, celebrations, friendships) so the perspective of marginalized people is more than an academic or helping exercise
	CULTURALLY APPROPRIATE INTERVENTION STRATEGIES
Attitudes and Beliefs	Values bilingualism and does not view another language as an impediment to counseling
Knowledge	Is aware of institutional barriers that prevent marginalized groups from using mental health services
Skills	Is able to exercise institutional intervention skills on behalf of clients. Help clients determine whether a "problem" stems from racism or bias in others so clients do not inappropriately personalize problems

From Arredondo et al. (1996). Multicultural counseling competencies and standards. *Journal of Multicultural Counseling and Development, 24*, 42–78.

After reviewing these competencies, the reader will note that having knowledge of self and clients is not obtained solely by reading information and watching videos about various cultures and identities (e.g., female, biracial, LGBT, people with disabilities, etc.). Moreover, it is not about having an understanding of how privilege, racism, discrimination, and oppression exist in the United States. In other words, a culturally skilled counselor must be a proactive participant in the process of developing competency that goes beyond "book knowledge." The competencies reflect this sentiment, as they include statements requiring counselors to actively seek a nonracist identity; contrast their own beliefs and attitudes with others in a nonjudgmental fashion; understand how they directly or indirectly benefited from individual, institutional, and cultural racism, as outlined in white identity development models. He or she must also be (a) *actively involved* with people from marginalized groups *outside* of the counseling setting; (b) *willing* to step outside of his or her comfort zone; (c) *motivated* to learn and grow as a cultural being; and (d) *determined* to continually reflect on self (which can be very difficult and create anxiety and/or confusing emotions, especially for those with privilege).

Cultural Competency Is Multidimensional

As indicated throughout this text, there are many identities and experiences impacting a client's life, and these aspects influence mental health status and substance use. In an effort to conceptualize clients and their problems, counselors must have a grasp on their own awareness of the attitudes and beliefs, knowledge, and skills related to various levels: (a) individual; (b) professional; (c) organizational; and (d) societal. In essence, cultural competency is multidimensional.

Dr. Derald Wing Sue (2001) created a visual representation of this philosophy by illustrating a multidimensional cube (see Figure 18.1 below). There are three dimensions: (1) race and culture-specific attributes;

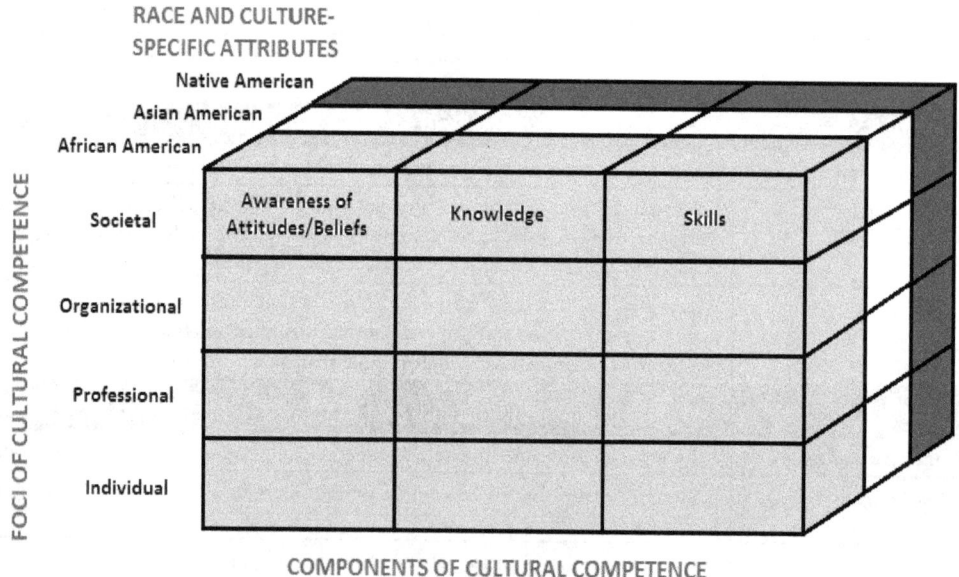

Figure 18.1: *A multidimensional model for developing cultural competence.* **Adapted from Sue, D. W. (2001). Multidimensional facets of cultural competence: A major contribution.** *Counseling Psychologist, 29,* **790–821.**

(2) awareness, knowledge and skills; and (3) various foci (i.e., societal, organizational, professional, and individual). Each cell of the cube symbolizes the interchange between the three dimensions. In this figure, the cube is specific to race, but this concept can be applied to other cultural-specific populations (e.g., LGBT or people with disabilities). Dr. Sue does, however, emphasize the importance of focusing on race. Often, other sociodemographic differences get pushed to the forefront in the counseling profession because racial and ethnic differences cause more discomfort for helpers than others. Moreover, it is worth noting that most counselors are white, while most of their clients are persons of color. Therefore, the emphasis on the multidimensional cube is on race.

The multidimensional model can assist a counselor to view competency in a more concrete manner without minimizing the complex nature of it. Part of being a culturally competent helper is to be able to use one's knowledge, skills, and awareness in order to address the differences between oneself and the client. In the next section, the author will discuss how talking about differences can actually build rapport and trust within the therapeutic relationship between two people of very different backgrounds and worldviews.

BROACHING

Premature termination of counseling services by clients is a concern for helping professionals in the mental health field. In fact, 50 percent of clients from a culturally diverse background terminate therapy prematurely (Sue & Sue, 2013). Termination is often attributed to the inability of the counselor to build a therapeutic alliance with the client. Distrust of those working in the health fields often exists, especially among people of color.

Historical events have impacted the willingness of marginalized groups to seek treatment due to the lack trust for those who provide treatment services. For instance, the Tuskegee syphilis experiment will undeniably be considered one of the most unethical and nontherapeutic experiments of our time. Hundreds of black men in Macon County, Alabama, were: (a) not provided informed consent to participate in the study; (b) not told they had syphilis; and (c) told they were provided medical treatment for their "bad blood," when, in fact, they were not given any medicine. This experiment lasted for 40 years (from 1932–1972). Penicillin became available in the 1940s, and it could have helped to save these men's lives; however, no penicillin was ever given, and many went blind and died due to their ailments. In addition, since the men did not know they had the disease, many women and children were also infected as a result.

A shorter study was conducted in Guatemala by American doctors from 1946 to 1948. Unlike the Tuskegee experiment, nearly 700 Guatemalans (who were mostly prison inmates and those with mental health issues) were purposely infected with venereal diseases to test the effectiveness of penicillin. Prostitutes who had syphilis were allowed to sleep with the prisoners, and if they did not contract the disease by direct contact, the prisoners were infected by having the syphilis bacteria poured onto scrapes on their penises, forearms, or faces.

In 1997, President Bill Clinton made a formal apology for the Tuskegee experiments, and Secretary of State Hillary Clinton and Health and Human Services Secretary Kathleen Sebelius made a statement in 2010 apologizing for the events in Guatemala. However, to what extent can an apology lessen the anger, distrust, and fear that resulted from these outrageous, inhumane acts by American health professionals? In what ways can counselors with privilege (and those without a history of racism, oppression, and daily microaggressions) build trust and rapport with clients who are marginalized? How can counselors attempt to eliminate "cultural miscommunication?"

One way to do so is to examine the racial and cultural factors with the client and how these factors may be influencing the client's presenting problem(s). This process is referred to as *broaching*. Broaching behaviors have been found to increase: (a) counselor credibility; (b) client satisfaction; (c) the extent of client disclosure; and (d) the likelihood of returning for subsequent counseling sessions (Day-Vines et al., 2007). Counselors must be consistent in their efforts to explore issues of diversity in sessions. Again, all counseling is multicultural; you will never be the same as your client in all aspects (e.g., age, gender, race, ethnicity, sexual orientation, religion, class, etc.). These differences have been referred to as the "so-called 5-ton pink elephant" in the room (Utsey, Hammar, & Gernat, 2005, p. 570). To illustrate this point, if multicultural aspects are not addressed, there will be a *dead* 5-ton pink elephant in the middle of the counseling room.. Counselors must take the time to discuss culture and be sensitive to how these differences can impact the therapeutic relationship.

Exercise

Take a moment and think about how you would broach differences of race in the counseling room. What would you say? How comfortable are you with such a discussion?

The following is an example of broaching. A counselor may say to a client, "You and I are similar in that we are both women, but we are also not alike in that we are of different races and ages. I think it's important to acknowledge culture and how our experiences within a culture can impact our worldview. These differences, as well as similarities, could potentially impact communication and the therapeutic process. How do you feel about working with a white woman, who is older than you?"

Counselors can exhibit five different broaching styles: (1) avoidant; (2) isolating; (3) continuing/incongruent; (d) integrated/congruent; and (5) infusing (Day-Vines et al., 2007). *Avoidant* style is one that ignores or minimizes race and other cultural differences; therefore, the counselor does not broach these differences in session. *Isolating* style is one in which the therapist does broach, but it is simplistic and superficial and only occurs once. Broaching is often seen as a technique or event which is not connected to other aspects of the client's experience as a cultural being. *Continuing/incongruent* style is when a counselor will inquire about diversity aspects and differences on several different occasions, and he or she may be eager to consider cultural factors. However, the skills to fully explore issues in a manner that empowers the client will be lacking. *Integrated/congruent* style incorporates broaching not only in session, but as part of one's professional identity. A counselor using this style distinguishes among and between culture-specific behaviors and unhealthy human functioning, as well as recognizes the complexity of the client's multiple identities, systemic factors, and personal experiences. *Infusing* style is a lifestyle orientation which transcends the bounds of professional identity and is one that is committed to social justice and advocacy on the clients' behalf.

Earlier in this text, the author discussed the white racial identity model by Helms and the status a counselor can have with regard to race (e.g., contact, disintegration, reintegration, etc.). According to Day-Vines et al. (2007), specific broaching behaviors and attitudes depend on which "eyeglasses" (or status) one views the world through and his or her racial identity. In Table 18.2 below, broaching attitudes and behaviors are outlined according to status. As the reader can see, counselors within the Contact status are typically color blind, view broaching as unnecessary, and refuse to consider contextual dimensions. Helping professionals

Table 18.2: Racial Identity Status and Broaching Attitudes and Behaviors

RACIAL IDENTITY STATUS	DESCRIPTION OF RACIAL IDENTITY	BROACHING ATTITUDES AND BEHAVIORS
Contact	• Oblivious to own racial identity • Uncritical acceptance of racism or color-blind perspective about race	• Avoiding broaching style • Refusal to broach • Broaching regarded as unnecessary • Refuses to consider contextual dimensions of race, ethnicity, and culture
Disintegration	• First acknowledgment of white identity • Conflict resulting from contradictions in belief system; current beliefs are compared with racial realities	• Vacillates between avoiding and isolating broaching styles • Broaches only once • May recognize the need for broaching but may avoid it because of discomfort, lack of skill, or concern about negative reactions from client
Reintegration	• Idealizes whites; denigrates people of color • Assumes original stereotypes	• Same as above; as listed in the Disintegration Status
Pseudo-Independence	• Intellectualized acceptance of own and others' races	• Continuing/incongruent broaching style • May broach the subject of race several times, but mechanically • Cannot translate recognition of cultural factors into effective counseling interventions
Immersion/Emersion	• Honest appraisal of racism and significance of whiteness	• Integrated/congruent broaching style • Conscious understanding of need for broaching • Incorporates broaching into counseling efforts as appropriate • Accepts risk involved in broaching • Identifies culturally appropriate interventions
Autonomy	• Internalizes a multicultural identity with nonracist whiteness at its core	• Infusing broaching style • Considers broaching integral to effective counseling efforts • Recognizes and acknowledges the impact of race on client's presenting problems • Maintains a commitment to social justice and equality that transcends bounds of professional identity

Adapted from Day-Vines et al. (2007). Broaching the subjects of race, ethnicity, and culture during the counseling process. *Journal of Counseling and Development, 85*(4), p. 407.

must be aware that these factors play a large part in the premature termination of services; thus, they must be accountable for striving toward Autonomy status and an Infusing broaching style.

Broaching is part of being a competent helper; nevertheless, researchers have found many white clinicians experience anxiety in cross-racial counseling dyads, and this anxiety results in countertransference concerns. This type of anxiety is also seen in multicultural courses and in supervision settings. Utsey et al. (2007) found that discussing race and racism beyond the surface level is still considered taboo. Thus, exploring oppression and the experiences of the oppressed (i.e., broaching) will be avoided due to this anxiety.

The following is a list of specific findings from the Utsey et al. study which are demonstrative of issues among white counselors with respect to race discussions.

- During focus groups, when the word *black* was used, their voice would lower
- Members had difficulty describing themselves as white
- Anxiety was manifested in expressions of anger, fear, and defense mechanisms
- Anxiety caused difficulty with articulation, faltering and/or trembling voices, and difficulty with pronunciation of simple words

In an effort to decrease this anxiety, racism, discrimination, oppression, privilege, and all *isms* must be continually discussed (both professionally and socially). They should be explored beyond the surface level, and must always be taken into account when providing therapy. Anxiety surrounding these topics will hinder one's ability to communicate effectively with clients of marginalized groups and most likely will lead to the inability to appropriately conceptualize their clients' problems. Ultimately, this anxiety will impact the rapport and therapeutic relationship with clients and can lead to premature termination of services.

Building rapport within the first couple of sessions is crucial, and there are several recommendations made among scholars in the area of multicultural counseling. Sue and Sue (2013) suggest broaching differences during the first session and inquiring about the client's comfort level when working with a counselor who is of a different race, age, gender, etc. In addition, counselors are urged to identify the client's expectations and worldviews, what they believe counseling entails, and their feelings about counseling. With mandated clients, discuss how counseling may be useful for them and explain confidentiality and your relationship with the referring agency (e.g., probation office). Sue and Sue also recommend discussing the clients' positive assets and strengths (also referred to as *recovery capital* in the substance abuse field). Throughout the counseling process, counselors must also determine any external factors related to the presenting problem. For example, explore whether and how clients have responded to oppression, discrimination, and/or racism. Furthermore, the various identities of clients (e.g., female, lesbian, Native American) should be examined in session, and the counselor should be aware of identity development status and assist clients in enhancing a positive self-identity.

With all of this being said about knowledge, skills, and awareness, therapists should be cautious about how competency is viewed according to the client. The helping role of a therapist is bound by certain ethical codes (created by North American entities), and often these codes (as well as the theoretical orientation of the counselor) can contrast with other (non–Euro-American) cultural values, norms, or behaviors. For instance, therapists are taught NOT to (a) give advice or suggestions, as that fosters dependency; (b) self-disclose, as that is unprofessional; (c) barter with clients; (d) be in dual roles with clients; and (e) accept gifts from clients (Sue, 2001). In many cultures, however, these are considered the normal acts of a helper, which build rapport (e.g., advice giving and self-disclosure), increase the likelihood of one to seek help (e.g., dual relationships), and are signs of appreciation (e.g., giving gifts). Therefore, a therapist may actually be considered less competent and may even offend someone who is not of a Euro-American background due to these discrepancies in expectations.

SOCIAL JUSTICE AND ADVOCACY

Historically, practitioners in the various helping professions have been socialized to be apolitical and have neglected the concerns of marginalized groups, both in and out of the counseling room. As far as people of color, D. W. Sue (2001) stated the behavioral health field has:

> failed to adequately address issues of racism, bias, and discrimination as major contributors to mental distress among people of color and has played a passive role in rectifying the inequities that affect the standard of living for racial minority groups in the United States. (p. 801)

Dr. Sue called upon counselors to be proactive agents of change and advocates for cultural democracy and social justice. Counselors must be critically conscious and speak out and push for the inclusion, fairness, collaboration, cooperation, and equal access and opportunity for clients. These efforts are to eradicate the inequities that impede the economic, academic, personal, and social development of marginalized groups. In fact, one of the AMCD competencies states, "Culturally skilled counselors should be aware of relevant discriminatory practices at the social and community level that may be affecting the psychological welfare of the population being served" (AMCD, 1996). Not only should counselors be *aware* of these discriminatory circumstances, but also must *advocate* for the elimination of cultural and systemic oppression. Once counselors realize how their biases and actions may contribute to the marginalization of others and the inequities that exist in our society, they can no longer evade the responsibility for change. As stated earlier, this requires more than an intellectual exercise.

Social justice has been perceived as an abstract, philosophical concept. In an effort to provide a tangible framework and designate specific strategies to employ, the American Counseling Association (ACA) has identified 43 advocacy competencies for the profession (Lewis et al., 2002). These 43 competencies have

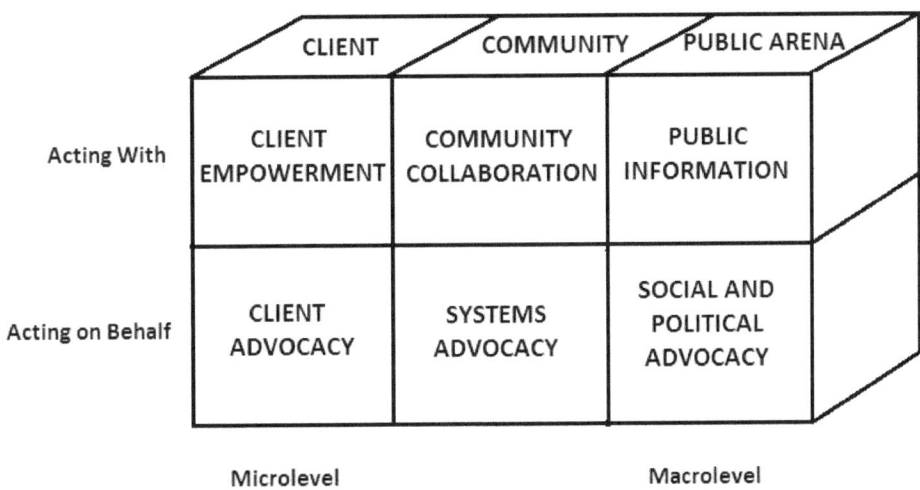

Figure 18.2: Adapted from *ACA Advocacy Competencies,* by J. A. Lewis, M. S. Arnold, R. House, & R. L. Toporek, 2002.

been categorized into six domains according to level of advocacy and the manner in which the advocacy is delivered. A counselor can advocate at the microlevel (i.e., client level), as well as more broadly at a higher level (i.e., community and public arena). Counselors provide advocacy at each of these levels in two manners: (1) acting with; and (2) acting on behalf. Figure 18.2 below illustrates the six domains based on a 2 x 3 multi-dimensional cube. *Acting on Behalf* – (1) Client Advocacy; (2) Systems Advocacy; (3) Social/Political Advocacy; and *Acting with* – (4) Client Empowerment; (5) Community Collaboration; and (6) Public Information.

As stated above, the ACA advocacy competencies are categorized according to domain. For instance, a counselor will *act with* and *empower* a client by identifying strengths and resources available. In substance abuse treatment, an example of this process could be the process of exploring a client's recovery capital. The following is a listing of a few advocacy competencies by domain; however, the reader is encouraged to review all of the 43 advocacy competencies. (Available at http://www.counseling.org/Resources/Competencies/ Advocacy_Competencies.pdf)

Acting with . . .

Client – Empowerment (Microlevel)

- Identify strengths and resources (e.g., recovery capital)
- Identify social, political, economic, and cultural factors and barriers affecting client
- Train clients in self-advocacy skills, help them develop self-advocacy plans, and assist them in carrying out action plans

Community – Collaboration

- Alert community groups with concerns related to environmental factors that negatively impact clients' development
- Develop alliances with groups working for change
- Identify and offer the skills the counselor can bring to the collaboration

Public Arena – Information (Macrolevel)

- Recognize the impact of oppression and other barriers to healthy development
- Prepare written and multimedia materials that provide clear explanations of the role of specific environmental factors in human development
- Communicate and disseminate information ethically and appropriately through a variety of media
- Identify and collaborate with other professionals who are involved in disseminating public information

Acting on Behalf . . .

Client – Advocacy (Microlevel)

- Negotiate services on behalf of clients and help them gain access to necessary resources
- Identify barriers to the well-being of clients—especially those of marginalized groups—and develop an initial plan of action to confront these barriers

- Identify potential allies for confronting these barriers and carry out the plan of action

Community –Systems Advocacy

- Provide and interpret data to show the urgency for change
- Analyze the sources of political power and social influence within the system
- Identify goals and develop a step-by-step plan for implementing the change process and develop a plan for dealing with probable responses to change
- Recognize and deal with resistance

Public Arena – Social and Political Advocacy (Macrolevel)

- Distinguish those problems that can best be resolved through social and political action
- Identify the appropriate avenues for addressing these problems
- Seek out and join with potential allies, while also supporting existing alliances for change
- With allies, prepare convincing data and rationales for change, and then lobby legislators and other policy makers

Researchers have recognized advocacy behaviors that go further than the ACA competency listing above. Chung and Bemak (2012) provide numerous counselor behaviors in their book, *Social Justice Counseling: The Next Steps Beyond Multiculturalism*. Many of these are similar to the ACA competencies, but the authors encourage therapists to also engage in advocacy using the Internet.

More specifically, therapists should use the Internet to:

- Market counseling services
- Access online audio- and video-based help
- Deliver multimedia-based assessment and information resources that match the ethnicity, age, and sex of the user
- Reach clients who have transportation difficulties or live in geographically remote areas
- Improve client access to self-help groups
- Expand opportunities for communication among counselors (Chung & Bemak, 2012)

Looking over the advocacy competencies, one can acknowledge that microlevel and microlevel advocacy must be provided for clients who struggle with addiction problems. For instance, substance abuse therapists will assist clients to learn how to advocate for their own services, negotiate for services on behalf of clients, prepare convincing data and rationales for change, and also lobby legislators/policy makers for such change. Change must happen at the programmatic/systemic levels. In a recovery-oriented system of care, persons working within health systems, institutions, government entities, etc., must get out of their silos and collaborate to assist in preventing and treating substance use. Therapists, physicians, psychiatrists, social workers, probation officers, child protective service workers, and others involved with a client's care must employ an *integrated* model of care. All of these people must make partnerships and make a concerted effort toward social justice.

Social justice and advocacy go beyond what occurs in the counseling room, and these counseling functions have been considered daunting by many practitioners (Lewis, 2011). Working toward environmental change should not be seen as separate work, an add-on, or going beyond their counseling responsibilities, but rather it must be viewed as a primary role as a therapist. Advocacy is not just a theoretical notion; it has practical strategies and interventions, and must be seen as a vital and central aspect to one's professional identity. In the next section, the author moves from the social justice and multicultural competency expectations of all counselors to the advocacy and competency expectations for those specifically working in the addictions field.

ADDICTION-RELATED COUNSELING COMPETENCIES

The Council for Accreditation of Counseling and Related Educational Programs (CACREP) is the accrediting body for master's level, counselor education programs (e.g., school counseling and clinical mental health counseling) in the United States. CACREP provides standards which these programs must meet in order to obtain and maintain accreditation. In 2009, a new edition of the CACREP standards was released, and for the first time, Addiction Counseling programs could be accredited. Addiction Counseling programs prepare graduates to work with persons and families affected by alcohol, drugs, gambling, sexual, and other addictive disorders (e.g., food related). These 60 semester-hour programs focus on models of prevention, treatment, and recovery. Graduates of Addiction Counseling programs may choose to work in private practice or may work in a variety of community agencies, offering counseling services for substance abuse concerns.

The Addiction Counseling program faculty must provide opportunities for Addiction Counseling students to learn the knowledge, skills, and awareness specific to working with clients with substance use disorders. Students should know about various content related to the history, philosophy, theories, and trends in addictions; ethical and legal considerations; co-occurring disorders, assessment, and diagnosis; prevention and intervention; and diversity and advocacy (CACREP, 2009). Not only are they to gain

Table 18.3: Addiction Counseling Standards (CACREP, 2009)

DOMAIN	COMPETENCY
Foundations; Knowledge	Understands factors that increase the likelihood for a person, community, or group to be at risk for or resilient to psychoactive substance use disorders.
Counseling, Prevention and Intervention; Skills and Practices	Individualizes helping strategies and treatment modalities to each client's stage of dependence, change, or recovery.
Diversity and Advocacy; Knowledge	Understands effective strategies that support client advocacy and influence public policy and government relations on local, state, and national levels to enhance equity, increase funding, and promote programs that affect the practice of addiction counseling.
Assessment; Skills and Practices	Screens for psychoactive substance toxicity, intoxication, and withdrawal symptoms; aggression or danger to others; potential for self-inflicted harm or suicide; and co-occurring mental and/or addictive disorders.
Diagnosis; Knowledge	Knows the principles of the diagnostic process, including differential diagnosis, and the use of current diagnostic tools such as the current edition of the *Diagnostic and Statistical Manual of Mental Disorders*.

knowledge, but also skills and awareness. Table 18.3 below is a sample of six out of the 57 competencies outlined in the 2009 CACREP Addiction Counseling Program standards.

In addition to the CACREP Addiction Counseling program standards, the Center for Substance Abuse Treatment (CSAT) has competencies for addiction counselors as well. This publication is titled, *Addiction Counseling Competencies: The Knowledge, Skills, and Attitudes of Professional Practice* (often referred to as Technical Assistance Publication [TAP] 21). TAP 21 identifies 123 competencies that are essential to the effective practice of counseling for substance use disorders and has become a benchmark (a) for curricula development; and (b) by which educational programs and professional standards are measured for the field of substance abuse treatment in the United States. The 123 competencies are divided into four areas: (1) Understanding Addiction; (2) Treatment Knowledge; (3) Application to Practice; and (4) Professional Readiness. Addiction counselors are encouraged to also look over the code of ethics for their particular helping profession (e.g., social work, counseling, psychology) and for their addiction-related certifications and licenses.

Over the years, the addiction counseling field has moved away from paraprofessionals and has required helpers to have more education, training, supervision, and clinical experience. Often, a counselor needs the state credential in order to bill for services like Medicaid. Credentials can vary by state. Some states offer certifications for addiction counseling and some offer licenses; most states do not have the same requirements or reciprocity. For instance, the credential given to master's level counselors by the Michigan Certification Board of Addiction Professionals (MCBAP) is the Certified Advanced Alcohol and Drug Counselor (CAADC) certification and requires completion of 180 hours of addiction-related education and training (which can be obtained in four college courses), the ICRC examination, six hours of addiction-related ethics training, 2,000 hours of field experience, and 300 hours of documented supervision. However, across the border in Indiana, an individual can become a Licensed Clinical Addiction Counselor (LCAC) after completing 27 semester hours of addiction-related graduate course work (equivalent to nine college courses), the ICRC examination, a 700-hour practicum in addiction work, 3,000 postgraduate clinical work over a two-year period, and 200 hours of documented supervision. Moreover, some states require up to 4,000 hours of clinical work and additional training in HIV/STD, veterans, elderly, and/or psychopharmacology. If the reader plans to obtain a credential in the field, the author recommends viewing the state requirements, even prior to starting clinical work, in an effort to gather all the necessary documentation and plan accordingly. In addition, if the reader has to take the ICRC examination, it may be most beneficial to plan on taking it shortly after one's education and training.

CONCLUSION

Diversity issues must be taken into account for any client who presents for counseling, and they must be broached in sessions. Counselors must continually strive for competency when working with those who have been marginalized, oppressed, and stigmatized. For a client who has a substance use disorder, the alcohol and/or other drug use should be conceptualized within the context of his or her culture and unique experiences. In an effort to obtain the knowledge and skills needed, helpers must also dig deep into their own biases, prejudices, worldviews, attitudes, and beliefs. Self-awareness is key, and once self-aware, one must act. The counseling field must unite to advocate for social justice in order to fully service the needs of clients. We must look to obtain a continuum of care that does not set up individuals to fail. We need to provide a recovery-oriented system of care within an integrated health care system which brings everyone to the table. Discrimination, racism, oppression, and inequities within our systems are to be recognized and brought into account in order to make systemic changes. To provide a recovery-oriented system of care and an integrated health system, counselors must have the strong voice of action for those who have no voice. You, the reader, will be that voice.

As this book was being written, on December 5, 2013, South African antiapartheid leader, philanthropist, and past president Nelson Mandela died. This author wishes to close with the following quote in his memory:

> *No one is born hating another person because of the color of [one's] skin, or [one's] background, or [one's] religion. People must learn to hate, and if they can learn to hate, they can be taught to love, for love comes more naturally to the human heart than its opposite.*
>
> —Nelson Mandela

Exercises

1. Look at the 31 AMCD Multicultural Counseling Competencies in the back of this text. Find two competencies that you could improve the most, and identify three methods (for each) to employ in an effort to strengthen these competencies.
2. Role-play a scenario in which you are broaching various differences in a counseling session. How would you articulate the consideration of cultural diversity? Notice your level of comfort during the role-play. Are you more comfortable addressing some differences, but not others?
3. After reading over the dimensions of social justice and advocacy by Lewis et al. (2002), think of a hypothetical (or real) client of a specific population and develop a written plan for addressing the various six domains of advocacy (e.g., empowerment, collaboration, public information). How do you propose to *act with* and *on behalf of* this client and this population in each of the domains?
4. Search the Internet for the addiction-related credentials in your state. What requirements must you complete? How interested are you in obtaining a license or certification in the field?

REFERENCES

Ang, S., & Van Dyne, L. (2008). *Handbook of cultural intelligence: Theory, measurement, and applications.* Armonk, NY: M. E. Sharpe, Inc.

Arredondo, P., Toporek, M. S., Brown, S. P., Jones, J., Locke, D., Sanchez, J., et al. (1996). Operationalization of the multicultural counseling competencies. *Journal of Multicultural Counseling and Development, 24,* 42–78.

Center for Substance Abuse Treatment (2006). *Addiction counseling competencies: The knowledge, skills, and attitudes of professional practice.* Technical Assistance Publication (TAP) Series 21. HHS Publication No. (SMA) 08-4171. Rockville, MD: Substance Abuse and Mental Health Services Administration.

Chung, R. C-Y., & Bemak, F. P. (2012). *Social justice counseling: The next steps beyond multiculturalism.* Thousand Oaks, CA: Sage Publications.

Council for Accreditation of Counseling and Related Educational Programs (2009). *2009 standards.* Retrieved from http://www.cacrep.org/doc/2009%20Standards%20with%20cover.pdf

Day-Vines, N. L., Wood, S. M., Grothaus, T., Craigen, L., Holman, A., Dotson-Blake, K., & Douglass, M. J. (2007). Broaching the subjects of race, ethnicity, and culture during the counseling process. *Journal of Counseling and Development, 85*, 401–409.

Lee, C. (2006). *Multicultural issues in counseling: New approaches to diversity* (3rd ed.). Alexandria, VA: American Counseling Association.

Lewis, J. A. (2011). Operationalizing social justice counseling: Paradigm to practice. *Journal of Humanistic Counseling, 50*, 183–191.

Lewis, J. A., Arnold, M. S., House, R., & Toporek, R. L. (2002). *ACA advocacy competencies*. Advocacy Task Force, American Counseling Association. Retrieved from http://www.counseling.org/Resources/Competencies/Advocacy_Competencies.pdf

Peterson, M. G. (2013). *Therapist cultural intelligence as a moderator of working alliance and outcome in multicultural counseling*. (Doctoral Dissertation). Retrieved from ProQuest. (UMI 3560591)

Sue, D. W. (2001). Multidimensional facets of cultural competence: A major contribution. *Counseling Psychologist, 29*, 790–821.

Sue, D. W., & Sue, D. (2013). *Counseling the culturally diverse: Theory and practice* (6th ed.). New York: Wiley.

Utsey, S. O., Hammar, L., & Gernat, C. A. (2005). Examining the reactions of White, Black, and Latino/a counseling psychologists to a study of racial issues in counseling and supervision dyads. *Counseling Psychologist, 33*, 565–573.

APPENDIX A

AMCD Multicultural Counseling Competencies

I. Counselor Awareness of Own Cultural Values and Biases

A. Attitudes and Beliefs
1. Culturally skilled counselors believe that cultural self-awareness and sensitivity to one's own cultural heritage is essential.
2. Culturally skilled counselors are aware of how their own cultural background and experiences have influenced attitudes, values, and biases about psychological processes.
3. Culturally skilled counselors are able to recognize the limits of their multicultural competency and expertise.
4. Culturally skilled counselors recognize their sources of discomfort with differences that exist between themselves and clients in terms of race, ethnicity and culture.

B. Knowledge
1. Culturally skilled counselors have specific knowledge about their own racial and cultural heritage and how it personally and professionally affects their definitions and biases of normality/abnormality and the process of counseling.
2. Culturally skilled counselors possess knowledge and understanding about how oppression, racism, discrimination, and stereotyping affect them personally and in their work. This allows individuals to acknowledge their own racist attitudes, beliefs, and feelings. Although this standard applies to all groups, for White counselors it may mean that they understand how they may have directly or indirectly benefited from individual, institutional, and cultural racism as outlined in White identity development models.
3. Culturally skilled counselors possess knowledge about their social impact upon others. They are knowledgeable about communication style differences, how their style may clash with or foster the counseling process with persons of color or others different from themselves based on the A, B, and C Dimensions and how to anticipate the impact it may have on others.

C. Skills
1. Culturally skilled counselors seek out educational, consultative, and training experiences to improve their understanding and effectiveness in working with culturally different populations. Being able to recognize the limits of their competencies, they (a) seek consultation, (b) seek further training or education, (c) refer out to more qualified individuals or resources, or (d) engage in a combination of these.

Derald Wing Sue, Patricia Arredondo, and Roderick J. McDavis, from "Multicultural Counseling Competencies and Standards: A Call to the Profession," *Journal of Counseling & Development*, vol. 70, no. 4, pp. 482-483. Copyright © 1992 by John Wiley & Sons, Inc. Reprinted with permission.

2. Culturally skilled counselors are constantly seeking to understand themselves as racial and cultural beings and are actively seeking a non-racist identity.

II. Counselor Awareness of Client's Worldview

A. Attitudes and Beliefs
1. Culturally skilled counselors are aware of their negative and positive emotional reactions toward other racial and ethnic groups that may prove detrimental to the counseling relationship. They are willing to contrast their own beliefs and attitudes with those of their culturally different clients in a nonjudgmental fashion.
2. Culturally skilled counselors are aware of their stereotypes and preconceived notions that they may hold toward other racial and ethnic minority groups.

B. Knowledge
1. Culturally skilled counselors possess specific knowledge and information about the particular group with which they are working. They are aware of the life experiences, cultural heritage, and historical background of their culturally different clients. This particular competency is strongly linked to the "minority identity development models" available in the literature.
2. Culturally skilled counselors understand how race, culture, ethnicity, and so forth may affect personality formation, vocational choices, manifestation of psychological disorders, help seeking behavior, and the appropriateness or inappropriateness of counseling approaches.
3. Culturally skilled counselors understand and have knowledge about sociopolitical influences that impinge upon the life of racial and ethnic minorities. Immigration issues, poverty, racism, stereotyping, and powerlessness may impact self-esteem and self-concept in the counseling process.

C. Skills
1. Culturally skilled counselors should familiarize themselves with relevant research and the latest findings regarding mental health and mental disorders that affect various ethnic and racial groups. They should actively seek out educational experiences that enrich their knowledge, understanding, and cross-cultural skills for more effective counseling behavior.
2. Culturally skilled counselors become actively involved with minority individuals outside the counseling setting (e.g., community events, social and political functions, celebrations, friendships, neighborhood groups, and so forth) so that their perspective of minorities is more than an academic or helping exercise.

III. Culturally Appropriate Intervention Strategies

A. Beliefs and Attitudes
1. Culturally skilled counselors respect clients' religious and/or spiritual beliefs and values, including attributions and taboos, because they affect worldview, psychosocial functioning, and expressions of distress.
2. Culturally skilled counselors respect indigenous helping practices and respect help giving networks among communities of color.

3. Culturally skilled counselors value bilingualism and do not view another language as an impediment to counseling (monolingualism may be the culprit).

B. Knowledge
1. Culturally skilled counselors have a clear and explicit knowledge and understanding of the generic characteristics of counseling and therapy (culture bound, class bound, and monolingual) and how they may clash with the cultural values of various cultural groups.
2. Culturally skilled counselors are aware of institutional barriers that prevent minorities from using mental health services.
3. Culturally skilled counselors have knowledge of the potential bias in assessment instruments and use procedures and interpret findings keeping in mind the cultural and linguistic characteristics of the clients.
4. Culturally skilled counselors have knowledge of family structures, hierarchies, values, and beliefs from various cultural perspectives. They are knowledgeable about the community where a particular cultural group may reside and the resources in the community.
5. Culturally skilled counselors should be aware of relevant discriminatory practices at the social and community level that may be affecting the psychological welfare of the population being served.

C. Skills
1. Culturally skilled counselors are able to engage in a variety of verbal and nonverbal helping responses. They are able to send and receive both verbal and nonverbal messages accurately and appropriately. They are not tied down to only one method or approach to helping, but recognize that helping styles and approaches may be culture bound. When they sense that their helping style is limited and potentially inappropriate, they can anticipate and modify it.
2. Culturally skilled counselors are able to exercise institutional intervention skills on behalf of their clients. They can help clients determine whether a "problem" stems from racism or bias in others (the concept of healthy paranoia) so that clients do not inappropriately personalize problems.
3. Culturally skilled counselors are not averse to seeking consultation with traditional healers or religious and spiritual leaders and practitioners in the treatment of culturally different clients when appropriate.
4. Culturally skilled counselors take responsibility for interacting in the language requested by the client and, if not feasible, make appropriate referrals. A serious problem arises when the linguistic skills of the counselor do not match the language of the client. This being the case, counselors should (a) seek a translator with cultural knowledge and appropriate professional background or (b) refer to a knowledgeable and competent bilingual counselor.
5. Culturally skilled counselors have training and expertise in the use of traditional assessment and testing instruments. They not only understand the technical aspects of the instruments but are also aware of the cultural limitations. This allows them to use test instruments for the welfare of culturally different clients.
6. Culturally skilled counselors should attend to as well as work to eliminate biases, prejudices, and discriminatory contexts in conducting evaluations and providing interventions, and should develop sensitivity to issues of oppression, sexism, heterosexism, elitism and racism.
7. Culturally skilled counselors take responsibility for educating their clients to the processes of psychological intervention, such as goals, expectations, legal rights, and the counselor's orientation.

CPSIA information can be obtained
at www.ICGtesting.com
Printed in the USA
LVHW062006280720
661765LV00005B/15